Praise for
THE MONUMENTS MEN

"Whether you're a fan of art, military history, or stories with real-life heroes, *The Monuments Men* is a treasure worth the hunt."

—**Howard Shirley,** *BookPage*

"This in-depth examination is a worthy legacy for the Monuments Men, who untangled countless mysteries and prevented what could have been an irreversible, international cultural catastrophe."

—**Betty Gorden,** *Atlanta Journal-Constitution*

"Edsel is particularly adept at capturing the quirky personalities of the individual Monuments Men."

—**Jonathan Lopez,** *Boston Sunday Globe*

"It's a terrific story, and it certainly is good to give these men (and that one remarkable woman) their due."

—**Jonathan Yardley,** *Washington Post*

"The hunters' exploits make a fascinating read. Edsel carefully and colorfully backgrounds *The Monuments Men* with vivid accounts of the war's progress."

—**Carl Hartman,** *Associated Press*

"This intriguing story, told largely through letters written by the rescuers and now in various government archives, will appeal to many general and military history readers." —*Library Journal*

"Not until 2007 was the work of the Monuments Men acknowledged. The National Endowment for the Humanities awarded to them a medal given to individuals or groups whose work has 'deepened the nation's understanding of the humanities.' And now comes this book, a recognition that is well justified—and highly readable."

—Thomas B. Allen, *Washington Times*

"Historical details come thick and fast, but Edsel manages to keep the narrative breezy."

—William Lee Adams, *TIME*

"There is certainly an astonishing amount of John Wayne-ism and derring-do on the part of the Monuments Men, all the more so because nearly all of them were middle-aged men who left comfortable jobs and families to enlist—and then found themselves traipsing through bombed-out Europe tracking down elusive paintings or statues."

—Jenni Frazer, *The Jewish Chronicle*

THE MONUMENTS MEN

ALLIED HEROES, NAZI THIEVES, AND THE GREATEST TREASURE HUNT IN HISTORY

Robert M. Edsel

with Bret Witter

Little, Brown and Company

New York   Boston   London

Little, Brown and Company
Hachette Book Group
237 Park Avenue
New York, NY 10017
littlebrown.com

The publisher is not responsible for websites (or their content) that are not owned by the publisher.

Printed in the United States of America

Originally published in hardcover by Center Street, September 2009
First Little, Brown and Company mass market edition, October 2013

10 9 8 7 6 5 4 3 2 1

Whatever these paintings may have been to men who looked at them a generation back—today they are not only works of art. Today they are the symbols of the human spirit, and of the world the freedom of the human spirit made.... To accept this work today is to assert the purpose of the people of America that the freedom of the human spirit and human mind which has produced the world's great art and all its science—shall not be utterly destroyed.

—President Franklin D. Roosevelt,
dedication ceremony of the National
Gallery of Art, March 17, 1941

It used to be called plundering. But today things have become more humane. In spite of that, I intend to plunder, and to do it thoroughly.

—Reichsmarschall Hermann Göring,
speaking to a conference of Reich
Commissioners for the Occupied
Territories and the Military
Commanders, Berlin, August 6, 1942

CONTENTS

III
GERMANY

IV
THE VOID

V
THE AFTERMATH

AUTHOR'S NOTE

Most of us are aware that World War II was the most destructive war in history. We know of the horrific loss of life; we've seen images of the devastated European cities. Yet how many among us have walked through a majestic museum such as the Louvre, enjoyed the solitude of a towering cathedral such as Chartres, or gazed upon a sublime painting such as Leonardo da Vinci's *Last Supper*, and wondered, "How did so many monuments and great works of art survive this war? Who were the people that saved them?"

The major events of World War II—Pearl Harbor, D-Day, the Battle of the Bulge—have become as much a part of our collective conscience as the names of the books and films—*Band of Brothers*, *The Greatest Generation*, *Saving Private Ryan*, *Schindler's List*—and the writers, directors, and actors—Ambrose, Brokaw, Spielberg, Hanks—who brought these epic events and the heroism of that time to life for us once again.

But what if I told you there was a major story about World War II that hasn't been told, a significant story at the heart of the entire war effort, involving the most unlikely group of heroes you've never heard of? What if I told you there was a group of men on the front lines who quite literally saved the world as we know it; a group that didn't carry machine guns or drive tanks, who weren't official statesmen; men who not only had the vision to understand the grave threat to the greatest cultural and artistic achievements of civilization, but then joined the front lines to do something about it?

These unknown heroes were known as the "Monuments Men," a group of soldiers who served in the Western Allied military effort from 1943 until 1951. Their initial responsibility was to mitigate combat damage, primarily to structures—churches, museums, and other important monuments. As the war progressed and the German border was breached, their focus shifted to locating movable works of art and other cultural items stolen or otherwise missing. During their occupation of Europe, Hitler and the Nazis pulled off the "greatest theft in history," seizing and transporting more than five million cultural objects to the Third Reich. The Western Allied effort, spearheaded by the Monuments Men, thus became the "greatest treasure hunt in history," with all the unimaginable and bizarre stories that only war can produce. It was also a race against time, for hidden in the most incredible locations, some of which have inspired modern-day popular icons like Sleeping Beauty's Castle at Disneyland and *The Sound of Music*, were tens of thousands of the world's greatest artistic masterpieces, many stolen by the Nazis, including priceless paintings by Leonardo da Vinci, Jan Vermeer, and Rembrandt, and sculptures by Michelangelo and Donatello. And some of the Nazi fanatics holding them were intent on making sure that if the Third Reich couldn't have them, the rest of the world wouldn't either.

In the end, 350 or so men and women from thirteen nations served in the Monuments, Fine Arts, and Archives section (MFAA)—a remarkably small number in a fighting force numbering into the millions. However, there were only sixty or so Monuments Men serving in Europe by the end of combat (May 8, 1945), most of whom were American or British. Monuments-laden Italy had just twenty-two Monuments officers. Within the first several months after D-Day (June 6, 1944), fewer than a dozen Monuments Men were on the ground in Normandy. Another twenty-five were gradually added until the end of hostilities, with the awesome responsibility of covering all of northern Europe. It seemed an impossible assignment.

My original plan for this book was to tell the story of the Monuments Men's activities throughout Europe, concentrating on events from June 1944 to May 1945 through the experiences of just eight Monuments Men who served on the front lines—plus two key figures, including one woman—using their field journals, diaries, wartime reports, and most importantly their letters home to wives, children, and family members during combat. Because of the vastness of the story and my determination to faithfully convey it, the final manuscript became so lengthy that it regrettably became necessary to exclude from this book the Monuments Men's activities in Italy. I have used northern Europe—mainly France, the Netherlands, Germany, and Austria—as a crucible for understanding the Monuments effort.

Monuments officers Deane Keller and Frederick Hartt, both American, and John Bryan Ward-Perkins, who was British, and others experienced incredible events during their difficult work in Italy. Our research unearthed insightful and moving letters home that detailed the sometimes overwhelming responsibility they faced to protect this irreplaceable cradle of civilization. I will be including these heroes' memorable experiences in Italy, using many of their own words, in a subsequent book.

I have taken the liberty of creating dialogue for continuity, but in no instance does it concern matters of substance and in all cases it is based on extensive documentation. I have at all times tried not only to understand and communicate the facts, but also the personalities and perspectives of the people involved, as well as their perception of events at the very instant they occurred. With the advantage of hindsight, these can be quite different from our opinions; thus one of the great challenges of history. Any errors in judgment are mine alone.

At its heart, *The Monuments Men* is a personal story: a story about people. Allow me then one personal story. On November 1, 2006, I flew to Williamstown, Massachusetts, to meet and interview Monuments Man S. Lane Faison Jr., who also served in the OSS (Office of Strategic Services), precursor to the CIA (Central Intelligence Agency). Lane arrived in Germany in the summer of 1945 and promptly went to Altaussee, Austria, to assist with the interrogations of key Nazi officials who had been detained by Western Allied forces. His particular assignment was to find out as much as possible about Hitler's art collection and his plans for the Führermuseum. After the war, Lane was an educator of art at Williams College for almost thirty years, training and sharing his gifted insights with students, both the strivers and the achievers. His professional legacy lives on through his students, in particular the leaders of many of the United States' leading museums: Thomas Krens (Solomon R. Guggenheim Foundation, 1988–2008), James Wood (J. Paul Getty Trust, 2004–present), Michael Govan (Los Angeles County Museum of Art, 2006–present), Jack Lane (Dallas Museum of Art, 1999–2007), Earl A. "Rusty" Powell III (National Gallery of Art, Washington, D.C., 1992–present), and the legendary Kirk Varnedoe (Museum of Modern Art, 1986–2001).

Although ninety-eight years old, Lane was in seemingly good health. Still, I was warned in advance by Gordon, one of his four sons, that "Pop hasn't been staying awake for periods much longer than thirty minutes, so don't be disappointed if you don't learn very much from your conversation." And what a conversation it was, lasting almost three hours as Lane flipped through my first book, *Rescuing Da Vinci*, a photographic tribute to the work of the Monuments Men, stopping periodically to stare intently at images that seemed to transport him back in time. Over and again, as his memory was jogged, the twinkle in his eye appeared, and his arms moved enthusiastically with the telling of each amazing story until we both needed to stop. Gordon was in disbelief, a sentiment each of his brothers later echoed.

As I rose to say goodbye, I walked to the side of his

recliner and extended my hand to thank him. Lane reached out and firmly clasped it with both of his hands, pulled me close, and said, "I've been waiting to meet you all my life." Ten days later, a week shy of his ninety-ninth birthday, he died. It was Veterans Day.

MAIN CHARACTERS

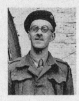

Major Ronald Edmund Balfour, First Canadian Army. Age in 1944: 40. Born: Oxfordshire, England. Balfour, a historian at Cambridge University, was what the British called a "gentleman scholar": a bachelor dedicated to the intellectual life without ambition for accolades or position. A dedicated Protestant, he began his life as a history scholar, then switched to ecclesiastic studies. His prized possession was his immense personal library.

Private Harry Ettlinger, U.S. Seventh Army. Age: 18. Born: Karlsruhe, Germany (immigrated to Newark, New Jersey). A German Jew, Ettlinger fled Nazi persecution in 1938 with his family. Drafted by the army after graduating from high school in Newark in 1944, Private Ettlinger spent much of his tour of duty lost in the army bureaucracy before finally finding his niche in early May 1945.

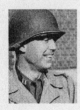

Captain Walker Hancock, U.S. First Army. Age: 43. Born: St. Louis, Missouri. Hancock was a renowned sculptor who had won the prestigious Prix de Rome before the war and designed the Army Air Medal in 1942. Warmhearted and optimistic, he wrote often to his great love, Saima Natti, whom he had married only two weeks before shipping to Europe for duty. His most common refrain was his joy in his work and his dreams of a house and studio where they could live and work together in Gloucester, Massachusetts.

Captain Walter "Hutch" Huchthausen, U.S. Ninth Army. Age: 40. Born: Perry, Oklahoma. Hutch, a boyishly handsome bachelor, was a practicing architect and design professor at the University of Minnesota. Stationed primarily in the German city of Aachen, he was responsible for much of the northwest portion of Germany.

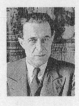

Jacques Jaujard, director of French National Museums. Age: 49. Born: Asnières, France. As the director of the French National Museums, Jaujard was responsible for the safety of the French state art collections during the Nazi occupation from 1940 to 1944. He was a boss, mentor, and confidant of the other great hero of the French cultural establishment, Rose Valland.

Private First Class Lincoln Kirstein, U.S. Third Army. Age: 37. Born: Rochester, New York. Kirstein was a cultural impresario and patron of the arts. Brilliant but prone to mood swings and depression, a founder of the legendary New York City Ballet, he is widely considered one of the most important cultural figures of his generation. Nonetheless, he was one of the lowest-ranking members of the MFAA, serving as the very capable assistant to Captain Robert Posey.

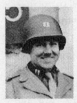

Captain Robert Posey, U.S. Third Army. Age: 40. Born: Morris, Alabama. Raised in poverty on an Alabama farm, Posey graduated from Auburn University with a degree in architecture thanks to funding from the army's Reserve Officers' Training Corps (ROTC). The loner of the MFAA, he was deeply proud of Third Army and its legendary commander, General George S. Patton Jr. He wrote frequently to his wife, Alice, and often picked up cards and souvenirs for his young son Dennis, whom he called "Woogie."

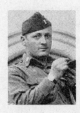

Second Lieutenant James J. Rorimer, Comm Zone and U.S. Seventh Army. Age: 39. Born: Cleveland, Ohio. Rorimer was a wunderkind of the museum world, rising to curator of the Metropolitan Museum at a young age. A specialist in medieval art, he was instrumental in the founding of the Met's medieval collections branch, the Cloisters, with the help of the great patron John D. Rockefeller Jr. Assigned to Paris, his bulldog determination, willingness to buck the system, and love of all things French endeared him to Rose Valland. Their relationship would be vitally important in the race to discover the Nazi treasure troves. Married to a fellow employee of the Metropolitan, Katherine, his daughter Anne was born while he was on active duty; he was not able to see her for more than two years.

Lieutenant George Stout, U.S. First Army and U.S. Twelfth Army Group. Age: 47. Born: Winterset, Iowa. A towering figure in the then obscure field of art conservation, Stout was one of the first people in America to understand the Nazi threat to the cultural patrimony of Europe and pushed the museum community and the army toward establishing a professional art conservation corps. As a field officer, he was the go-to expert for all the other Monuments Men in northern Europe and their indispensable role model and friend. Dapper and well-mannered, with a fastidiousness and thoroughness that shone in the field, Stout, a veteran of World War I, left behind a wife, Margie, and a young son. His oldest son served in the U.S. Navy.

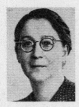

Rose Valland, Temporary Custodian of the Jeu de Paume. Age: 46. Born: Saint-Etienne-de-Saint-Geoirs, France. Rose Valland, a woman of modest means raised in the countryside of France, was the unlikely hero of the French cultural world. She was a longtime unpaid volunteer at the Jeu de Paume museum, adjacent to the Louvre, when the Nazi occupation of Paris began. An unassuming but determined single woman with a forgettable bland style and manner, she ingratiated herself with the Nazis at the Jeu de Paume and, unbeknownst to them, spied on their activities for the four years of their occupation. After the liberation of Paris, the extent and importance of her secret information, which she fiercely guarded, had a pivotal impact on the discovery of looted works of art from France.

THE MONUMENTS MEN

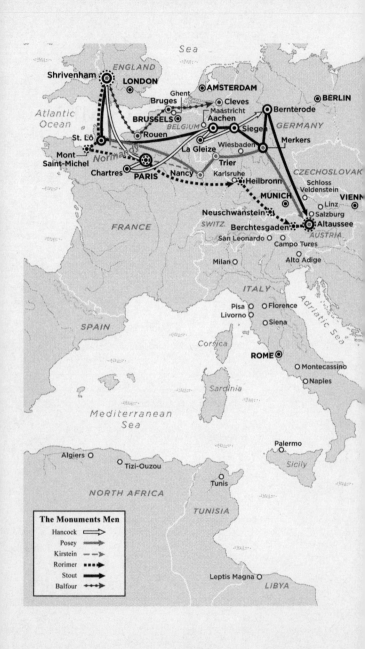

The Monuments Men

Hancock
Posey
Kirstein
Rorimer
Stout
Balfour

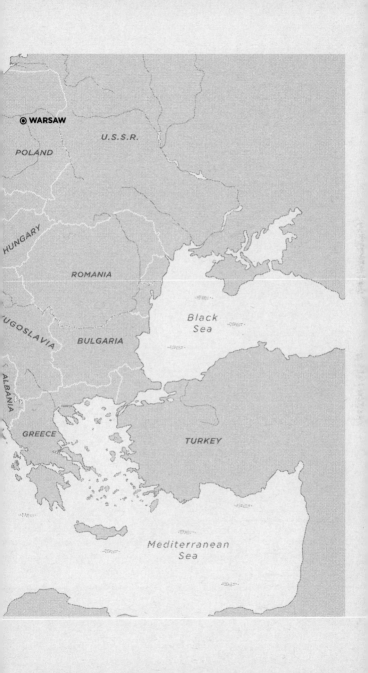

SECTION

I

The Mission

1938–1944

This is a long road we have to travel. The men that can do things are going to be sought out just as surely as the sun rises in the morning. Fake reputations, habits of glib and clever speech, and glittering surface performance are going to be discovered and kicked overboard. Solid, sound leadership . . . and ironclad determination to face discouragement, risk, and increasing work without flinching, will always characterize the man who has a sure-enough, bang-up fighting unit. Added to this he must have a darn strong tinge of imagination—I am continuously astounded by the utter lack of imaginative thinking. . . . Finally, the man has to be able to forget himself and personal fortunes. I've relieved two seniors here because they got to worrying about "injustice," "unfairness," "prestige," and—oh, what the hell!

—SUPREME COMMANDER GENERAL DWIGHT
DAVID EISENHOWER IN A LETTER TO
GENERAL VERNON PRICHARD, AUGUST 27, 1942

*"I think we got some work done, back at the start,
because nobody knew us, nobody bothered us—and we
had no money."*

> —JOHN GETTENS, FOGG MUSEUM CONSERVATION
> DEPARTMENT, DESCRIBING SCIENTIFIC
> BREAKTHROUGHS HE MADE WITH
> GEORGE STOUT, 1927–1932

THE MONUMENTS MEN

The Monuments Men were a group of men and women from thirteen nations, most of whom volunteered for service in the newly created Monuments, Fine Arts, and Archives section, or MFAA. Most of the early volunteers had expertise as museum directors, curators, art scholars and educators, artists, architects, and archivists. Their job description was simple: to save as much of the culture of Europe as they could during combat.

The creation of the MFAA section was a remarkable experiment. It marked the first time an army fought a war while comprehensively attempting to mitigate cultural damage, and it was performed without adequate transportation, supplies, personnel, or historical precedent. The men tasked with this mission were, on the surface, the most unlikely of heroes. Of the initial sixty or so that served in the battlefields of North Africa and Europe through May 1945, the primary period covered by our story, most were middle-aged, with an average

age of forty. The oldest was sixty-six, an "old and inde-structible"[1] World War I veteran; only five were still in their twenties. Most had established families and accomplished careers. But they had all *chosen* to join the war effort in the Monuments, Fine Arts, and Archives section, and to a man they were willing to fight and die for what they believed. I am proud to introduce them to you and to tell, as best I can, their remarkable stories.

CHAPTER 1

Out of Germany

Karlsruhe, Germany
1715–1938

The city of Karlsruhe, in southwestern Germany, was founded in 1715 by the Margrave Karl Wilhelm von Baden-Durlach. Local legend held that Karl Wilhelm walked into the woods one day, fell asleep, and dreamt of a palace surrounded by a city. Actually, he left his previous residence at Durlach after a fight with the local townspeople. Still, always the optimist, Karl Wilhelm had his new settlement laid out like a wheel, with his palace in the center and thirty-two roads leading out from it like spokes. As in the dream, a town soon grew around his palace.

Hoping the new city would grow quickly into a regional power, Karl Wilhelm invited anyone to come and settle where they pleased, regardless of race or creed. This was a rare luxury, especially for Jews, who were relegated to Jewish-only neighborhoods throughout most of Eastern Europe. By 1718, a Jewish congregation was established in Karlsruhe. In 1725, a Jewish merchant named Seligmann immigrated there from Ettlingen, the nearby town where his family had lived since 1600. Seligmann thrived in Karlsruhe, perhaps because it wasn't until 1752, when the town finally felt itself a legitimate regional power, that anti-Jewish laws became the fashion. Around 1800, when inhabitants of Germany became legally obligated to take a surname, Seligmann's descendants chose the last name Ettlinger, after their city of origin.

The main street in Karlsruhe is Kaiserstrasse, and on this road in 1850 the Ettlingers opened a women's clothing store, Gebrüder Ettlinger. Jews were forbidden by then to own farmland. The professions, like medicine, law, or government service, were accessible to them but also openly discriminatory, while the trade guilds, such as those for plumbing and carpentry, barred their admission. As a result, many Jewish families focused on retail. Gebrüder Ettlinger was only two blocks from the palace, and in the late 1890s the regular patronage of Karl Wilhelm's descendant, the Grand Duchess Hilda von Baden, wife of Friedrich II von Baden, made it one of the most fashionable stores in the region. By the early 1900s the store featured four floors of merchandise and forty employees. The duchess lost her position in 1918, after Germany's defeat in World War I, but even the loss of their patron didn't dent the fortunes of the Ettlinger family.

In 1925, Max Ettlinger married Suse Oppenheimer, whose father was a wholesale textile merchant in the nearby town of Bruchsal. His primary business was uniform cloth for government employees, like policemen and customs officials. The Jewish Oppenheimers, who traced their local roots to 1450, were well known for their integrity, kindness, and philanthropy. Suse's mother had served as, among others things, the president of the local Red Cross. So when Max and Suse's first son, Heinz Ludwig Chaim Ettlinger, called Harry, was born in 1926, the family was not only well-off financially, but an established and respected presence in the Karlsruhe area.

Children live in a closed world, and young Harry assumed life as he knew it had gone on that way forever. He didn't have any friends who weren't Jewish, but his parents didn't either, so that didn't seem unusual. He saw non-Jews at school and in the parks, and he liked them, but buried deep within those interactions was the knowledge that, for some reason, he was an out-sider. He had no idea that the world was entering an economic depression, or that hard times bring recriminations and blame. Privately, Harry's parents worried not just about the economy, but about the rising tide of nationalism and anti-Semitism. Harry noticed only that perhaps the line between himself and the larger world of Karlsruhe was becoming easier to see and harder to cross.

Then in 1933, seven-year-old Harry was banned from the local sports association. In the summer of 1935, his aunt left Karlsruhe for Switzerland. When Harry started the fifth grade a few months later, he was one of only two Jewish boys in his class of forty-five. His father was a decorated veteran of World War I, wounded by shrapnel outside Metz, France, so Harry was granted a temporary exemption from the 1935 Nuremberg Laws that stripped Jews of German citizenship and, with it, most of their rights. Forced to sit in the back row, Harry's grades dropped noticeably. This wasn't the result of ostracism or intimidation—that did occur, but Harry was never beaten or physically bullied by his classmates. It was the prejudice of his teachers.

Two years later, in 1937, Harry switched to the Jewish school. Soon after, he and his two younger brothers received a surprise gift: bicycles. Gebrüder Ettlinger had gone bankrupt, felled by a boycott of Jewish-owned businesses, and his father was now working with Opa (Grandpa) Oppenheimer in his textile business. Harry was taught to ride a bicycle so he could get around Holland, where the family was hoping to move. His best friend's family was trying to emigrate to Palestine. Almost everyone Harry knew, in fact, was trying to get out of Germany. Then word came that the Ettlingers' application was denied. They weren't going to Holland. Shortly thereafter, Harry crashed his bicycle; his admission to the local hospital was also denied.

There were two synagogues in Karlsruhe, and the Ettlingers, who were not strictly observant Jews, attended the less orthodox. The Kronenstrasse Synagogue was a large, ornate hundred-year-old building. The worship center soared four floors into a series of decorated domes—four floors was the maximum allowable height, for no building in Karlsruhe could be higher than the tower of Karl Wilhelm's palace. The men, who wore pressed black suits and black top hats, sat on long benches in the bottom section. The women sat in the upper balconies. Behind them, the sun streamed in through large windows, bathing the hall in light.

On Friday nights and Saturday mornings, Harry could look out over the whole congregation from his perch in the choir loft. The people he recognized were leaving, forced overseas by poverty, discrimination, the threat of violence, and a government that encouraged emigration as the best "solution" for both Jews and the German state. Still, the synagogue was always full. As the world shrunk—economically, culturally, socially— the synagogue drew more and more of the fringes of the Jewish community into the city's last comfortable embrace. It wasn't unusual for five hundred people to fill the hall, chanting together and praying for peace.

In March 1938, the Nazis annexed Austria. The public adulation that followed cemented Hitler's control of power and reinforced his ideology of "*Deutschland über alles*"—"Germany above all." He was forming, he said, a new German empire that would last a thousand years. German empire? Germany above all? The Jews of Karlsruhe believed war was inevitable. Not just against them, but against the whole of Europe.

A month later, on April 28, 1938, Max and Suse Ettlinger rode the train fifty miles to the U.S. consulate in Stuttgart. They had been applying for years to Switzerland, Great Britain, France, and the United States for permission to emigrate, but all their applications had been denied. They weren't seeking papers now, only answers to a few questions, but the consulate was crammed with people and in complete disarray. The couple was led from room to room, unsure of where they were going or why. Questions were asked and forms filled out. A few days later, a letter arrived. Their application for emigration to the United States was being processed. April 28, it turned out, was the last day the United States was taking requests for emigration; the mysterious paperwork had been their application. The Ettlingers were getting out.

But first, Harry had to celebrate his bar mitzvah. The ceremony was scheduled for January 1939, with the family to leave thereafter. Harry spent the summer studying Hebrew and English while the family's possessions disappeared. Some were sent to friends and relatives, but most of their personal items were boxed for passage to America. Jews weren't allowed to take money out of the country—which made the 100 percent tax paid to the Nazi Party for shipping all but meaningless—but they were still allowed to keep a few possessions, a luxury that would be stripped from them by the end of the year.

In July, Harry's bar mitzvah ceremony was moved forward to October 1938. Emboldened by his success in Austria, Hitler proclaimed that if the Sudetenland, a small stretch of territory made part of Czechoslovakia after World War I, was not given to Germany, the country would go to war for it. The mood was somber. War seemed not only inevitable, but imminent. At the synagogue, the prayers for peace became more frequent, and more desperate. In August, the Ettlingers moved up the date of their son's bar mitzvah ceremony, and their passage out of Germany, another three weeks.

In September, twelve-year-old Harry and his two brothers took the train seventeen miles to Bruchsal to visit their grandparents for the last time. The textile business had failed, and his grandparents were moving to the nearby town of Baden-Baden. Oma (Grandma) Oppenheimer fixed the boys a simple lunch. Opa Oppenheimer showed them, one last time, a few select pieces from his collection of prints. He was a student of the world and a minor patron of the arts. His art collection contained almost two thousand prints, primarily ex libris bookplates and works by minor German Impressionists working in the late 1890s and early 1900s. One of the best was a print, made by a local artist, of the self-portrait by Rembrandt that hung in the Karlsruhe museum. The painting was a jewel of the museum's collection. Opa Oppenheimer had admired it often on his visits to the museum for lectures and meetings, but he hadn't seen the painting in five years. Harry had never seen it, despite living four blocks away from it his whole life. In 1933, the museum had barred entry to Jews.

Putting the prints away at last, Opa Oppenheimer turned to the globe. "You boys are going to become Americans," he told them sadly, "and your enemy is going to be"—he spun the globe and placed his finger not on Berlin, but on Tokyo—"the Japanese."[1]

A week later, on September 24, 1938, Harry Ettlinger celebrated his bar mitzvah in Karlsruhe's magnificent Kronenstrasse Synagogue. The service lasted three hours, in the middle of which Harry rose to read from the Torah, singing the passages in ancient Hebrew as had been done for thousands of years. The synagogue was filled to capacity. This was a ceremony to honor his passage into adulthood, his hope for the future, but to so many the chance for a life in Karlsruhe seemed lost. The jobs were gone; the Jewish community was shunned and harassed; Hitler was daring the Western powers to oppose him. After the ceremony, the rabbi took Harry's parents aside and told them not to delay, to leave not tomorrow but that very afternoon, on the 1:00 p.m. train to Switzerland. His parents were stunned. The rabbi was advocating travel on Shabbat, the day of rest. It was unheard of.

The ten-block walk home seemed long. The celebratory meal of cold sandwiches was eaten quietly in an empty apartment. The only guests were Oma and Opa Oppenheimer, Harry's other grandmother Oma Jennie, and her sister Tante (Aunt) Rosa, both of whom had moved in with the family around the time Gebrüder Ettlinger went bankrupt. When Harry's mother told Opa Oppenheimer what the rabbi had advised, the veteran of the German army went to the window, looked onto Kaiserstrasse, and saw dozens of soldiers milling about in their uniforms.

"If the war would start today," the canny veteran said, "all these soldiers would be off the street and in their barracks. The war will not start today."[2]

Harry's father, also a proud veteran of the German army, agreed. The family left not that afternoon, but the next morning on the first train to Switzerland. On October 9, 1938, they arrived in New York harbor. Exactly one month later, on November 9, the Nazis used the assassination of a diplomat to put into full force their crusade against German Jews. *Kristallnacht*, the Night of Broken Glass, saw the destruction of more than seven thousand Jewish businesses and two hundred synagogues. The Jewish men of Karlsruhe, including Opa Oppenheimer, were rounded up and put in the nearby Dachau internment camp. The magnificent hundred-year-old Kronenstrasse Synagogue, where only weeks before Heinz Ludwig Chaim Ettlinger had celebrated his bar mitzvah, was burned to the ground. Harry Ettlinger was the last boy ever to have his bar mitzvah ceremony in the old synagogue of Karlsruhe.

But this story isn't about the Kronenstrasse Synagogue, the internment camp at Dachau, or even the Holocaust against the Jews. It is about a different act of negation and aggression Hitler perpetrated on the people and nations of Europe: his war on their culture. For when Private Harry Ettlinger, U.S. Army, finally returned to Karlsruhe, it wasn't to search for his lost relatives or the remains of his community; it was to determine the fate of another aspect of his heritage stripped away by the Nazi regime: his grandfather's beloved art collection. In the process he would discover, buried six hundred feet underground, something he had always known about but never expected to see: the Rembrandt of Karlsruhe.

CHAPTER 2

Hitler's Dream

Florence, Italy
May 1938

In early May 1938, a few days after Harry Ettlinger's parents accidentally signed their applications for emigration to America, Adolf Hitler made one of his first trips outside Germany and Austria. The trip was a state visit to Italy, to meet his Fascist ally Benito Mussolini.

Rome, so vast, so monumental, so redolent of empire with its massive, columned ruins, almost certainly humbled him. Its splendor—not its current splendor but the reflection of ancient Rome—made Berlin seem a mere provincial outpost. Rome was what he wanted his German capital to become. He had been moving toward conquest for years, planning his subjugation of Europe, but Rome sparked the idea of *empire*. Since 1936, he had been discussing with his personal architect, Albert Speer, a plan to rebuild Berlin on a massive scale. After Rome, he told Speer to build not just for today, but for the future. He wanted to create monuments that over the centuries would become elegant ruins so that a thousand years into the Reich, humankind would still be looking in awe at the symbols of his power.

Hitler found the smaller-scale Florence, the art capital of Italy, similarly inspiring. Here, in the intimate cluster of buildings that marked the birthplace of the Italian Renaissance, was the cultural heart of Europe. Nazi flags fluttered; the citizens cheered; but the artwork moved him. He spent more than three hours in the Uffizi Gallery, staring in wonder at its famous works of art. His entourage tried to keep him moving. Behind him, Mussolini, who had never willingly stepped foot in an art museum in his life,[1] muttered in exasperation, "*Tutti questi quadri...*"—"All these paintings..."[2] But Adolf Hitler would not be hurried.

As a young man, he had dreamed of being an artist and an architect. That dream had been crushed when his application to the Academy of Fine Arts Vienna was rejected by a panel of so-called art experts he believed to be Jews. He had wandered in the wilderness for a decade, almost destitute and virtually living on the streets. But his true destiny had finally revealed itself. He was not destined to create, but to remake. To purge, and then rebuild. To make an empire out of Germany, the greatest the world had ever seen. The strongest; the most disciplined; the most racially pure. Berlin would be his Rome, but a true artist-emperor needed a Florence. And he knew where to build it.

Less than two months earlier, on Sunday, March 13, 1938, Adolf Hitler had placed a wreath on his parents' grave in his adopted hometown of Linz, Austria. The afternoon before, March 12, had seen the fulfillment of one of his great ambitions. He, who had once been rejected and ignored, had crossed from Germany, which he now ruled, into his native Austria, which he had just annexed into the Reich. At every town, the crowds cheered his convoy and mobbed his touring car. Mothers cried with joy at the sight of him; children showered him with flowers and adulation. In Linz, he was hailed as a conquering hero, a savior of his country and his race.

The next morning, he had been forced to linger in Linz. So many trucks and tanks in the German convoy had broken down that the road to Vienna was completely blocked. All morning he cursed his commanders for ruining his moment, for embarrassing him before his people and the world. But that afternoon, alone in the cemetery, his soldiers and hangers-on at a respectful distance, the bigger moment descended on him again, like an eagle plunging from the sky to grasp a fish.

He had done it. He wasn't just a mournful son kneeling before his mother's iron cross. He was the Führer. He was, as of that day, the emperor of Austria. He didn't have to cower at the sight of Linz's haphazard industrial riverfront; he could rebuild it. He could pour money and prestige into this small industrial town until it toppled the dominance of the Jewish-tinged (but at the same time virulently anti-Semitic) Vienna, a city he despised.

Perhaps on that day, he had thought of Aachen. For eleven hundred years the city, burial place of Charlemagne, Holy Roman Emperor and founder of the First German Reich in AD 800, had stood as a monument to that man's glory. Upon its ancient foundations, Charlemagne had built an enduring seat of power, centered on the magnificent Aachen Cathedral. Adolf Hitler would rebuild Berlin on the blueprint of Rome.

But he would rebuild Linz, this rural backwater of factories and smoke, in his own image. It wasn't just a dream; he had the power now to forge an enduring testament to his own fierce leadership and artistic soul. Two months later, in the Uffizi Gallery in Florence, he saw clearly what Linz was destined to become: the cultural center of Europe.

In April 1938, Hitler had begun to consider the idea of an art museum in Linz, a place to house the personal collection he had begun amassing in the 1920s. His visit to one of the epicenters of Western art showed that his thinking had been far too small. He would not give Linz a mere museum. He would remodel the city's riverfront along the Danube into a cultural district like the one in Florence, but with wide avenues, walking paths, and parks, and with every viewing point considered and controlled. He would build an opera house, a symphony hall, a cinema, a library, and of course a giant mausoleum to house his tomb. And nearby, in the center of it all, would stand the Führermuseum, *his* Aachen Cathedral, the largest, most imposing, most spectacular art museum in the world.

The Führermuseum. It would be his artistic legacy. It would vindicate his rejection from the Academy of Fine Arts Vienna. It would give form and purpose to his purge of "degenerate" works of art by Jews and modern artists; his new museums, like the Haus der Deutschen Kunst (House of German Art) in Munich, the first public project financed by his government; his huge yearly art exhibitions for the edification of the German people; his advocacy of art collecting among the Nazi elite; his decade-long pursuit of a world-class personal art collection. He had spent his life searching for artistic purity and perfection. The Führermuseum, the most spectacular art museum in history, culled from the riches of the entire world, gave that pursuit a defining rationale.

The foundation for culling those riches had already been laid. By 1938, he had already purged the German cultural establishment. He had rewritten the laws, stripping German Jews of their citizenship and confiscating their collections of art, their furniture, all their possessions right down to their silverware and their family photos. Even at the moment he knelt before his mother's grave on his second day as ruler of Austria, Nazi SS troops under the command of Heinrich Himmler were using those laws to arrest the Jewish patriarchy of Vienna and seize their property for the Reich. The SS knew where the artwork was hidden; they had a list of everything. Years earlier, German art scholars had begun visiting the countries of Europe, secretly preparing inventories so that when Hitler conquered each country—oh yes, he had been preparing for conquest even then—his agents would know the name and location of every important object of artistic and cultural value.

In the years to come, as his power and territory grew, these agents would spread like tentacles. They would force their way into every museum, hidden bunker, locked tower, and living room to buy, trade, confiscate, and coerce. The racially motived property seizures of Nazi leader Alfred Rosenberg would be turned into an art plundering operation; the insatiable ambition of Nazi Reichsmarschall Hermann Göring would be bent into an engine of exploitation. Hitler would use new laws, *his* laws, to gather the great artwork of Europe and sweep it back into the Fatherland. Once there, he would jam it into every available storage facility until the day it could be displayed in the world's most magnificent museum. Until then it would be chronicled in enormous catalogues so that perhaps in the not-so-distant future, after a long day of ruling the world, he could relax at home, his faithful dog and a steaming pot of tea by his side, and select from the greatest art collection ever assembled, *his* art collection, a few choice pieces to brighten his day. In the coming years, Adolf Hitler would sketch this vision over and over again. He would contemplate it, turn it over in his mind, until with the help of architects Albert Speer, Hermann Giesler, and others, the Führermuseum and the Linz cultural district—the symbols of his artistic soul—would become a set idea, then a twenty-foot-long architectural rendering, and finally a three-dimensional scale model, large enough to fill an entire room, showing every building, bridge, and tree that would ever grow and prosper under his mighty hand.

June 26, 1939
Letter from Hitler directing Dr. Hans Posse to supervise the construction of the Führermuseum in Linz

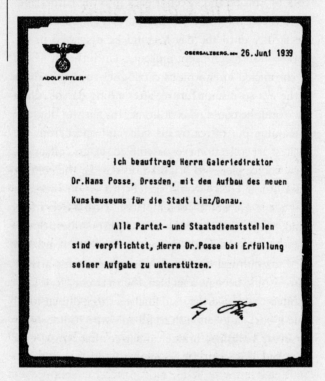

OBERSALZBERG, DEN 26. Juni 1939

ADOLF HITLER

Ich beauftrage Herrn Galeriedirektor Dr. Hans Posse, Dresden, mit dem Aufbau des neuen Kunstmuseums für die Stadt Linz/Donau.

Alle Partei- und Staatsdienststellen sind verpflichtet, Herrn Dr. Posse bei Erfüllung seiner Aufgabe zu unterstützen.

"I commission Dr. Hans Posse, Director of Dresden Gallery, to build up the new art museum for Linz Donau. All Party and State services are ordered to assist Dr. Posse in fulfillment of his mission."

—signed: Adolf Hitler

CHAPTER 3

The Call to Arms

New York City
December 1941

The Christmas lights sparkled defiantly in New York City in mid-December 1941. The windows of Saks and Macy's blazed, and the giant tree at Rockefeller Center glared out at the world with a thousand wary eyes. At the Defense Center, soldiers trimmed Christmas trees, while around them citizens made preparations to feed 40,000 enlisted men in the largest feast the city had ever seen. In stores, "as usual" signs hung in the windows, a sure indication this was anything but an ordinary Christmas. On December 7, the Japanese had bombed Pearl Harbor, shocking the nation and catapulting it into war. While most Americans shopped and fumed and decided for the first time in years to spend a few days with their families—bus and train travel set a record that year—spotters stared up at the sky on both coasts, looking for signs of enemy bombers.

Much had changed since Hitler's annexation of Austria in 1938. By the end of that year, Czechoslovakia had capitulated. On August 24, 1939, Germany and the Soviet Union had signed a nonaggression pact. A week later, on September 1, the Germans invaded

Poland. In May 1940, the Nazi blitzkrieg (lightning war) turned west, routed a combined British-French force, and overran Belgium and Holland. By June, the Germans had taken Paris, catching the shocked French in the midst of evacuation. The Battle of Britain began in July, followed in September by a fifty-seven-day aerial bombardment of London that became known as the "Blitz." By the end of May 1941, the bombs had killed tens of thousands of British civilians and damaged or destroyed more than a million buildings. On June 22, confident that Western Europe had been subdued, Hitler turned on Stalin. By September 9, the German Wehrmacht (Armed Forces) had stormed through western Russia to Leningrad (formerly the capital, St. Petersburg). The Leningrad Blockade, which would last nearly nine hundred days, had begun.

The result, at least for the officially neutral Americans, had been a gradual heightening of tension, a slow tightening of the cords that over the course of three years had created a great store of pent-up energy. The American museum community, like so many others, had buzzed with activity. Much of it centered on protection plans, from evacuations to the creation of climate-controlled, underground rooms. When the Nazis took Paris, the director of the Toledo Museum of Art wrote to David Finley, director of the not yet opened National Gallery of Art in Washington, D.C., to encourage the creation of a national plan, saying, "I know [the possibility of invasion] is remote at the moment, but it was once remote in France."[1] It had taken the British almost a year to retrofit an enormous mine in Manod, Wales, for the safe storage of evacuated artwork. Did the U.S. art community really have another year to prepare?

Now, in the aftermath of Pearl Harbor, the worst attack ever on U.S. soil, the tension had turned into an almost desperate need to act. An air raid on a major American city seemed likely; an invasion by Japan or Germany, or even both, not out of the question. At the Museum of Fine Arts, Boston, the Japanese galleries were closed for fear of attacks by angry mobs. At the Walters Gallery in Baltimore, small gold and jeweled items were removed from the display cases so as not to tempt firemen with axes who might enter for an emergency. In New York City, the Metropolitan Museum of Art was closing at dusk for fear of visitors running into things or stealing pictures in a blackout. Every night, the Museum of Modern Art (MoMA) was moving paintings to a sandbagged area, then rehanging them in the morning. The Frick Collection was blacking its windows and skylights so that enemy bombers couldn't spot it in the middle of Manhattan.

All this weighed on the minds of America's cultural leaders as they stepped from their taxis and up the stairway entry of the Metropolitan Museum of Art on the freezing cold morning of December 20, 1941. They had been summoned, via Western Union telegram, by Francis Henry Taylor, director of the Metropolitan Museum of Art and president of the Association of Art Museum Directors, and David Finley, the director of the National Gallery of Art. The forty-four men and four women who filed through the Met that morning were mostly museum directors, representing the majority of the leading American institutions east of the

Rocky Mountains: the Frick, Carnegie, Met, MoMA, Whitney, National Gallery, Smithsonian, and the major museums of Baltimore, Boston, Detroit, Chicago, St. Louis, and Minneapolis. Included were major names in the field like Jere Abbott, William Valentiner, Alfred Barr, Charles Sawyer, and John Walker.

Among them strode Paul Sachs, the associate director of Harvard's Fogg Art Museum. The Fogg was a relatively small institution, but Sachs had outsized influence within the museum community. He was the son of one of the early partners in the investment banking firm Goldman Sachs (the founder, Marcus Goldman, was his maternal grandfather), and was the museum community's primary conduit to the wealthy Jewish bankers of New York. More importantly, Sachs was the museum community's premier educator. In 1921, Sachs had created at Harvard his "Museum Work and Museum Problems" course, the first academic program specifically designed to cultivate and train men and women to become museum directors and curators. In addition to the connoisseurship of art, the "Museum Course" taught the financial and administrative aspects of running a museum, with a focus on eliciting donations. The students met regularly with major art collectors, bankers, and America's social elite, often at elegant dinners where they were required to wear formal dress and observe the social protocol of high culture. By 1941, Sachs's students had begun to fill the leadership positions of American museums, a field they would come to dominate in the postwar years.

How influential was Paul Sachs? Because he was short, about five foot two, he hung paintings low on the wall. When American museums rose to prominence after the war, many of the directors hung their paintings lower than their counterparts in Europe. Sachs's students had simply accepted it as the norm, and the other museums followed their lead.

Sachs, at the urging of George Stout, the dapper head of the Fogg's obscure but groundbreaking Department of Conservation and Technical Research, had taken a strong interest in the condition of the European museum community. The men, along with others at the Fogg, had created a short slide presentation to highlight this predicament. On the afternoon of the first day, as the overhead lights dimmed and Sachs's slide show flickered to life on the wall before them, the directors of America's great museums were subjected to a series of horrible reminders of the artistic toll of the Nazi advance. England's National Gallery in London deserted, its great works buried at Manod. The Tate Gallery filled with shattered glass. The nave of Canterbury Cathedral filled with dirt to absorb the shock of explosions. Slides of the Rijksmuseum in Amsterdam, the most famous national museum of the Netherlands, showed the paintings of the great Dutch masters stacked like folding chairs against empty walls. Perhaps its most famous holding, Rembrandt's monumental painting entitled *The Night Watch*, was rolled like a carpet and sealed in a box that appeared unnervingly like a coffin. In Paris, the Grande Galerie of the Louvre, reminiscent in its size and majesty of a Gilded Age train station, contained nothing but empty frames.

The images conjured other thoughts: of the stolen masterworks of Poland, which had not been seen in years; of the obliteration of the historic center of Rotterdam, destroyed by the Luftwaffe because the pace of peace negotiations with the Dutch had been too slow for Nazi tastes; of the great patriarchs of Vienna, imprisoned until they agreed to sign over to Germany their personal art holdings; of Michelangelo's *David*, entombed in brick by worried Italian officials, even though it stood inside a world-famous museum in the heart of Florence. Then there was Russia's state museum, the Hermitage. The curators had managed to evacuate 1.2 million of its estimated two million-plus works of art to Siberia before the Wehrmacht cut the rail lines out of Leningrad. It was rumored the curators were living in the basement with the remaining masterpieces, eating animal-based glue and even candles to keep from starving.

Paul Sachs's presentation had its desired effect: It focused the energies of the museum community. By that evening, they had unanimously agreed that America's museums would remain open as long as humanly possible. Defeatism was not an option, but neither was complacency. During the next two days, charged with an uncommon nervous energy, the museum leaders argued the practical and strategic concerns of operating in wartime: Should they open their doors to citizens for protection in the event of air raids? Should the most valuable works be permanently stored and replaced with lesser works? Should special events and exhibits continue, even if they drew crowds too large for efficient evacuation? Should works be sent from museums on the coasts to museums in the interior states, where the dangers were few? What about incendiary bombs? Blackouts? Broken glass?

The final resolution, introduced the next day by Paul Sachs, was a call to arms:[2]

> If, in time of peace, our museums and art galleries are important to the community, in time of war they are doubly valuable. For then, when the petty and the trivial fall way and we are face to face with final and lasting values, we...must summon to our defense all our intellectual and spiritual resources. We must guard jealously all we have inherited from a long past, all we are capable of creating in a trying present, and all we are determined to preserve in a foreseeable future.
>
> Art is the imperishable and dynamic expression of these aims. It is, and always has been, the visible evidence of the activity of free minds....Therefore be it resolved:
>
> 1) That American museums are prepared to do their utmost in the service of the people of this country during the present conflict
> 2) That they will continue to keep open their doors to all who seek refreshment of spirit
> 3) That they will, with the sustained financial help of their communities, broaden the scope and variety of their work
> 4) That they will be sources of inspiration illuminating the past and vivifying the present; that they will fortify the spirit on which victory depends.

Despite the high-flown words, most of the major East Coast museums continued making preparations for war. The Metropolitan quietly closed its less important galleries, replacing the curatorial staff with firemen. On New Year's Eve, in the dead of night, the National Gallery loaded seventy-five of its best works and secretly slipped them out of Washington, D.C. When the museum opened for the first time in 1942, lesser works hung in their places. On January 12, the masterpieces arrived at the Biltmore, the great Vanderbilt estate in the mountains of North Carolina, where they would remain hidden until 1944.

But all the energy of that December meeting wasn't spent on evacuations. Sensing an opportunity, Paul Sachs and his dapper conservator George Stout invited the museum directors to the Fogg for a series of seminars on museum safety. Dozens came to be educated by Stout, who had been in close contact with leading conservators in Europe for years, about the difficulties that lay ahead. Stout taught about molds and fungus, the virtues of wire mesh, and heat damage. He explained why bombs blew out windows, and how best to crate paintings to avoid punctures from flying glass. For the December meeting at the Met, he had prepared a pamphlet on countering the effects of air raids. In the spring of 1942, he expanded that pamphlet into an article in his monthly trade journal, *Technical Issues*, providing the first attempt at a systemic approach to preservation of works of art in times of war.

At the same time, Stout pushed for a concerted, industry-wide response. In April 1942, he elucidated the problems of wartime conservation in a pamphlet sent to Francis Henry Taylor, the man behind the December 1941 meeting. American museums, he suggested, were unprepared to handle a crisis because "there [is] no collected body of knowledge; there [are] no accepted standards of procedure." Museums must "be willing to pool all of their experiences, to share their losses as well as their gains, to expose their doubts as well as their convictions, and to maintain a regular method of co-operative work.... The good of all [will] have to be definitely and practically considered as the good of any one."[3]

Stout's solution, beyond the sharing of information, was the immediate training of a large new class of conservators, "special workmen" who could handle the largest, most dangerous upheaval in the history of Western art. Stout suggested the training would take five years, even as he admitted the art world was in crisis. Already more than two million European works had been moved from their cozy museums to barely adequate temporary storage, often across bumpy roads and under bombardment by the enemy. And those were just the official evacuations; the number didn't account for the rumors of mass plundering by the Nazis. It was going to take an extraordinary amount of effort and intelligence to put the art world right again. And what about the inevitable, and no doubt brutally destructive, aerial and ground attacks necessary to win the freedom of Europe?

In the summer of 1942, in a pamphlet entitled *Protection of Monuments: A Proposal for Consideration During War and Rehabilitation*, Stout laid out in explicit terms the challenges that lay ahead:[4]

As soldiers of the United Nations fight their way into lands once conquered and held by the enemy, the governments of the United Nations will encounter manifold problems....In areas torn by bombardment and fire are monuments cherished by the people of those countrysides or towns: churches, shrines, statues, pictures, many kinds of works. Some may be destroyed; some damaged. All risk further injury, looting or destruction....

To safeguard these things will not affect the course of battles, but it will affect the relations of invading armies with those peoples and [their] governments.... To safeguard these things will show respect for the beliefs and customs of all men and will bear witness that these things belong not only to a particular people but also to the heritage of mankind. To safeguard these things is part of the responsibility that lies on the governments of the United Nations. These monuments are not merely pretty things, not merely valued signs of man's creative power. They are expressions of faith, and they stand for man's struggle to relate himself to his past and to his God.

With conviction that the safeguarding of monuments is an element in the right conduct of the war and in the hope for peace, we...wish to bring these facts to the attention of the government of the United States of America and to urge that means be sought for dealing with them.

And who was best able to handle such safeguarding? The highly trained corps of "special workmen" Stout had previously proposed, of course.

September 17, 1940
German Feldmarschall Keitel's order concerning seizure of cultural property

COPY

The Chief of the Supreme Command of the
Armed Forces Berlin W 35, Tirpitzufer 72-76,
17 Sept 1940 Tel: 21 81 91

2 f 28.1.4 W. Z. No. 3812/ 40 g
To the Chief of Army High Command for the
Military Administration in Occupied France.

In supplement to the order of the Führer
transmitted at the time to Reichsleiter Rosenberg
to search lodges, libraries and archives in the
occupied territories of the west for material
valuable to Germany, and to safeguard the latter
through the Gestapo, the Führer has decided:

The ownership status before the war in France,
prior to the declaration of war on 1 September
1939, shall be the criterion.

Ownership transfers to the French state or
similar transfers completed after this date are
irrelevant and legally invalid (for example,
Polish and Slovak libraries in Paris, possessions
of the Palais Rothschild or other ownerless Jewish
possessions). Reservations regarding search,
seizure and transportation to Germany on the
basis of the above reasons will not be recognized.

Reichsleiter Rosenberg and/or his deputy
Reichshauptstellenleiter Ebert has received
clear instructions from the Führer personally
governing the right of seizure; he is entitled to
transport to Germany cultural goods which appear
valuable to him and to safeguard them there. The
Führer has reserved for himself the decision as
to their use.

It is requested that the services in question
be informed correspondingly. Signed : KEITEL For
information : Attention : Reichsleiter Rosenberg

CHAPTER 4

A Dull and Empty World

Harvard and Maryland
Winter 1942–1943

George Stout was not a typical museum official. Unlike many of his peers, who were the product of the eastern elite establishment, Stout was a blue-collar kid from the small town of Winterset, Iowa (also the hometown of actor John Wayne). From there, he went straight into the army, where he served during World War I as a private in a hospital unit in Europe. On a lark, he decided to study drawing after returning from war. Following his graduation from the University of Iowa, Stout spent five years in hand-to-mouth jobs, saving for the tour of the cultural centers of Europe that was the unspoken prerequisite of a career in the arts. By the time he arrived at Harvard to begin graduate studies in 1926, the year Harry Ettlinger was born in Karlsruhe, Germany, Stout was a twenty-eight-year-old husband with a pregnant wife. His Carnegie Fellowship paid him a stipend of $1,200 a year (his monthly rent was $39), which his young family soon found was enough to stay "only a little above starvation level."[1]

In 1928, Stout joined the small art conservation department at the Fogg Art Museum as an unpaid graduate assistant. Conservation, the technical art of preserving older or damaged works, was the least popular field in the art history department, and Stout was probably its most diligent and self-effacing disciple. In fact, in a department based on braggadocio, where a student's prospects were often based on personal relationships with superstar professors like Paul Sachs, Stout was perhaps the most anonymous student. But he was also meticulous, a trait that carried over to his personal appearance: carefully swept-back hair, trim worsted suits, and a fine pencil mustache in the style of one of the great film stars of the day, Errol Flynn. George Stout was dapper, debonair, and resolutely unflappable. But beneath his placid exterior was a brilliant and restless mind, capable of great leaps of understanding and far-reaching vision. He also possessed another essential quality: extraordinary patience.

Soon after joining the conservation department, Stout noticed an abandoned card catalogue from the university library. The rows of tiny drawers gave him an idea. The conservation department contained an astonishing array of the raw materials of painting: pigments, stones, dried plants, oils, resins, gums, glues, and balsams. With the help of the department chemist, John Gettens, Stout placed samples in each of the card catalogue's drawers, added various chemicals, and observed the results. And took notes. And observed. And waited. For years. Five years later, using only piles of scraps and a discarded chest of drawers, Stout and Gettens had pioneered studies in three branches of the *science* of art conservation: rudiments (understanding raw materials), degradation (understanding the causes of deterioration), and reparations (stopping and then repairing damage).

"I think we got some work done, back at the start," Gettens commented shortly before his death in 1974, "because nobody knew us, nobody bothered us—and we had no money."[2]

The breakthrough led Stout—still known only to the handful of practitioners in his field—to a new mission. For centuries, conservation had been considered an art, the domain of restorers trained by masters in the techniques of repainting. If it was going to become a science, as Stout's experiments suggested, then it needed a body of scientific knowledge. Throughout the 1930s, Stout corresponded regularly with the great conservators of the day, sharing information and slowly compiling a set of scientific principles for the evaluation and preservation of paintings and visual arts.

Things began to change in July 1936, when the Spanish Fascists, supported by powerful German armaments and military training, plunged their country into a civil war. By October, incendiary bombs were landing close to El Escorial, the great monastery-museum thirty miles northwest of Madrid. Two weeks later, the windows were blown out of Spain's national museum, the Prado. In the spring of 1937, Germany entered the conflict and unleashed, for the first time, its corps of tanks and airplanes, the foundation of its evolving doctrine of "lightning warfare."

The art world realized that Germany's powerful weapons, and especially its use of massive aerial bombardment, had suddenly made the bulk of the continent's great artistic masterpieces susceptible to destruction.

The Europeans and British quickly began to develop plans for protection and evacuation, and George Stout began to slowly, letter by letter, reshape his storehouse of knowledge for a world at war. For the meeting at the Metropolitan Museum in December 1941, he created a pamphlet about air raid techniques. It was only a few pages long, but it was culled from a decade of research. It was typical George Stout: detailed, timely, and understated. Here was a man who never hurried. Who was careful. Punctual. Precise. *An expert and a precisionist makes his analysis first*, he always said, *then his decision.*[3]

He spent most of the next year and a half training curators and pushing for a national conservation plan. But nothing came together, and by the fall of 1942 the unflappable George Stout was discouraged. He had spent his entire career developing expertise in an obscure subset of art history, and suddenly world events had thrust that expertise to the forefront. This was *the* moment for art conservation; there was not a second to lose if the world's cultural patrimony was going to be preserved—and nobody would listen to him. Instead, the wartime conservation movement was being controlled by the museum directors, the "sahibs" of the art world, as Stout called them. Stout was a workman, a toiler in the trenches, and he had the nuts-and-bolts technician's distaste for the manager's world of committees, conversations, and the cultivation of clients.

"I got damned good and tired of the personal, playhouse point of view that seemed to hold in the museum administration a fair share of the time," he wrote a friend at Harvard's Fogg Art Museum. "I tried to buck it, but that was useless....I figure to have about 20 years more of useful time. That's enough to work with but not enough to play with and I'm through with all that smirking and primping for rich people and making paper dolls out of policies and principles just to please them."[4]

Stout was convinced that only his dedicated corps of "special workmen," trained in art conservation and working through the army, could accomplish anything of lasting value in the coming war. But the museum directors were, in his opinion, smirking and primping, trying to land an endorsement from President Roosevelt for a high-level cultural committee to advise the military—a committee that no doubt would be comprised of the directors themselves.

In early 1943, unable to make any headway in America, Stout and fellow conservator W. G. Constable of the Museum of Fine Arts, Boston, turned to the British. In a letter to Kenneth Clark, director of the National Gallery in London, the men laid out their plan for a conservation corps. Clark thought the concept ludicrous. "I find it hard to believe," he wrote back, "that any machinery could be set up which would carry out the suggestions contained in your petition, e.g. even supposing it were possible for an archeologist to accompany each invading force, I cannot help feeling that he would have great difficulty in restraining a commanding officer from shelling an important military objective just because it contained some fine historical monuments."[5]

Stout may never have seen the reply. By January 1943, with the nation at war and in need of men, he had given up on the conservation program and applied for active duty in the navy, in which he had been a reservist since the end of World War I. "In these last months," he admitted in a letter home after his arrival at Patuxent River Naval Air Station in Maryland, "I have not felt worthy. I was failing to get done what in these times a man ought to do. The work was hemmed in by other people and it was small and secondary. Now there is a chance to do work that needs doing, and a good deal more than any man can do."[6]

Although he couldn't tell his wife what he was doing because of the military censors—he was testing camouflage paint for airplanes—he assured her that he was happy. "[The job] has so much to it and so much responsibility that I am scared and pleased. If we can do what we hope to do, or any decent part of it, I'll have no doubt about what is called 'making a contribution.'"[7]

Soon after, his friend Constable wrote that Colonel James Shoemaker, head of the United States Military Government Division, had unexpectedly taken an interest in Stout's work, requesting all his information on monuments and conservation. Constable cautioned that "though all signs point to the creation of some kind of conservation corps being in the military mind, I have not the least idea whether the idea has crystallized, and it may never do so."[8]

Stout wrote back that "this move of the nebulous scheme into definite shape in army hands is most satisfying.... Francis Taylor telephoned me some days ago. He was on another trip to get his big scheme started. But he sounded out of sorts and fed up, as if the business wasn't going too well. Perhaps the modest, steady effort will do more."[9]

Stout assured Constable, however, that his navy billet was "distinctly my cup of tea" and that he had no interest in leaving it. "I'll do anything I can to help," he wrote, "but it's hard to imagine what that would be, or where I'd get the time for it."[10]

Still, the decision to enlist in the navy gnawed at him—not because of the conservation program (he considered that a dead issue), but because of his family. Stout was forty-five, married, the father of two sons. He had held out for the higher pay grade of a lieutenant's rank, but he knew his modest military pay would barely support his family, even in the modest means to which they were accustomed by his long toils in an obscure specialty. He was a man of his time, and although Margie worked as a teacher, he believed it was his duty to provide. And he hated the idea of leaving her.

"This seems a dull and empty world after the great experience of being at home those precious hours," he wrote Margie after a brief furlough in July 1943. "I was so deeply touched by you and [his seven-year-old son] Tom, your valor and your incomprehensible love for me. I do not deserve it but I return it all and I swear to do my best to be worthy. I have to keep on teaching myself...that this is right and that I have not left you to struggle because of a romantic whim."[11]

November 5, 1940
Reichsmarschall Hermann Göring's order concerning distribution of Jewish art treasures

In carrying out the measures taken to date for the safeguarding of Jewish art property by the Chief of Military Administration in Paris and the Einsatzstab Rosenberg (Chef OKW. 2 f 28.14. W. Z. Nr 3812/ 40 g), the categories of art objects moved to the Louvre will be established as follows:

1. Those art objects for the further disposition of which the Führer has reserved for himself the right of decision;
2. Those art objects which will serve to complete the collection of the Reichsmarschall;
3. Those art objects and library material which appear useful for building up the Hohe Schule and for the task of Reichsleiter Rosenberg;
4. Those art objects that are appropriate for turning over to German museums; will immediately be inventoried, packed and transported to Germany by the Einsatzstab with all due care and with the assistance of the Luftwaffe.
5. Those art objects which are appropriate for transfer to French museums and to the French and German art trade will be sold at auction at a date yet to be fixed; and the proceeds will be assigned to the French State for benefit of the French dependents of war casualties.

6. Further seizure of Jewish art property in
   France will be effected in the heretofore
   efficient manner by the Einsatzstab Rosenberg,
   in co-operation with the Chief of the Military
   Administration Paris.

Paris, 5 November 1940

I shall submit this suggestion to the Führer,
pending whose approval this procedure will
remain effective.

Signed: GÖRING

CHAPTER 5

Leptis Magna

North Africa
January 1943

While the Americans worried and planned, the British were actively engaged in combat operations against the Axis powers. In Europe, the Allied war machine consisted mainly of underground saboteurs and the brave pilots battling the German Luftwaffe over the English Channel; in the USSR, the Red Army was fighting a defensive entrenchment against an aggressive Nazi offensive; but across the Mediterranean the battle swung back and forth over the great desert of North Africa. The British held Egypt; a combined German-Italian force held Libya and Algeria to the west. For two years, starting with an Italian assault on Egypt in 1940, the battle went back and forth across the desert. It wasn't until October 1942, and the decisive defeat of the German-Italian forces at the Second Battle of El Alamein, that the British finally broke through and began to push their way toward Tripoli, the Libyan capital.

By January 1943, they had reached Leptis Magna, a sprawling Roman ruin only sixty-four miles east of Tripoli. It was here that Lieutenant Colonel Sir Robert

Eric Mortimer Wheeler, Royal Artillery, British North African Army, beheld the majesty of Emperor Lucius Septimius Severus's imperial city: the imposing gate of the basilica, the hundreds of columns that marked the old marketplace, the enormous sloping amphitheater, with the blue waters of the Mediterranean sparkling in the background. At the height of its power at the turn of the third century AD—when Emperor Severus had showered money on his hometown in an attempt to make it the cultural and economic capital of Africa— Leptis Magna had been a port, but in the last seventeen hundred years the harbor had silted up and become a hardpan of clay, a dull and empty world.

Here, Mortimer Wheeler thought, *is power. And a reminder of our mortality.*

The city was broken, wearing down and sliding back into the Sahara Desert that had been encroaching on it for the last two thousand years. Most of the columns and blocks were dull, already mirroring the color of reddish sand, but amid the ruins he could make out a few gleaming white additions, some of the many "improvements" made by the Italians over the last decade. *A new empire is rising from the ruins of the old*, Mussolini told the Italians time and again. *We are building another Roman empire.* Wheeler took a drink from his canteen and scanned the enormous sky for signs of enemy planes. Nothing, not even a cloud. For the second time, the Italians had forsaken this cornerstone of their "empire" without even putting up a fight.

The first time was 1940, when 36,000 British and Australian troops turned back an advance on Egypt by the 200,000-man Italian Tenth Army.

The British lost the ruins in 1941 when the Italians, buttressed by crack German troops and under the command of the German general Erwin Rommel, pushed them back to Egypt. Soon after, the Italians published the great cultural propaganda piece *Che cosa hanno fatto gli Inglesi in Cirenaica—What the English Have Done in Cyrenaica*. The pamphlet showed plundered artifacts, smashed statues, and defaced walls at the Cyrene Museum, the work, the Italians claimed, of British and Australian soldiers. Only with the recent recapture of Cyrene, four hundred miles east of Leptis Magna, had the British learned the Italian claims were false. The statues had been broken for hundreds of years; the pedestals were empty because the Italians had removed the statues; the graffiti was not on the walls of the museum galleries, but in a back room filled with similar graffiti by Italian troops.

But what a black eye the whole episode had caused the War Office: For almost two years, the British had to defend themselves against charges they had no way to confirm or deny. They had no archeologists in North Africa, and no one had examined the site while it was in British hands. In fact, no one in the army had considered the historic and cultural value, and therefore propaganda value, of Cyrene at all.

Now Wheeler stood in the center of Leptis Magna, watching in amazement as the British army repeated that mistake. To his left, equipment trucks were grinding over the ancient Roman paving stones. To his right, troops were climbing on fallen walls. An Arab guard, Wheeler noticed, could do nothing more than wave his arms as a tank drove right past him and into the temple.

The gunner popped out and started waving. His mate snapped a picture. *Perfect day in North Africa, Mum, wish you were here.* Had the British army learned nothing from the debacle of Cyrenaica? At this rate, they really were going to give the Italians something to complain about.

"Can't we do something, sir?" Wheeler asked the deputy chief Civil Affairs officer (CAO). Civil Affairs was assigned to administer a captured area once the fighting had stopped. It kept the peace, as it were, even if that peace was only a mile or two from the front line.

The officer shrugged. "Just soldiers being soldiers," he said.

"But this is Leptis Magna," Wheeler protested. "The great city of the Roman emperor Lucius Septimius Severus. The most complete Roman ruin in all of Africa."

The man just looked at him. "Never heard of it," he said.

Wheeler shook his head. Every officer had been told about Cyrenaica. But a CAO of the British North African Army had never been briefed on Leptis Magna, even though the army was sure to be fighting there. Why? Because they hadn't yet been accused of desecrating it? Was the whole war an exercise in understanding mistakes only after they had been made?

"Are they important?" the officer asked.

"What?"

"The broken buildings."

"They're classical ruins, sir. And yes, they're important."

"Why?"

"They're irreplaceable. They're history. They're…
It's our duty as soldiers to protect them, sir. If we don't,
the enemy will use that against us."

"Are you a historian, Lieutenant?"

"I'm an archeologist. Director of the London
Museum."[1]

The Civil Affairs officer nodded. "Then do something about it, Director."

When Wheeler realized the CAO was serious, he
swung into action. By good fortune, he soon discovered that an archeological colleague from the
London Museum, Lieutenant Colonel John Bryan
Ward-Perkins, happened to be serving as an artillery
captain in a unit near Leptis Magna. With the support of the CAO, the two men rerouted traffic, photographed damage, posted guards, and organized repair
efforts at the ruined city. *If nothing else*, they thought,
it keeps the troops busy.

In London, their reports met with a quizzical stare.
Leptis Magna? Preservation? "Send it to Woolley,"
someone finally said. "He'll know what to do."

Woolley was Sir Charles Leonard Woolley, a world-
famous archeologist who in the years before World War
I had been a close companion of Sir Thomas Edward
Lawrence, better known as Lawrence of Arabia. Now
in his sixties, he was serving in the British War Office
in a completely unrelated capacity. Woolley did indeed
care about the world's ancient treasures, and by the
spring of 1943, the three men had found time around
their regular duties to prepare preservation plans for all
three of Libya's ancient sites.

It was Wheeler and Ward-Perkins who insisted that,

in addition to being protected, "the ancient sites and the Museums [of Greek and Roman North Africa] should be made accessible to troops and the interest of the antiquities be brought home to them."[2] An informed army, in other words, is a respectful and disciplined army. And a respectful and disciplined army is much less likely to cause cultural harm. Without realizing it, the British were inching their way toward the goal George Stout was pushing so earnestly back in the United States: the world's first front line monuments protection program.

CHAPTER 6

The First Campaign

Sicily
Summer 1943

In January 1943, as Wheeler and Ward-Perkins formalized their plans for Leptis Magna and George Stout reported for naval duty in Maryland, U.S. President Roosevelt and British Prime Minister Winston Churchill met for a secret summit in Casablanca, Morocco. (Soviet premier Joseph Stalin was invited, but could not attend.) North Africa lay in Allied hands, the Italians having been routed by Free French and British forces in Algeria, but Fortress Europe remained unbreached. Roosevelt, under the advice of his military commanders, in particular General George C. Marshall, wanted to attack immediately across the English Channel; Churchill and his military advisors, with the support of the American General Dwight D. "Ike" Eisenhower, argued that the Allies weren't ready. After ten days of meetings, the two powers agreed on an invasion of Europe, but not across the English Channel. They would go in through the back door: the island of Sicily, just off the toe of the Italian mainland.

The Sicilian campaign would be a joint operation, unprecedented in history, with the United States and

Great Britain sharing command on everything from air combat missions to laundry duty at the preparations base in Algiers. Needless to say, it was not going to be easy to integrate two independent armies. Almost immediately, the troops in North Africa noticed the home powers had gotten a few assignments muddled: The food was British and the toilets French, when it should have been the other way around. It was a harbinger of things to come.

Among the thousands of responsibilities that became "allied" between the two powers that spring was the nascent conservation program begun by Wheeler and Ward-Perkins in the ruins of Leptis Magna. In late April 1943, it was decided that two officers, one American and one British, should be sent to Sicily to inspect all monuments in the occupied territories "as soon as practicable after occupation."[1] Paul Sachs and the museum directors got their first crack at policy when the U.S. Army asked them to recommend someone to become the American Advisor on Fine Arts and Monuments. They suggested one of their own, Francis Henry Taylor, the Met director and maker of "big schemes" so derided by George Stout, but he was rejected for military duty because he was...well, too fat. Pressed for time, and needing someone already enlisted in the military, the directors chose Captain Mason Hammond, a Harvard classics professor working in Army Air Forces Intelligence.

Unfortunately, nobody told Hammond, who arrived in Algiers for his mysterious new assignment knowing only that he would be working on conservation issues. His first days were filled with more shocks than just terrible food and despicable toilets.

He arrived in June. He was told the invasion was set for early July.

Invasion? He had assumed he would be serving in North Africa. No, he was told, he was going to Sicily.

Then he better get to the library in Algiers and brush up on his knowledge. Sicily was not his area of expertise. Sorry, he was told, no public research. It could tip German spies to the army's next destination.

Then he would study the army's research on Sicily. None was available, for the same reason.

Then could he study the lists and descriptions of the monuments he was supposed to protect? Unfortunately, the lists were still being worked on by Paul Sachs and his colleagues in New York. They might not be finished for weeks. And even if they arrived before the invasion, they would be off-limits, too. Same reason: German spies. The lists would be shipped to Sicily and given to commanders *after* the landing.

Then he needed to speak to his fellow art officers immediately.

Art officers? There was only one. And he was British. And he...wasn't there. Lord Woolley, who was running the British side, had wanted Wheeler or Ward-Perkins, but both had been reassigned since Leptis Magna. Once he found out they weren't available, he had begun to drag his feet on assigning his officer.

Dragged his feet?

There wasn't another officer. At least not yet.

Then what about staff for the deployment?

No staff.

Transportation?

None assigned.

Typewriters? Radios? Lanterns? Maps? Scratch paper? Pencils?

No supplies assigned either.

What about orders?

Didn't have any. He was free to go where he chose.

Hammond, confronted with the reality on the ground, realized that in essence there was no mission at all. Freedom, it seemed, was another word for nothing important to do. Which didn't bother Hammond. "I doubt if there is need for any large specialist staff for this work," he wrote from North Africa to a friend, "since it is at best a luxury and the military will not look kindly on a lot of art experts running around trying to tell them what not to hit."[2] Even the first "Monuments Man," as the conservation experts came to be known, initially thought the manner in which the army was going about the mission was utterly foolish and a waste of time.

The Allies landed in Sicily on the night of July 9–10, 1943. Hammond, low on the priority list for transportation and considered part of the occupation force, didn't arrive until July 29, long after the troops had left the beachhead. In Syracuse, his first headquarters, the weather was warm but pleasantly breezy. Local cultural officials greeted him enthusiastically—the mainland Italians and Germans had treated them terribly, they were happy to be free of them—and took him on a sightseeing tour of the local monuments. Despite being in the path of the army, they had received little damage. The southern coast, his next destination, was tranquil, nothing but hills sloping quietly to the sea. As he looked over the great Roman ruins at Agrigento a few days later, striped with shadow in the relentless Sicilian sun, he saw plenty of damage, but none that had been done in the last thousand years. His prediction seemed prescient; other than consult with a few local Sicilian experts, there wasn't much for a Monuments Man to do.

The walls of reality came crashing in at Palermo, the Sicilian capital. The Allies had bombed the city relentlessly as part of a diversionary air campaign, destroying the old harbor section, numerous churches and cathedrals, the state library, state archives, and the botanical gardens. Every official in the area, it seemed, was demanding action from the Allied Military Government (AMG), and everyone was directed to the one poor captain sitting in a folding chair in a threadbare corner of a shared office. The Sicilians were willing to help, but they needed explanations, assessments, financing for repairs, equipment, supplies, and skilled craftsmen for emergency work on buildings in danger of collapse. The archbishop wanted special attention paid to the churches...and to his personal palazzo. General Patton, whose U.S. Seventh Army troops had taken the city, wanted money to redecorate his barracks, the former palace of the king of Sicily.

Hammond didn't have time to listen to all the questions, much less answer them. For more than a month, he wasn't able to get out of the office to inspect any sites. Using his personal typewriter he had carried with him from home, he sent reports to the War Department, and long letters home, begging for information and reinforcements. Nothing came until September, when the British Monuments officer Captain F. H. J.

Maxse finally arrived. But by then it was too late. When the Allies leapt from the toe of Sicily to mainland Italy on September 3, 1943, Hammond was still frustrated, confused, and hopelessly mired hundreds of miles away in Palermo. Even small, mostly rural Sicily had proven too much for the initial MFAA effort.

———

On September 10, 1943, a week after the Allied landing in mainland Italy, a jubilant Paul Sachs wrote to George Stout: "I should have written to you some time ago to tell you that your 'brain child' has finally taken shape in an official kind of way and, as you know, the President has appointed an American Commission for the Protection and Salvage of Artistic and Historic Monuments in Europe with Mr. [Supreme Court] Justice Roberts as Chairman, and I have been asked to be a member of that Commission and I have accepted.... It seemed to me...that I ought to post you at once because not only is this commission the result of your great thinking and clear statements at the time of the Metropolitan meeting just after Pearl Harbor, but in a very true sense you seem to me the real father of the whole show...it is my deliberate opinion that the appointment of this Commission is due to your initiative, imagination and energy."[3]

Stout must have read the announcement with bemusement. Sure, he was the father, but what exactly had he birthed? Not the frontline, specialist force he had envisioned, but another layer of bureaucracy? Paul Sachs and the museum directors had, after more than two years of effort, pushed through their vision, not his.

On September 13, as U.S. Fifth Army fought desperately to hold on to its Italian beachhead at Salerno, Stout sent Sachs a reply. "I congratulate the U.S. Government and the chairman of the American commission on getting you to serve," he told Sachs in his usual self-deprecating, biting, and slyly humorous style. "You are kind to give me so much credit in getting this work under way, but you magnify it one hell of a lot. Something far below the average set of brains is needed to figure out what ought to be done. Getting it done is what counts."[4]

March 20, 1941
Report to the Führer by Alfred Rosenberg, head of the main Nazi looting organization, known as the ERR

I report the arrival of the principal shipment of ownerless Jewish "cultural property" [Kulturgut] in the salvage location Neuschwanstein by special train on Saturday the 15th of this month. It was secured by my staff for Special Purposes [Einsatzstab] in Paris. The especial train, arranged for by Reichsmarschall Hermann Göring, comprised 25 express baggage cars filled with the most valuable paintings, furniture, Gobelins, works of artistic craftsmanship and ornaments. The shipment consisted chiefly of the most important parts of the collections Rothschild, Seligmann, Bernheim-Jeune, Halphen, Kann, Weil-Picard, Wildenstein, David-Weill, Levy-Benzion.

My Staff for Special Purposes started the confiscatory action in Paris during October 1940 on the basis of your order, my Führer. With the help of the Security Service (SD) and the Secret Field Police [Geheime Feldpolizei] all storage—and hiding—places of art possessions belonging to the fugitive Jewish emigrants were systematically ascertained. These possessions were then collected in the locations provided for by the Louvre in Paris. The art historians of my staff have itemized scientifically the complete art-material and have photographed all works of value. Thus, after completion, I shall

be able to submit to you shortly a conclusive
catalogue of all confiscated works with exact
data about origin plus scientific evaluation
and description. At this time the inventory
includes more than 4000 individual pieces of art,
partly of the highest artistic value. Besides
this special train the masterpieces selected by
the Reichsmarschall—mainly from the Rothschild
collection—have been forwarded in two special
cars to Munich already some time ago. They have
been deposited there in the air raid shelters of
the Führer-building. . . .

Over and above the main shipment there are
secured in Paris a large number of additional
abandoned Jewish art possessions. These are
being processed in the same sense and prepared
for shipment to Germany. Exact accounts about
the extent of this remaining shipment are
at the moment not available. However, it is
estimated that the work in the Western areas
will be finished entirely within two to three
months. Then a second transport can be brought to
Germany.

Berlin, 20 March 1941 A. Rosenberg

CHAPTER 7

Monte Cassino

Southern Italy
Winter 1943–1944

U.S. Fifth Army landed on mainland Italy near Salerno on September 9, 1943. It was supposed to be a surprise landing, with no air or naval support, but as the troop carriers approached the shore near Salerno the Germans shouted out over a loudspeaker in English, "Come on in and surrender. We have you covered." The Americans came in firing anyway, and the battle was one of the bloodiest of the war. The campaign hadn't been much easier since. The battle for the major airfields at Foggia was so intense, for instance, that afterward the decimated 82nd Airborne Division had to be merged with the British X (Tenth) Corps.

Nonetheless, Fifth Army took its primary objective, the southern port city of Naples, on October 1. They pushed on immediately, taking the high ground south of the Volturno River on October 6. Before them stretched several hundred miles of rugged, mountainous terrain, dug through with fortifications and strung with four major defensive lines. The Italian surrender, offered on September 3, the day of the first Allied landing on the mainland, had been announced on September 8, but Hitler had not been caught off guard. He had anticipated Italy's lack of resolve and stationed German troops throughout the country. As the Italian soldiers laid down their weapons, hardened German troops had swarmed in to take their place. They were well-trained, battle-tested, determined... and everywhere. The weather deteriorated. Drenching rain turned the mud roads into bogs, then freezing cold turned those bogs into ice. Rivers skipped their banks; troop bivouacs flooded. The treacherous mountain terrain north of the Volturno allowed the Germans to engage and retreat with deadly efficiency. German observers on the mountain peaks called in nearly continuous artillery fire. Allied commanders had hoped to be in Rome before the onset of winter. When the sleet started falling, they weren't even halfway there.

On December 1, Fifth Army entered the Liri Valley. Flanking units fought the Germans on the snowy peaks, while the main body of troops moved through the valley in a driving rain, mostly under cover of darkness, always under fire. Forty-five days later, they finally reached the other end of what was already being referred to as Purple Heart Valley, because of the vast number of soldiers wounded or killed in action there. Before them lay the town of Cassino, the anchor of the Gustav Line, the Germans' main defensive entrenchment south of Rome. The mountain ridge above the town offered a commanding view of the valley, allowing the Germans to turn back an Allied assault on January 17, 1944. For weeks, the rain pounded the huddled men, and the temperature froze them in their boots. Another Allied assault was turned back, with high casualties, and still the shells poured down as steady as the rain.

The mountain was bad, but far worse for the weary soldiers was what stood atop it: the formidable, towering, thousand-year-old abbey of Monte Cassino. The monastery had been founded by Saint Benedict around AD 529, during the last days of the Roman Empire, partly because its excellent defensive position offered protection from a pagan world. It was at Monte Cassino that the saint wrote the Benedictine Rules, establishing the tradition of monasticism in the Western world. It was there he died and was buried. The abbey was sacred ground, an intellectual center and "a symbol of the preservation and cultivation of the things of the mind and the spirit through times of great stress."[1] Now the grand and imposing abbey seemed to glare down at the weary and bloodstained Allied troops, a symbol of Nazi strength.

Western Allied commanders didn't want to destroy the abbey. Only weeks earlier, in one of his last acts before leaving Italy, General Dwight D. Eisenhower had issued an executive order stating that important artistic and historical sites were not to be bombed. Monte Cassino, one of the great achievements of early Italian and Christian culture, was clearly a protected site. Eisenhower's order had provided exceptions. "If we have to choose between destroying a famous building and sacrificing our own men," he wrote, "then our men's lives count infinitely more and the buildings must go."[2] But he had also drawn a line between military necessity and military convenience, and no commander wanted to be the first to test that line.

So for a month, the Allied commanders vacillated, and for a month the Allied soldiers hunkered down in the valley of death. The weather was brutally cold. There seemed no end to the rain. Many days, the clouds were so thick the troops couldn't see the monastery, and the world was nothing but the blackened trunks of shell-damaged trees. Then the clouds would lift, and the abbey would stare down at them. Day after day, the troops slogged through grasping, freezing mud, wet to the bone and hounded by German shells. The press picked up on the misery, reporting not just on the squalid conditions but the growing list of dead and wounded men. The more the press and soldiers looked to the mountain, the more they saw the abbey not as a world treasure but as a leering death trap, bristling with German guns. The name Monte Cassino echoed around the world: the mountain of death, the valley of sorrow, the one building keeping Western Allied forces from Rome.

The citizens back home, appalled by the suffering of their boys, wanted Cassino destroyed. The British commanders wanted Cassino destroyed. The soldiers wanted Cassino destroyed. But some American and French commanders were opposed, unconvinced the Germans were inside. Brigadier Butler, deputy commander of U.S. 34th Division, remarked, "I don't know, but I don't believe the enemy is in the convent [*sic*]. All the fire has been from the slopes of the hill below the wall."[3] Finally the British, and especially the Indian, Australian, and New Zealand forces designated for the first wave of assault on the entrenched Germans, won out. Major General Howard Kippenberger, leader of the New Zealand forces at Monte Cassino, summarized the need for bombing this way: "If not occupied today, it [the abbey] might be tomorrow and it did not appear it would be difficult for the enemy to bring reserves into it during an attack or for troops to take shelter there if driven from positions outside. It was impossible to ask troops to storm a hill surmounted by an intact building such as this."[4]

On February 15, 1944, amid the cheers of Allied soldiers and war correspondents, a massive aerial bombing destroyed the magnificent abbey at Monte Cassino. General Eaker of the U.S. Army Air Forces hailed it as a great triumph, an example of what the Germans could expect for the rest of the war.

The rest of the world did not cheer. Instead, the Germans and Italians turned the tables on the Allies, suggesting that if this was what the world could expect then the Allies were the barbarians and the traitors. Cardinal Maglione, speaking for the Vatican, called the destruction of the abbey "a colossal blunder" and "a piece of gross stupidity."[5]

Two days later, after several smaller attacks, Western Allies launched a massive assault on the mountain. Once again, the troops were turned back by heavy fire. As Brigadier Butler had suspected, the Germans hadn't been in the abbey—they had actually been respecting its cultural importance—and the bombing had not weakened their position. In fact, it had strengthened it by allowing them to drop paratroopers into the ruins and incorporate them into their defenses. It would take another three months, and an estimated 54,000 of their own men dead and wounded, for the Allies to capture Monte Cassino.

On May 27, 1944, a week after its capture and more than three months after its destruction, the first Monuments Man to visit the town of Cassino, Major Ernest DeWald, arrived for an inspection tour of the ruins of Monte Cassino. He found the foundations and underground chambers of the complex intact, but almost everything aboveground was destroyed. The seventeenth-century church was gone; the library, art galleries, and monastery were nothing more than rubble. He located the debris that had once been the basilica, but found no trace of its famous eleventh-century bronze doors or mosaic tile. He didn't know if the monastery's magnificent library and celebrated art collection had been buried or destroyed, or if it had been removed by the Germans prior to the bombing. The only things of value Major DeWald saw that afternoon, as he picked through the rubble, were the faces of the angels that had adorned the choir stall, most broken but some still whole, their wide eyes staring unblinking at the great blue sky.

April 16, 1943
Rosenberg's transmittal letter to Hitler accompanying
albums of photographs of works of art stolen for the
Führermuseum

Mein Führer:

In my desire to give you, my Führer, some joy for
your birthday I take the liberty to present to
you a folder containing photographs of some of
the most valuable paintings which my Einsatzstab,
in compliance with your order, secured from
ownerless Jewish art collections in the occupied
Western territories. These photos represent an
addition to the collection of 53 of the most
valuable objects of art delivered some time ago
to your collection. This folder also shows only
a small percentage of the exceptional value and
extent of these objects of art, seized by my
Dienststelle (service command) in France, and put
into a safe place in the Reich.

I beg of you, my Führer, to give me a chance
during my next audience to report to you orally
on the whole extent and scope of this art seizure
action. I beg you to accept a short written
intermediate report of the progress and extent
of the art seizure action which will be used as a
basis for this later oral report, and also accept
3 copies of the temporary picture catalogues
which, too, only show part of the collection you
own. I shall deliver further catalogues which
are now being compiled, when they are finished.

I shall take the liberty during the requested
audience to give you, my Führer, another 20
folders of pictures, with the hope that this
short occupation with the beautiful things of art
which are nearest to your heart will send a ray
of beauty and joy into your revered life.

                              Heil, mein Führer
                              A. Rosenberg

CHAPTER 8

Monuments, Fine Arts, and Archives

Shrivenham, England
Spring 1944

Geogre Stout, dapper Fogg conservator turned navy man, breathed the first warm air of a British spring. It was March 6, 1944, a month after the destruction of Monte Cassino but still a few months before the planned invasion of northern France. Already, southern England was teeming with British and American soldiers. More than a million if rumors were right, which didn't make for the easiest situation in a country bombed to tatters by four years of Luftwaffe raids and perilously low on food and basic materials. "The trouble with the Yanks is that they are overpaid, oversexed, overfed, and over here" went a popular saying making the rounds of London.[1] But what did they expect from young men, many still just boys in their teens? No doubt they were cocksure, but only to hide their terror. After all, they would soon be throwing themselves against the beachheads of Fortress Europe, and everyone knew that many among them would never go home.

In Shrivenham, a small rural village about halfway

between Bristol and London, the mood was different. The joint United States–British Civil Affairs corps had taken over the American School (an American-style university) for a Civil Affairs training center, and despite the occasional formation of older soldiers marching in uniform, the stone walls and wide lawns seemed very far from the horrors of war.

What George Stout mostly noticed, whenever he left the grounds, were the green sprouts. The first spring buds were on the trees, and although Stout suspected they were too early and a late frost would nip them out, he was heartened by their optimism. Recently the winter doldrums had lifted, and the previous night he had walked five miles to a local pub with a couple of his colleagues, an Englishman and an American. The pub was a timeless British watering hole: ruddy farmers with pints of ale, wood beams, stone walls, a dartboard in the corner, not another soldier in sight. The beer was mild and bitter; the company cheerful. He missed the boards of the ship that brought him across the Atlantic, their tight formation, the simple and precise rhythm of the sea. The walk back to Shrivenham through the dark and orderly Oxfordshire countryside, with its carefully prescribed fields and neat little flower and vegetable gardens, was just the thing to help Stout forget that he had already been here two weeks, and he had yet to receive a letter from home.

A navy man assigned to the army, he thought to himself. *The ultimate fish out of water. Even the postmaster can't find me.*

Walking now to a neighboring village in the fresh light of a Sunday morning, he could see the messiness of the world around him. Boxwood and other trees covered with ivy. The ambling, tumbling stone walls. The chaotic sprouts, some shooting up greenly, some smashed by heels in the mud. The fields torn by hooves. The grasping trees. The meandering road. It was disjointed somehow, but beneath the surface he could sense order, an appropriateness in both time and space, a composition that appeared messy until, suddenly, you saw beneath the strokes the system at work.

Still, he would have preferred the boats. And home. And some space for his work in a world at peace. But he was a soldier now, and he had to admit this assignment was exactly, as the English said, his cup of tea. Monuments, Fine Arts, and Archives. He almost laughed to think of it. They were actually putting together a unit of skilled technicians, commissioned as officers in the army, to tackle issues of conservation.

The Monuments, Fine Arts, and Archives (MFAA) subcommission had been formalized in late 1943 as an official joint operation between the United States and Britain, run by the Civil Affairs branch of the Allied Military Government for Occupied Territories (AMGOT) and answering primarily to the M-5 division of the British War Office. The bureaucratic train wreck was a hint at the priority of the operation, which was buried so far down the military chain of command it was almost invisible. Everyone knew of the failures in Italy. Hammond's office had been dissolved and replaced by a new hierarchy, but the MFAA operation in Italy—a completely separate operation run by a separate chain of command, under the Allied Control Commission (ACC)—was still struggling to become relevant. There had been no Monuments Men north of Naples, for instance, when the decision was made to destroy the abbey at Monte Cassino. That failure not only catapulted the handful of Monuments officers in Italy into action, it proved how difficult it was to create an organization in the middle of a military campaign.

The situation, hopefully, would be different in northern Europe. Civil Affairs had every intention of having a trained group of officers in place before the landings in France. The Roberts Commission had given Paul Sachs, Stout's boss at the Fogg Museum, the responsibility of picking the Americans who would serve in that officer corps, and George Stout had been one of the first people asked to join. That was in September 1943. Stout didn't hear anything else for months, which didn't surprise him. These projects, Stout knew, were usually a "flash in the pants," as a navy colleague had ingeniously (if accidentally) remarked.[2] And he never trusted anything run by museum directors.

Still, he had laid out for Sachs his thoughts on the operation. Each army, he wrote, would need a team of conservators. Each team would need a specialized staff, ten people at least, and sixteen would be preferable, including packers, movers, taxidermists (yes, taxidermists), secretaries, drivers, and, most importantly, photographers. The staff couldn't be acquired in the field, because Stout knew from his World War I experience that in the field no men were superfluous, and no commander would give up his men. They had to be *assigned* to conservation duty, and they had to be equipped: jeeps, covered trucks, crates, boxes, packing materials, cameras, aerometers to check air quality, all the tools of the conservator's trade.

In December, with no word from Sachs, rumors reached Stout that the operation was dead. He continued with aircraft camouflage, assuming the museum boys had gotten it thoroughly fouled. A pity, he thought, that the army had left it all in the hands of the sahibs.

Even when his transfer came through in January 1944, Stout remained unconvinced. "What you feel about the salvage duty is exactly what I feel," he wrote his wife, Margie. "If it's set up decently, it can go along and be of some substantial service. If it's not, there will be infuriating difficulties, delays, and frustrations. I expect a certain amount of those anyway. And whether I like it or not, I'll probably be in for it if the Army decides to go through with the program.... One thing certain: it will be, if it develops, a military job. It will not be run by civilian museum people but by the Army and the Navy. If this were civilian museum command, I'd ditch. [But] my associates will be military men, as I understand it. In the Army and the Navy, efficiency is the rule and plain honesty holds in relations with people. Bluff does not usually get very far. And so we'll see."[3]

George Stout underestimated the sahibs. The civilian museum community, in the form of the Roberts Commission (and in time their counterparts in England, the Macmillan Commission), had been both a catalyst for the creation of a conservation corps and a guiding force in its development. It is doubtful the U.S. Army would have tolerated the MFAA if not for the prestige of the Roberts Commission, which had been formed with Roosevelt's explicit backing, and no one was better suited to assemble George Stout's corps of "special workmen" than the men who ran America's cultural establishment. They were able to take the two primary lessons of North Africa and Sicily—that the army would listen to conservation officials, *as long as they were military officers*, and that those officers needed to arrive at the front lines during or immediately after the fighting, not weeks or even months later—and form from them the basis of a workable plan. And for Stout, at least, there was something else just as promising: They had not assigned a single museum director to the officer corps of the MFAA.

No, it wasn't the character of the men or scope of the mission that worried George Stout as his thoughts drifted ahead to the coming invasion on that unseasonably warm March morning. It was the ad hoc nature of the operation. There was no formal mission statement, or even set chain of command. Nobody seemed clear how many men were needed for the job, how they would be distributed on the continent, even when or if more soldiers would arrive. Men simply showed up for duty with their transfer papers, seemingly at random. A general guidebook to conservation procedures had been culled from Stout's expertise and writings on the subject. But the Monuments Men had no formal training. Most of the effort was being put into basics like listing the protected monuments in the various countries of Europe. As far as Stout could tell, there was no one even handling the military side of the operation, such as procuring weapons, jeeps, uniforms, or rations. To say the race to put together a conservation unit before the invasion of France had started slowly was an understatement.

And then there was the size of the operation. Stout had recommended to Sachs a staff of sixteen men per officer; it was becoming increasingly clear there might not be sixteen men in the entire MFAA operation for northern Europe. Stout knew it wasn't easy to negotiate transfers through the military bureaucracy, especially one planning the most important operation in world history. And he was sure Paul Sachs knew more qualified men. He had taught most of America's young museum men, after all. But Stout could count the men reserved for monuments fieldwork on two hands. Rorimer. Balfour. LaFarge. Posey. Dixon-Spain. Methuen. Hammett. Eventually, if officers kept showing up with their papers, the MFAA might have twelve men. Total. There were more men sitting at his mess table on the crossing to England—and that was one boat out of a thousand, and it fed a hundred mess tables a day.

He thought of the current Monuments Men, sitting for an imaginary portrait on a sunny hillside outside their base at Shrivenham.

Geoffrey Webb, their commanding officer, tall and lean, past fifty, a Slade Professor at Cambridge and one of the most distinguished art scholars in the British Isles.

Beside him, Lord Methuen and Squadron Leader Dixon-Spain, both older British veterans of the First World War.

The youngest of the British contingent was Ronald Balfour, small and balding, in his forties, a historian at King's College, Cambridge—Geoffrey Webb's colleague from Cambridge, in fact, brought into the MFAA at his suggestion. Stout and Balfour were rooming together at Shrivenham, and Stout had taken instantly to his clearheaded, generous, and gracious nature. An avid Protestant, the scholar focused his studies on ecclesiastical matters, having made the move from history, which of course had its share of religious implications and images. Having simply stayed on at Cambridge after his undergraduate education, he was what the English often called a "gentleman scholar," a professional university man uninterested in publishing or career advancement, but rather enamored of intellectual pursuits and long, leisurely conversations and debates with those of a similar intellectual bent.

He had become over the years, Stout thought, a man besotted by paper. He could be considered the archives and manuscripts expert of the group, the one among them more concerned with the safety of historical papers than the visual arts, and his greatest triumph—as Balfour himself had said on more than one occasion—was the accumulation of an eight-thousand volume library by the age of thirty-five. All quality books, too, as he was also quick to point out. But while he was a man of paper, Ronald Balfour was no paper man. He might not look like a soldier with his small frame and scholar's wire-rimmed glasses, but he had a backbone of iron and a desire to fight. He had been raised by a military man in central England—Buckinghamshire, to be precise—and he knew and respected military culture. Besides, it had taken decades of careful collecting to accumulate his library, and he had no intention of letting it be destroyed by German bombs.

Then there was the American side. Marvin Ross, a Harvard graduate and expert on Byzantine art, was second in command to Webb. Ralph Hammett and Bancel LaFarge, both architects and experts on buildings.

Walker Hancock, early forties, was a renowned sculptor of monumental works. *Sacrifice*, his soldiers' memorial in his hometown of St. Louis, Missouri, seemed particularly relevant now. Even more than other soldiers, Hancock was a man of sacrifice. He had sacrificed for his father in attending the Virginia Military Academy, briefly, during World War I. He would no doubt have sacrificed more, if asked. But the war had ended, and art, his true calling, had lured him back to his hometown to study at Washington University, then to the Pennsylvania Academy of the Fine Arts, and finally, in the late 1920s, to the American Academy in Rome. He was the artist of the group, and perhaps, George Stout realized, its most decorated member. In 1925, Walker Hancock had won the prestigious Prix de Rome. In 1942, while in basic training, he received word that he had won a competition to design the Air Medal, one of the military's highest honors. That award had unknowingly been his ticket out of a front-line infantry unit.

Happy-go-lucky. Easy to talk to. Relentlessly upbeat. And yet Walker Hancock's personal sacrifice was clear. Only a few weeks before shipping for England, he had married his sweetheart, Saima, in a small chapel at the National Cathedral in Washington, D.C. He was deeply in love with her, that much was obvious, because he seemed to think of nothing but her. And yet he had sacrificed his career and his marriage to come overseas.

He had *volunteered* for it, in fact, when the army had wanted to keep him near home in the Pentagon, and he had done so gladly. He was almost too attentive, too gracious and kind. Stout couldn't see him on the battlefield. He always pictured him instead curled up with Saima in their Massachusetts art studio and home—Hancock was conscientiously putting away part of his pay for its purchase—a fire in the hearth and a large bust of Atlas half completed in the background. Hancock would be laughing, of course. Nothing could get him down for long. He was such a positive, good-natured character that he even claimed to like the army's food.

The recently arrived James Rorimer, only thirty-nine, was the polar opposite of the easygoing Hancock: a hard-charging, ambitious man carved out of the fire of the high-stakes museum world. Here was a man, short and powerfully broad, clearly suited for war. He had joined the staff of the Metropolitan Museum of Art just after graduating from Harvard, and while still in his twenties had been instrumental in planning a vast expansion of the museum's medieval collection. By 1934, only seven years into his career, he had risen to the position of curator of medieval art. When the new home of the Met's medieval collection, the Cloisters, opened in upper Manhattan in 1938, Rorimer had been one of its most prominent developers and curators. Only a man of singular talent and drive could climb through the ranks of the Met that quickly. Perhaps that's why it didn't surprise Stout that Rorimer had come from a blue-collar town like Cleveland, Ohio, and that his father had changed the spelling of the family name from the Jewish Rorheimer because of his concerns about anti-Semitism in American life.[4]

Of course, Rorimer wasn't even officially a Monuments Man. He was officially assigned to Civil Affairs, which ran the Shrivenham training complex. Rorimer had been given his board hearing on March 3, and Stout had it on good authority that he had expressed a keen interest in monuments work. And Stout knew MFAA commander Geoffrey Webb wanted him. Why wouldn't he? Rorimer was an art scholar of the highest order, spoke French, had an extensive knowledge of Paris, and was even taking classes at Shrivenham six days a week to become fluent in German.

Stout had to hand it to him, the kid was a bulldog. No one at Shrivenham had worked harder to get into the MFAA, and no one was working harder to hone his skills. If you put a job in front of James Rorimer, he would kill himself to get it done. Stout suspected he was looking at a future star of the American cultural establishment. If Rorimer survived the war.

Then there was Robert Posey, the outsider of the group. Stout didn't know much about Posey. He mostly kept quiet, and kept to himself. He wasn't a member of Paul Sachs's Harvard circle, and as far as anyone could tell he wasn't particularly well known in his field, which was architecture. He had grown up desperately poor in Alabama, that much Stout had gleaned, and had graduated from Auburn University, an honor paid for almost entirely by the army's Reserve Officers' Training Corps. He was clearly a military man by training and by temperament, as well as an expert in his cultural field, which made him ideal for the unit. But nobody quite knew how he became assigned to the MFAA. He was rumored to have been posted to England straight from the Arctic Circle, which seemed too strange not to be true. He also claimed, in a lighter moment, to be the only person ever to destroy a tank in Pennsylvania. It turned out that, in his earlier military duties, he had designed an experimental bridge. It didn't work, and the first tank to try to cross it had plunged straight into the river and sank. The other Monuments Men, Stout knew, didn't know quite what to make of Robert Posey, but George Stout understood him. Posey was a quiet, blue collar, by-the-book farmboy from the hinterlands of America: much like Stout himself.

But with that, the portrait was complete. Balfour the British scholar. Hancock the good-natured artist. Rorimer the bulldog curator. Posey the Alabama farmboy. And, lurking somewhere in the back, dapper, pencil-mustached George Leslie Stout. Stout laughed at the thought as he rounded a bend in the road. Old impeccable George Stout. Not this time. The weight of the dirty laundry over his shoulder, one reason for this Sunday excursion from the barracks, reminded him that the grooming facilities at the army training school were rather substandard, and that he was already a bit more disheveled than he preferred.

Ah well. The operation might be his "brain child," as Paul Sachs had written, but over here George Stout was just another grunt, with no authority over anyone. And that was the way he liked it. Even in the military, Stout had an inherent distrust of managers. He preferred to get his hands dirty with real work—and then to wash them meticulously soon after.

It was a good group, he had to admit. A group he himself might have chosen, if given the chance. Only eleven men, unfortunately, but eleven good men. Not trained conservators, but the next best thing: scholars, artists, museum curators, and architects, men who worked for a living, not ordered others to work. They were established professionals. Almost all had wives, and most had children. They were old enough to understand what was at stake, and perhaps young enough to survive the rigors of the battlefield.

Survive. It wasn't a word George Stout wanted to think about. He was going to war with these men, and he knew that meant some of them probably wouldn't survive. It was a crime to send them out, he thought again, without the proper equipment and staff.

He blamed Lord Woolley, that old archeologist at the War Office. A good bloke, as Ronald Balfour would say, but he was starving the group. Woolley took inordinate pride in the fact that only three people ran the command office for the whole conservation operation—and one of them was Lady Woolley, his wife. With that staff, how could the effort be taken seriously? "We protected the arts at the lowest possible cost."[5] That was Woolley's motto. Taken from Pericles' Funeral Oration. Stout was sure the military brass appreciated the historical reference. That cleverness, no doubt, would come in handy in the field.

If it's all set up properly, he had told his wife. That was the key. Was it really too much, in a million-man army, to ask for a spare one hundred men? Was it really too much to provide a few thousand dollars for cameras, radios, and other basic equipment?

"What say, George, there she is," Ronald Balfour said in his clipped British accent.

The words broke into Stout's thoughts, bringing him back to England, to spring, to 1944. He looked up. Before him was a neat cluster of stone houses roofed with thatch. Beyond them, he could see a church tower, one of the reasons they had come to this small village. Stout looked at the sun, high overhead now, and then at his watch. The service would have let out long ago.

"Quick stop for these," Stout said, indicating his bag of laundry, "and then we'll go up."

"Right-oh," Balfour replied, smiling at the pat British expression the Americans seemed so fond of. Balfour, Stout thought, was difficult not to like. But more importantly, he was a man you could trust. A good thing, since it was men like Balfour who would make the difference. Stout was a scientist, a modernizer, but he never put his faith in machines. The skilled observer, not the machine, was the essence of conservation. That was the secret, he believed, to success in any endeavor: to be a careful, knowledgeable, and efficient observer of the world, and to act in accordance with what you saw. To be successful in the field, a Monuments officer would need not just knowledge; he would need passion, smarts, flexibility, an understanding of military culture: the way of the gun, the chain of command. In Balfour, Stout saw that mix of keen intellect, practical instincts and respect for the uniform. And it gave him confidence.

Just get us over there, he thought, *and we'll do this job*.

As a young man, Stout had spent a summer with his uncle in Corpus Christi, Texas. They had worked six days a week; on the seventh day, they fished. One day, they caught a Gulf flounder, a bottom-dweller with both eyes on the same side of its head. It was hard for an Iowa boy to believe that the world contained fish so unexpected and strange. That afternoon, on the way back to port, the motor died. Stout paddled for hours, but the boat was stranded, floating listlessly in the shallow waters of the Gulf of Mexico, until a schooner under sail came along and towed it to shore. Since then, Stout had seen too much of the world to put his faith in motors. He was always prepared to rely on the tide and row. And he was always confident he would make it back to shore.

He knew the Monuments Men weren't going to France empty-handed. They had maps of important structures and museums, created under the direction of the museum directors and other advisors, then over-laid onto aerial reconnaissance photographs. The lists of protected monuments, compiled by civilians and vet-ted by Civil Affairs officers, were beyond reproach. And he couldn't fault the handbooks on conservation tech-niques, which were based on his own work.

But still, he could see the Band-Aids holding the operation together. The museum directors didn't understand the military; the military still wasn't confi-dent this was a good idea. The Monuments Men were only advisors; they couldn't force any officer, of any rank, to act. They were allowed freedom of movement, but they would have no vehicles, no offices, no support staff, and no backup plan. The army had given them a boat, but not the motor. The men in the field, George Stout could already see, were going to have to row, and he had a strong suspicion they would be rowing against the tide. But once you're on the water, he knew, if you keep paddling a schooner just might pass.

Just get us over there, Stout thought, still not convinced the operation wasn't about to collapse. *Just give us a chance.*

"Romanesque revival," Ronald Balfour said over Stout's shoulder. "Small but well-built, probably late 1800s. What do you think, George?"

George Stout looked up at the country church. It was simple, solid, and handsomely detailed. There wasn't anything overtly beautiful, but there was nothing out of place, nothing extravagant or shabby, and that held a beauty all its own. It could well have been a Romanesque revival church, but the word that sprang to his mind was "romantic." As in a romantic location, a place for lovers, where he and his wife, Margie, would have laughed in years gone by. Or was it romantic as in overly optimistic and well-intentioned, like his romantic notion that you could save buildings such as this on the battlefields of a modern war?

"We'll be lucky to find one like it on the continent," Stout said, peering up at the unspoiled church.

Balfour smiled. "Ah George, you old dog. Always a pessimist."

Stout thought of the two life insurance policies he had taken out before sailing for England, his hedge against the hedgerows. Always be prepared.

"I'm an optimist, Mr. Balfour. A cautious optimist, but an optimist nonetheless."

CHAPTER 9

The Task

Southern England

Late May 1944

On May 26, 1944, General Eisenhower, Supreme Commander of the Allied Expeditionary Forces, issued the following order.[1] Unlike in Italy, where his order was issued almost six months after the start of the invasion of Sicily, this came eleven days before the invasion of northern Europe.

> Shortly we will be fighting our way across the Continent of Europe in battles designed to preserve our civilization. Inevitably, in the path of our advance will be found historical monuments and cultural centers which symbolize to the world all that we are fighting to preserve.
>
> It is the responsibility of every commander to protect and respect these symbols whenever possible.
>
> In some circumstances the success of the military operation may be prejudiced in our reluctance to destroy these revered objects. Then, as at Cassino, where the enemy relied on our emotional attachments to shield his defense, the lives of our men are paramount. So, where military necessity dictates, commanders may order the

required action even though it involves destruction to some honored site.

But there are many circumstances in which damage and destruction are not necessary and cannot be justified. In such cases, through the exercise of restraint and discipline, commanders will preserve centers and objects of historical and cultural significance. Civil Affairs Staffs at higher echelons will advise commanders of the locations of historical monuments of this type, both in advance of the frontlines and in occupied areas. This information, together with the necessary instruction, will be passed down through command channels to all echelons.

EISENHOWER

The following day, the MFAA forwarded to General Eisenhower's headquarters at SHAEF (Supreme Headquarters Allied Expeditionary Forces) a list of protected monuments in France. Everyone, military and civilian, was on edge. The whole war hinged on one great leap into the unknown: Operation Overlord, the landing in France. After being briefed on the plans, Winston Churchill had grasped Eisenhower's hand and told him, with tears in his eyes, "I am with you to the end, and if it fails we will go down together."[2] A defeat would mean at best another two years to regroup and replan, and at worst the fall of Britain. Nobody, least of all the field officers approving the "Off-Limits" lists in the upcoming battle zone, wanted to stand in the way of success. The MFAA list of Protected Monuments was rejected by field officers as too comprehensive and detrimental to battlefield maneuvers.

MFAA leaders had a decision to make: Would they bow to military pressure or stand for their mission and their beliefs? Instead of modifying the list, Woolley decided to explain it. Of the 210 protected buildings in Normandy, he told SHAEF, eighty-four were churches. Most of the others were Roman or medieval ruins, prehistoric stone circles, fountains, and similar structures that would do the army little good. In the whole of Normandy, he estimated, only thirty-five buildings that could be used for legitimate military purposes were being denied by MFAA restrictions. The army brass read the explanation, and the list was promptly approved. By June 1, the MFAA had reached its battle-ready number. Fifteen men would be serving on the continent, excluding Italy: eight Americans and seven British (another American and three British had arrived since Stout's "group portrait" in March, assigned to the "country units" of France, Belgium, and Germany). Seven of the men would serve at SHAEF headquarters in a strictly organizational capacity. The other eight men were assigned to British and American armies and the Communications Zone. To emphasize the joint nature of the operation, they served across lines, with one American in the British Twenty-first Army Group and one British in U.S. First Army. As impossible as it seems, it was the duty of these eight officers to inspect and preserve every important monument the Allied forces encountered between the English Channel and Berlin.

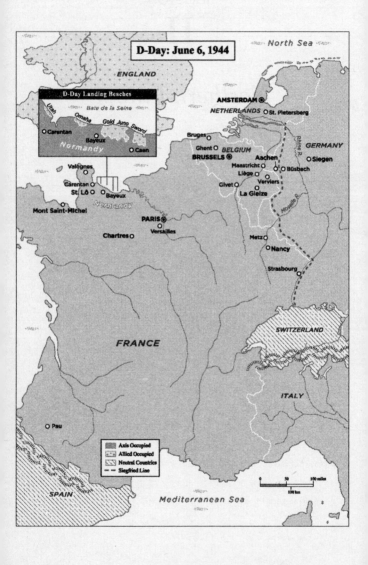

D-Day: June 6, 1944

ENGLAND

North Sea

D-Day Landing Beaches

Bate de la Seine

Utah
Omaha
Gold Juno Sword

Carentan
Bayeux
Caen

Normandy

AMSTERDAM
NETHERLANDS
St. Pietersberg

Bruges

Ghent
BELGIUM
BRUSSELS

Aachen

Rhine R.
GERMANY

Siegen

Maastricht
Liège
Verviers
Büsbach

Givet
La Gleize

Valognes

Carentan
St. Lô
Bayeux

Mont Saint-Michel

Normandy

PARIS
Versailles

Chartres

Metz
Nancy

Moselle R.

Strasbourg

FRANCE

SWITZERLAND

ITALY

Pau

Axis Occupied
Allied Occupied
Neutral Countries
Siegfried Line

0   50   100 miles
100 km

SPAIN

Mediterranean Sea

Dear Ones:

We are told that the invasion of Western Europe
by overwhelming forces is underway. I read the
morning paper and was delighted to know that Rome
has been spared. Now I am thinking of the combat
troops and the task which is theirs. We older
men are anxious on the one hand to help deal the
death blow to tyranny, and on the other we think
of our families at home and the obligations which
we have as husbands, fathers, sons, and members
of the peace-time community.

My status has changed but little. I have no idea
as to what the future holds in store. I do hope
that I can be useful. I am convinced my low
rank alone is making an assignment difficult.
Knowledge of Europe and Europeans, ability to
make and keep friends, a sense of *real* values,
a successful career, a useful mind and body,
connections—none of these including a will to
be useful—what is called of service to humanity—
seem to make things click. I expect to continue
as a Monuments and Fine Arts officer—but there is
no indication of what kind of work I'll have.

Love,

Jim

CHAPTER 10

Winning Respect

Normandy, France
June–August 1944

The naval bombardment of Omaha Beach began at 5:37 a.m. on the morning of June 6, 1944. Near dawn, the aerial bombardment began. The first wave of Allied troops hit Omaha Beach at "H-Hour": 6:30 a.m. It didn't take them long to realize the naval and aerial bombardments hadn't worked. Flying in a heavy fog and fearful of dropping short on their own troop carriers, the bombers had dropped their bombs too far inland, leaving the dug-in German coastal forces untouched. The eastern and westernmost American units on Omaha took heavy casualties before they could crawl halfway up the beach. The second wave, coming in thirty minutes later, found the survivors pinned down on the small sandbank that marked the high-tide line. They were soon pinned down too, their equipment jammed on the overcrowded beach, their wounded drowning in the incoming tide. After six hours of fighting and dying, the Americans held a perilously small strip of land. The tide was eating up their beachhead almost as quickly as they could secure it.

Still the troops came, wave after wave. With the

natural conduits from the beach cut off by German crossfire, small groups began to scale the bluffs. Colonel George A. Taylor rallied survivors with the cry, "Two kinds of people are staying on this beach, the dead and those who are going to die. Now let's get the hell out of here."[1] Forty-three thousand troops were ferried across the English Channel to "Bloody Omaha" that day; more than twenty-two hundred died there. They were mostly enlisted men and volunteers, trained and drilled for this battle but still bearing the marks of their lives as teachers, mechanics, laborers, and office workers. They died at Sword Beach, Gold Beach, Juno Beach, and Pointe du Hoc, too. They came in waves at Utah Beach, more than 23,000 men, rising out of the fog and surf, moving endlessly inland toward the German lines. The 101st and 82nd Airborne divisions had parachuted 13,000 men behind enemy lines, and if the soldiers coming ashore didn't rendezvous with them by nightfall the paratroopers could be wiped out. And even if they met the airborne units, or what was left of them, these soldiers knew the battle was far from over, that the beachhead was precarious, and that a million German fighters lay hidden in the hedgerows, ready to bury them forever in the soil of France.

The Germans had miscalculated. They thought the Western Allies could never supply an army without a port, but the soldiers poured onto the beach at Utah carrying ammunition, weapons, and cans of gasoline. They came not just the first morning, but day after day, mostly infantry troops but also tankers, gunners, chaplains, ordnance officers, engineers, medics, reporters, typists, translators, and cooks. They landed from every manner of watercraft, but especially the LSTs (Landing Ship, Tanks). For miles there were "LSTs at every beach, their great jaws yawning open, disgorging tanks and trucks and jeeps and bulldozers and big guns and small guns and mountains of cases of rations and ammunition, thousands of jerry cans filled with gasoline, crates of radios and telephones, typewriters and forms, and all else that men at war require."[2] Overhead, the roar of Allied aircraft was continual—14,000 sorties were flown on D-Day alone, with almost as many on every succeeding clear day. The English Channel was so full of ships that for more than a month the one day crossing took three days. And within that tempest, just a few yards off Utah Beach, stood a small, quiet, four-hundred-year-old church.

Who knows what the soldiers thought of the church? Most of the men at three-mile-wide Utah Beach probably never saw it. Many others rushed right by it, for it is rarely mentioned in memoirs or histories of the war. It probably served first as a resting point, then perhaps a meeting point to organize before moving inland. Doubtless, men died there, brought by comrades or felled by German mortars, bullets, or mines. The roof took artillery fire, the beams splintered, but the small chapel stood and, in time, began to house daily services for some of the thousands of men coming ashore, and the hundreds more returning from the front.

In the first days of August, for the first time, a soldier noticed the stones. "Chapel called Ste-Madeleine," he wrote. "Fr. McAvoy has posted a sign calling for daily services at 1700. Good sixteenth-century Renaissance architecture in *Maison Carrée* style. Fragments which can be used for restoration are in and about the immediate area which is off the highway. Main portal damaged by fragmentation from south or west. Wooden roof in good condition except for minor damage."[3] Then he took a photograph to file and send to England. The soldier was Second Lieutenant James Rorimer, the dogged curator of the Metropolitan Museum, and unlike the thousands of other troops who had crossed Utah Beach, he wasn't in France to use the little chapel for whatever purposes war required. As a Monuments Man, he was there to save it.

———————

As with most things at Normandy, Lieutenant Rorimer's deployment didn't go exactly as planned. He was supposed to land earlier, but his passage was delayed as the army rushed higher priority personnel to the front lines. Even when finally assigned passage, he missed his boat—the duty captain wasn't expecting a Monuments Man, one of the few soldiers crossing not assigned to a unit, and left early. Given a choice of ships the next day, he chose to cross with a shipload of French veterans from the North African campaign. He wanted to land on French soil with Free French troops.

By late July, the Allies thought they would be racing across France; but after eight weeks, they had advanced only twenty-five miles inland, on a front of less than eighty miles. In many places, progress was worse. In early August, the British Second Army and its Monuments officer Bancel LaFarge were only a few miles past Caen, their objective on the first day. Five other Monuments Men had arrived in France, but they too found their areas of operation limited by the slow advance. A planned sprint had turned into a quagmire, and the press was beginning to utter the dreaded word "stalemate." James Rorimer, coming ashore August 3, was the last Monuments Man to land during major combat operations at Normandy.

The reason was instantly obvious: there wasn't room for anyone else. Beyond Utah Beach, Rorimer found not the tranquil French countryside that had existed only two months before, but a teeming city of soldiers. In the channel behind him, the scene was "stupefying and impressive," according to John Skilton, a Civil Affairs officer who later became a Monuments Man. The channel was full to the horizon with vessels waiting to dock. The beaches were crawling with troops; the water teemed with soldiers wading ashore. Overhead, thousands of silver balloons formed a security wall against enemy aircraft. Beyond them were the Allied fighters. In front, off the beach, there was traffic. "Never had I seen such a multitude of vehicles of all types and sizes," wrote Skilton. "As far as the eye reaches the roads form one uninterrupted ribbon of vehicles."[4]

But it wasn't until he was riding in a convoy toward Advance Section headquarters that Rorimer realized the magnitude of the situation. Around him was a moonscape of blown-open pillboxes, mutilated hedgerows, and rutted land. Destroyed vehicles were being moved off to dumps by giant wreckers, while shattered guns and fortifications rusted alongside the road. Airplanes roared continuously overhead. The explosions of their bombs mixed with the detonations of nearby mines. Most of the mines were being blown by mine-sweepers, but others were being tripped by unlucky troops or civilians. "The attempt to record [cultural] damage amid the gaping craters and fire-swept hulks of buildings," Rorimer wrote of his first sight of Normandy, "would be like trying to scoop up wine with a broken keg."[5]

Advance Section headquarters (Ad Sec), strung out for miles in farm buildings and tents, appeared no more organized than the beaches. Rorimer, having missed his crossing the day before, was only vaguely expected. He had to walk several miles, and back again, just to be sworn in. His commanding officer simply warned him about booby traps, which had turned up in safes, church pews, and even on dead bodies, then turned back to his maps. That was it. James Rorimer was on his own. So he set up a little office, sat back, and wondered what to do first.

He didn't sit long. It is one thing to be an eighteen-year-old soldier and to know you are heading into a life-and-death struggle with another eighteen-year-old soldier as far removed from the reason for this battle as you are. Even the majors and sergeants knew they were battling not monsters but career military men like themselves who happened to be wearing a different-colored uniform. To most soldiers, war was circumstance. But to someone like James Rorimer, it was the mission of a lifetime. Hitler had fired a shot across the bow of the art world in 1939, when the blitzkrieg of Poland included units tasked with the deliberate theft of art and destruction of that country's cultural monuments. The watershed event came soon after, when the

Nazis seized the Veit Stoss Altarpiece—a Polish national treasure—and transported it to Nuremberg, Germany. Then they stole Leonardo da Vinci's *Lady with an Ermine*, one of only fifteen or so paintings solely attributed to the hand of the master, along with masterpieces by Raphael and Rembrandt. These works, all but the Veit Stoss altarpiece part of the famed Czartoryski Collection, were the most important in Poland. None had been seen or heard of since. A year later, when Western Europe fell, facts gave way to rumor and innuendo. But even that was enough for the art world to know that museums and collections, large and small, were being systematically dismantled and transported to Germany. The landing at Normandy was the first chance for the museum professionals in America and England not only to discover what had occurred behind the Nazi veil, but to begin to right the wrongs. James Rorimer had no intention of sitting at a desk while art history was unfolding before him.

And yet that is almost exactly what happened.

Rorimer volunteered for military duty in 1943. At thirty-seven years old, he was a rising star at the Metropolitan Museum of Art, having recently been promoted to curator of the Cloisters, the branch of the Met dedicated to medieval art and architecture. But like many other successful professionals, Rorimer was inducted as a buck private and stationed at Fourth Infantry Training Battalion, Camp Wheeler, Georgia. In February 1944, his daughter Anne was born. "At last, I am a proud father," he wrote his wife, Katherine, whom he called Kay, at the news, "the pictures are the most valued possessions I have with me."[6] Soon after, he shipped out for England. He would not see his daughter for more than two years.

Assigned to training in Civil Affairs at Shrivenham, the determined Rorimer soon got himself assigned to monuments work. "Gradually I meet more art 'historians' here," he wrote his wife after his posting to the MFAA. "We will be held in a pool for duty when, where and if needed.... I keep in the background while others play politics."[7]

With a background in French art and knowledge of the language, Rorimer expected to be working on preparations for the invasion of his "favorite European country."[8] But the MFAA was a muddle. By April, with an official monuments posting but no assignment, Rorimer went in search of a useful job. He finally found one on April 9—teaching officers to drive army trucks. With his usual diligence and hard work, he was soon an expert on trucks and teaching classes eight hours a day. But he admitted to Kay that "I have been carrying monuments work into the field as often as I had a spare moment."[9]

Still, when an opportunity arose on April 30 to be a public relations officer and historian for another unit, he immediately embraced the opportunity. But MFAA head Geoffrey Webb refused to release him from service. "My actual assignment depends on circumstances, moods, politics and Webb," he groused to Kay.[10] He believed in monuments work, but like the dapper Fogg conservator George Stout, who had spent years trying to get the unit off the ground, he had little faith the effort would ever crystallize. "Tell Sachs that all I had feared had happened," he wrote just more than a month before D-Day, "and that I had a good job teaching motor vehicles and maintenance."[11] A week later, on May 7, he had changed his mind. "Some days, or hours—once in a while—one thinks that Civil Affairs is the most wonderful assignment in all the world...we [Monuments Men] have an extraordinary job to perform and I am satisfied that things are being as well handled as possible."[12]

The fact is, James Rorimer wasn't conditioned for the army's bureaucratic runaround. At the Metropolitan Museum, he had risen rapidly through the ranks. Despite his youth, he had bulldozed through the difficulties of creating a new museum branch like the Cloisters, cultivating a great patron in John D. Rockefeller Jr., and organizing a disparate staff. In the army, Rorimer was at the bottom of a huge bureaucracy and completely powerless; a promotion to second lieutenant still meant he was the lowest-ranking commissioned man in the army and in the MFAA. "War disrupts many things," he wrote his wife in April, "particularly if one is a junior officer after years of a continued successful civilian career. I only hope that my desire to serve will in due time not be hampered by the little fellows who play politics and show brass."[13] He didn't receive his assignment in the MFAA until more than four weeks *after* the Normandy invasion; soon after, he was on the continent. Once clear of the bureaucratic tangle of England, with his dream assignment, there was no way James Rorimer was going to fail—no matter how difficult and unsure the task at hand.

In Normandy, each Monuments Man had a battle zone for which he was responsible. Most corresponded with individual battle groups, such as U.S. First Army, U.S. Third Army, or British Second Army. Rorimer's was Communications Zone, the area behind the front lines where roads were built and supplies ferried through. Unfortunately, the information on the boundaries of the "Comm Zone" was changing so rapidly that it was almost impossible to keep track of them— or sometimes even the exact location of the front lines. Normandy was crisscrossed by hedgerows, enormous earthen dams topped with trees and bushes that separated the fields and sheltered the roads. There were often eight or ten a mile, limiting visibility to the empty field in front of you and, across it, the ominous wall of the next hedgerow. After two or three hedgerows, all running at lopsided angles, commanders didn't know whether they were heading forward or back.

"Just stick to the road," a harried officer advised Rorimer as he was about to head out from headquarters for his first day in the field. "And keep your head down. A dead Monuments officer is of no use at all."[14]

At the motor pool, a soldier checked his orders and shook his head. "Sorry, Lieutenant, Monuments section isn't on the list. You'll have to hitch a ride. Trucks are always leaving—repairing wires, transporting supplies, burying the dead. You shouldn't have any trouble."

Rorimer headed out in the first convoy that could take him. He had dozens of sites to visit, but no plan and no defined objective. He had only the desire for action, to be of service. His first stop was Carentan, the strategic link between Omaha and Utah beaches. The town had been nearly obliterated by aerial bombardment and Allied artillery, but in the midst of the carnage Rorimer was surprised to find the one building on the protected monuments list, its cathedral, almost untouched. Only the tower had been damaged, and even that was minor. Rorimer lowered his binoculars. His first task was to record the condition of the monuments after the battle; his second was to supervise emergency repair work if needed. With the tower in no immediate danger of collapse, there was no reason to linger in Carenten. He press-ganged the elderly French departmental architect of Cherbourg, who was also inspecting the ruins, into taking responsibility for reinforcing the tower, then motioned to a boy watching him from the shadows across the street.

"*Tu veux aider?*" Rorimer asked. "Do you want to help?" The boy nodded. Rorimer reached into his pack. "When that man comes down from the tower," he instructed the boy in French, "tell him I moved on to another town. Then ask him to put these on the building." He handed the boy several signs. They said, in both English and French:[15]

OFF LIMITS
To all Military Personnel
HISTORIC MONUMENT
Trespassing on or Removal of any Materials or
Articles from These Premises is Strictly Forbidden
By Command of the Commanding Officer

A Monument Man's third, and perhaps most important, task was to see that no further damage occurred, from soldiers or local citizens. Protected monuments, even in ruins, were not to be disturbed. He watched as the boy moved off toward the cathedral, a small ragged spot against the background of shattered stones and broken glass. He wasn't even wearing shoes. Rorimer chased after him a few steps, grabbed him by the shoulder. "*Merci*," he said, holding out a stick of gum. The boy took it and smiled, then turned and ran toward the cathedral.

A few minutes later, Rorimer was gone, off in another convoy to check another monument. Within a few days, he couldn't even have begun to tell where he'd been without the help of his field journal and checklist of monuments. The towns blurred together as he backtracked and crisscrossed his own path in search of transportation. He'd be an hour on a road packed with tanks, all outfitted by their crews with pointed metal battering rams. "Rhino tanks," they called them, perfect for driving through the hedgerows instead of over them. Then the jeep would turn a corner and there would be no one for miles. In one stretch, the hedgerows would be burned out and chopped through, the ground pitted with bomb craters and muddied by boots. In the next, the cows lolled in the shade of the tree line, as peaceful as the summer before. Some towns were destroyed; others untouched. Even in the towns, one block would be decimated while the next looked completely whole—until you noticed the one broken window on a second floor where a stray bullet had struck. War did not come like a hurricane, Rorimer realized, destroying everything in its path. It came like a tornado, touching down in patches, taking with it one life while leaving the next person unharmed.

There was only one constant, it seemed, in that

wilderness of destruction and reprieve: the churches. In almost every town Rorimer saw the sight he had first seen in Carentan: intact church, broken tower. Normandy was flat ground, and the highest point for miles was usually a cathedral tower. The Western Allies wouldn't violate the sanctity of a cathedral; the Germans showed no such scruples. In violation of the Rules of Land Warfare set forth in the Hague Conventions, German snipers and observers regularly hid in the towers, picking off troops and calling down mortar fire on advancing units. The Allies learned to call in their own concentrated fire, collapsing the towers while leaving the rest of the cathedral largely unscathed. Rorimer didn't know if the Allies were looking at the protected monuments lists or not, but it didn't matter. The army commanders understood, inherently, that some structures were worth saving.

Not that every cathedral was spared. At La-Haye-du-Puits, Rorimer had to dislodge the huddled peasants who had been coming there every day to pray; the structure was badly damaged, and he feared the shaking caused by the armored vehicles and artillery pieces rolling by in the street outside would collapse the tower. Allied bulldozers had pushed the rubble of the central section of the church of Saint-Malo at Valognes into the nave to clear a supply route—which, unfortunately, went right through the remains of the church. The citizens cried and begged for relief, but when Rorimer told them there was no other way, they understood. This was the price of freedom.

There were closer calls. The historic abbey of St. Sauveur-le-Vicomte, a German munitions depot, was destroyed by Allied aerial bombardment. When Rorimer arrived, American GIs were feeding children out of their own rations; there had been fifty-six orphans and thirty-five nuns inside. "The abbey is blessed," the mother superior told him. "It was destroyed, but everyone escaped unharmed."

The château of Comte de Germigny had been set ablaze by Allied bombers. As he approached, Rorimer could see the shards of wall, blackened on the edges, sticking up like enormous shoulders of stone. In their shadow, a bulldozer was backing, preparing to knock down one of the last nearly complete walls. It was common practice to knock down damaged walls; the army used the stone as base material for roads. But this château was on the protected monuments list, and this particular wall was part of the château's private chapel. On the back side, Rorimer noticed two large eighteenth-century statues.

"Stop the bulldozer," he yelled at the startled engineer, who no doubt had spent the last few days knocking down other walls at the damaged château. "This is a historic home." He held up his list of protected monuments. "It is not to be destroyed."

A few minutes later, the commanding officer came stomping through the rubble. "What's the trouble here...Second Lieutenant." The mention of Rorimer's rank, the lowest commissioned-officer rank in the army, was intentional. The Monuments Men had no authority to give orders; their role was purely advisory, and this officer knew it.

"This is a historic monument, sir. It's not to be damaged."

The officer looked at the broken wall and the fragments of stone. "The flyboys should have thought of that."

"It's private property, sir. It must be respected."

The officer buttonholed the junior man—junior in rank, at least, if not in age. "We have a war to win here, Lieutenant. My job in that war is to see that this road goes through."

The officer turned to leave. In his mind, the conversation was over, but James Rorimer was a bulldog: short, squarely built, and not afraid of a challenge. Through persistence and hard work he had advanced to the highest levels of the Metropolitan Museum, America's greatest cultural institution, in less than ten years. He had that potent mixture of ambition and belief: in himself and in his mission. He had no practice in failure, and he had no intention of starting now.

"I've photographed this wall for an official report."

The officer stopped and turned around. The cheek of this bastard. Who did he think he was? Rorimer held out a copy of Eisenhower's proclamation on monuments and war. "Only in the event of necessity, sir. Supreme Commander's orders. Do you want to spend the rest of your tour explaining why this demolition was a military necessity, not a convenience?"

The officer stared the little man in the eye. He looked like a soldier, but damned if he didn't act like a fool. Didn't this screwball know there was a war on? But he could see, just looking at James Rorimer, that it was no use. "Okay," the officer grumbled, signaling the bulldozer back from the wall, "but this is a helluva way to fight a war."[16]

Rorimer thought about the abbey of St. Sauveur-le-Vicomte, where he had found American GIs feeding children out of their rations. The soldiers had been camped out in the rain, ordered out of the monks' warm, dry beds by a combat general who understood the historic and cultural value of the abbey. That general probably wasn't too popular with the troops, but Rorimer knew it was men like that who won the respect of the French.

"I disagree, sir," Rorimer said to the officer at Comte de Germigny. "I think this is exactly the way to fight a war."

Dear Margie:

Luck struck me three days back and I've a billet under a roof. It is a great comfort and I'm making the most of it while it lasts.

Put me down as saying that I take my hat off to the people of France. I don't mean the important political people. They may be alright but I don't know about them. The valor of the simple country people is touching. Everyone sees it as he moves about the roads. Crippled and battered and seemingly unchanged they keep about their jobs. They are kind to us—more kind than we deserve—and are most friendly. Their own tri-color is hung out at hundreds of cottage doors, and a staggering number of stars and stripes. Where they got them is beyond imagination. They must have been sewn in the linings of their clothes. Some plainly were home-made, the stripes sewn out of white and something approaching red, the stars stitched on. Going about the roads we are waving to them all the time, and often they stand in front of crushed houses. No victory parade could match this for meaning. . . .

Writing now makes me feel as if I had lost at least one of my senses. I can't hear you or see you and I wonder if you hear me. One thing is quite sure. I love you.

Yours,
George

CHAPTER 11

A Meeting in the Field

Normandy, France
August 1944

An ancient crossroads, the town of Saint-Lô sat on high ground commanding a view of a main east-west highway in Normandy. Since early June, the 29th Infantry Division (the "29ers") had been bogged down there in a deadly showdown with the German 352nd Division. By mid-July, hardly a man was alive on either side who had fought on D-Day.

On July 17, an hour before dawn, the 29ers began an all-out assault on Saint-Lô, no reinforcements held in reserve. It was a surprise attack; the men jumped into the German trenches using primarily bayonets and hand grenades. They broke through the enemy lines at dawn and took the high ground less than a mile from town. The Germans counterattacked, but a massive Allied artillery and fighter-bomber strike broke their charge. In the smoky haze of a French morning, the 29ers pushed over the final hill and saw for the first time the objective for which they had fought and died. "St.-Lô had been hit by B-17s on D-Day, and every clear day thereafter," wrote the historian Stephen Ambrose. "The center of the place was a lifeless pile of rubble 'in which roads and sidewalks could scarcely be distinguished.' "[1]

But the city wasn't lifeless. Behind every pile of stones, a German soldier was waiting. The Allied advance soon turned into a running battle, with much of the fighting centered on the cemetery near the collapsed church of Sainte-Croix. Bullets shattered headstones as rhino tanks equipped with homemade battering rams ran over tombs like hedgerows, forcing the Germans back into the decimated town. When the battle finally ended in Allied victory, the 29ers wrapped the body of Major Tom Howie, a former schoolteacher and one of its most popular officers, in an American flag and hoisted it to the top of a pile of stones that had once been the church of Sainte-Croix. The city was finally in Allied hands, but at a tremendous cost. The 29th Division had lost more men at Saint-Lô than they had on Omaha Beach.

James Rorimer was sent to Saint-Lô to assess the damage. He found a city in ruins, the dead lying unburied in the rubble, the homeless residents stumbling through piles of splintered wood and ashes in search of food and water. "The Germans set fire to homes with gasoline," one man told him, as he picked his way through the debris. "They set mines on every major street." Somewhere nearby a mine exploded; another building collapsed. The city architect wept at his first sight of the town's historic district. The Germans had built trenches and underground concrete forts around and within the city's most important monuments, and the Allies had bombed them flat. The main government buildings were cratered by bombs, then devoured by flames. The Hotel de Ville, whose library contained the charter of William the Conqueror, was gutted. The nearby museum and its centuries of accumulated treasures were reduced to dust. The center of the church of Notre-Dame was a pile of rubble twenty feet high. The parts of the church still standing, Rorimer noted, were "filled with grenades, smoke bombs, ration boxes, and every conceivable sort of debris. There were booby traps on the pulpit and on the altar."[2]

The officers at headquarters found Rorimer's report so unbelievable the colonel in charge of Civil Affairs made his own inspection. He found the scene, if anything, even more terrible than Rorimer described. Later estimates put the destruction at 95 percent, a scale of annihilation rivaled only by the worst of the firebombed German towns. The great Irish writer Samuel Beckett, an expat in France, described Saint-Lô as "the Capital of the Ruins."[3] Rorimer's inventory of destroyed objects included not just the town's ancient architecture but hundreds of years of archives, an astonishing collection of ceramics, numerous private art collections, and, perhaps most sadly, a large selection of illuminated manuscripts prepared and collected by the monks at the monastery of Mont Saint-Michel. The priceless manuscripts, handwritten in script, decorated with illustrations, and dating in some cases to the eleventh century, had been moved to the Departmental Archives at Saint-Lô for safekeeping.

But the destruction, while unfortunate, was far from wanton. The capture of Saint-Lô was a linchpin of Allied success, giving them the high ground from which they could pinpoint artillery and aerial strikes on the heart of the German defenses. A few weeks later, after the largest aerial bombardment in military history, U.S. First Army and U.S. Third Army funneled through the break at Saint-Lô, finally smashing the German "Ring of Steel" that had kept the Allies hemmed into Normandy for two months. If ever a city symbolized the complexity of the Monuments Men's mission, the difficulty of balancing preservation and strategic advancement, it was Saint-Lô.

————

It was fitting then that the Monuments Men in the field met as a group for the first time outside the ruins of Saint-Lô. The meeting took place on August 13, just as General Patton, who had been driving east from the town, turned his Third Army northwest in an attempt to surround the German army. Although the battle for Normandy was not officially over, victory seemed inevitable, and it was time both to assess the past and consider the future. It had been a hard few months, and the weariness in their bones spoke to the difficulty of the mission. James Rorimer, hitching a ride from headquarters, was practically asleep in his mud-stained boots. He was accompanied by the architect Captain Ralph Hammett, a fellow Monuments Man serving in Comm Zone. Major Bancel LaFarge, the New York buildings expert and first Monuments Man ashore, arrived in a small car provided by his colleagues in British Second Army. In February, LaFarge would leave the field to become the MFAA's second in command. Captain Robert Posey, the Alabama architect and outsider of the group, who was assigned to George Patton's hard-charging Third Army, couldn't secure transportation from the front and missed the meeting.

From an outside vantage, it didn't appear much of a group: three middle-aged men in wrinkled brown uniforms, less than half of the eight MFAA officers who had been expected in Normandy. They hadn't seen each other since Shrivenham, and in each other's faces they saw how much they had changed from the polished career men they had so recently been. There was no laundry in Normandy, no shower, no leave. They had spent weeks scrambling across endless battlefields and through brutalized towns, often in driving summer rains that turned every dirt patch into a sucking, muddy mess. They were exhausted, dirty, frustrated… but alive, both physically and spiritually. They could see it in each other's eyes. After all those months and years of waiting, it was good to be doing something, *anything*, to help the Allied cause.

"I think that I have never been happier," James Rorimer had written his wife. "I work from morning until night and with the most splendid cooperation from my Colonel and his staff. I not only have the proper credentials from higher authority but the fact that I am a slave to work and am Infantry trained are now redounding full fold. My French is always anything but hesitating and I am doing all the things I have wanted to do since war was declared."[4]

This was not to say the job was easy: far from it. The men had all realized that they really were on their own in the field. There were no set procedures to follow; no proper chain of command; no right way of dealing with combat officers. They had to feel each situation out; to improvise on an hourly basis; to find a way to finish a job that seemed more daunting every day. They had no real authority, but served merely as advisors. When they were in the field, no one was there to help except the enlisted men and officers they convinced of the rightness of their cause. Those who expected clear guidelines, power, proper tools, or even visible success were going to wash out of the service quickly. But for those, like James Rorimer, who thrived on muscling through progress in a difficult and sometimes deadly environment, it was an adrenaline rush that no civilian job could provide. As Rorimer wrote, "These are not the days for personal considerations....Kay, you were right, it's a thrilling experience."[5]

There was no use complaining. These were the parameters of their war, and in the scope of all the other duties in the combat zone, it wasn't a bad war to fight. Rorimer had never been a complainer; he had always been a doer. That's why he was here. And that's what he expected to do from now until Hitler was dead in the ground and the German army was buried with him.

Nonetheless, despite everyone's best intentions, the conversation soon turned to problems. There weren't enough "Off Limits" signs, someone said, for all the damaged churches, much less the other buildings. Cameras had supposedly been ordered for Hammett and Posey, but they still hadn't arrived. And nobody had a radio. Theirs was a solitary task. They weren't a unit; they were individuals with individual territories and individual goals and methods. How were officers wandering the field alone supposed to communicate with headquarters, much less each other, if they didn't have a radio?

Rorimer was just about to bring up the subject of permanently assigned transportation—or the lack thereof—when he noticed the dilapidated German Volkswagen bouncing across a nearby field. Behind the wheel, with his foot firmly pressed to the gas pedal, was an American in standard officer uniform: a metal helmet, woolen OD (olive drab) shirt, green or OD trousers, and field boots beneath a pair of over-shoes. Although it was warm, he wore a field jacket for protection against the rain, which had been rising at a moment's notice all summer. The car had no wind-shield, so the officer wore rakish goggles, similar to those used by World War I pilots. Around his helmet was a blue stripe; on the front of his jacket were the large white letters "USN," the unmistakable marks of a navy man. It was that more than anything that told Rorimer the man behind the wheel was their colleague George Stout.

Stout stepped out of the car, snapped off his goggles, and brushed the road dirt carefully from his face and clothes. When he took off his combat helmet, which came down almost over his eyes, they noticed his hair was crisply cut and carefully combed. His laundry folds were just as crisp. Tom Stout would later describe how his father, in his twilight years, would amble the country lanes near his Massachusetts home dressed in a sporting jacket, an ascot, and a beret, his walking stick in hand, stopping frequently to engage in conversation with acquaintances. He seemed to exude the same casual confidence at Saint-Lô, an air of gentility spoiled only by the Colt .45 on one hip and the dagger on the other. What was marvelous in civilian life, however, was magical on the battlefield. The dapper George Stout, unlike the rest of the Monuments Men, appeared no worse for wear.

The first thing everyone wanted to know was where he had acquired the car. "It has no horn, a sprung transmission, a weak brake, a loose steering column, and no top," Stout told them, "but I am most grateful to the Germans for leaving it behind."

"You requisitioned it, then?"

"I found it," Stout said simply. Here was a man who had changed the field of conservation with an old library card catalogue; he wasn't about to spend time complaining, not when there were plenty of supplies lying around.

"Stout was a leader," Craig Hugh Smyth, a later arrival to the Monuments Men, once wrote of him, "quiet, unselfish, modest, yet very strong, very thoughtful and remarkably innovative. Whether speaking or writing, he was economical with words, precise, vivid. One believed what he said; one wanted to do what he proposed."[6]

It was George Stout who had called the meeting, and like any good leader (although he was not in the chain of command above any of these men) his intentions weren't merely to swap notes. He had been one of the first Monuments Men ashore, arriving in Normandy on July 4, and in the last six weeks he had probably traveled more miles and salvaged more monuments than anyone. He had not come to Saint-Lô for congratulations or complaints. He had come to identify problems and find ways to solve them.

Not enough "Off Limits" signs? Rorimer would handle having five hundred printed immediately. There wasn't much electricity in Normandy, but the army had a printing press in Cherbourg they turned on at night. In the meantime, the rest of the men could make them in the field.

Soldiers and civilians tended to ignore handwritten signs? Stout had the solution for that one, too: use white engineering tape around important locations. No soldier would scavenge in a site clearly marked "DANGER: MINES!"

The general MFAA directive called for the use of French civilians to hang signs when possible, to counter the impression that the Allies were invaders. Children, Rorimer suggested, were often the most useful. They were eager to please, and usually wanted nothing more than a stick of gum or piece of chocolate. "The local cultural authorities are good, too," he said. "A little direction and encouragement, and they can handle all but the most complicated tasks."

As for cameras, everyone agreed the job couldn't be done without them, but for now they would try.

Communication was another issue. They were isolated in the field, with no way to contact headquarters and no way to share information among themselves. Their official reports took weeks to reach anyone, and by then they were not good for much but the files. Too many times, after hard and dangerous hours on the road, a Monuments Man had arrived to find the protected site already inspected, photographed, placed off-limits, and in the midst of emergency repairs. And what if a sudden German counterattack moved the front lines while a Monuments Man was out in the field?

"It's worse with the British," murmured Rorimer, who had become quite frustrated by the errant wandering of the British Monuments Man Lord Methuen. "They don't stay in their zones. And there's no communication."

"The British are working on it," Captain LaFarge said.

"As to the reports," Stout suggested, "let's start making additional copies for each other when we send them to Ad Sec."

That brought up the subject of assistants. Every man needed at least one qualified enlisted assistant, Stout still thought, and preferably a pool of specialists at headquarters to select from, too.

The most pressing problem, though, was the lack of transportation. LaFarge had his beat-up car and Stout his topless VW, but everyone else was wasting precious hours hitching rides, and even more time stuck in the inefficient routes hitchhiking required.

"The army always has the same reply," Rorimer grumbled. "The Roberts Commission in Washington should have arranged adequate tables of organization and equipment."

"And the Roberts Commission says the army will brook no interference," Stout replied, summing up the ad hoc, between-the-cracks situation of the whole mission. Still, always optimistic, Hammett and Stout had managed to arrange a meeting for August 16 with the duty officers of U.S. Twelfth Army Group, at which they would address all the issues discussed.

With the basics covered, the conversation drifted

to more general observations. Everyone agreed that, despite the obvious problems, the mission had been a surprising success. They were lucky: The area to cover was small and Normandy, although beautiful, had relatively few monuments designated for protection. It was a perfect place to start. They would have to be much more efficient in the future, they knew, but for now they were satisfied. The French were valorous, stoic, and appreciative. The Allied soldiers were considerate of French culture and open to suggestions. There was a bottleneck one level up from the field; the army bureaucracy simply refused to support the mission. But the commanders on the ground were, despite the occasional pain in the ass, largely respectful of the work. Their experiences confirmed George Stout's original belief that a man on the ground, talking face-to-face, was the only way for the mission to succeed.

Their real worry now was the Germans. The more the Monuments Men learned of their behavior, the more worried they became. The Germans had fortified churches. They had stockpiled weapons in areas inhabited by women and children. They had burned houses and destroyed infrastructure, sometimes for strategic purposes but often simply because they could. Their commanders, it was rumored, shot their own troops if they threatened to retreat. James Rorimer, after a moment of searching, produced a business card. On the front was a name: J. A. Agostini, a French cultural official in the town of Countances. On the back, the man had scrawled, "I certify that German military personnel used Red Cross trucks for pillaging and that sometimes they were accompanied by their officers."[7]

"An ominous warning," George Stout said, putting voice to all their thoughts. No one even bothered to agree.

———

"You idiot," James Rorimer's new and much less understanding commanding officer replied a few days later when the Monuments Man requested permission to travel a hundred miles out of the way to inspect Mont Saint-Michel, a medieval fortress on a rocky tidal island off the coast of Brittany. "This is twentieth-century war. Who gives a damn about medieval walls and boiling pitch?"[8]

This was another problem. The army was always shifting commanders, and Rorimer never knew who his CO would be when he returned to HQ—or their attitude toward cultural preservation. Still, the Monuments Men had the backing of General Eisenhower, the Supreme Commander, something the officer suddenly seemed to remember.

"All right," he huffed. "Get going. But let me tell you, Rorimer, you'd better get there in a hurry and come back fast. If you get left behind..."[9]

Rorimer turned so the officer wouldn't see his smile. He imagined the end of that sentence was *that would be no loss*, and he enjoyed the thought. He always took a bit of pleasure in tweaking the brass.

Unable to secure official transportation, but intrepid as always, Rorimer hired a civilian car—the French driver had hidden it in a haystack during the German occupation—to take him to the Brittany coast. A German counteroffensive had nearly cut through Patton's lines outside the town of Avranches, but the battle for Normandy was now all but over and the countryside west of Avranches was quiet. As they drove, Rorimer thought of the Mont Saint-Michel he had visited in years past. "The Mount," as the rocky island was known, was connected to mainland France only by a narrow, mile-long causeway. Around the edges of the island clung a small village; at the top sat the monastery of Mont Saint-Michel, the renowned medieval "City of Books." Rorimer cringed at the thought of how many of those books were lost at Saint-Lô. If the monastery was gone too... He remembered the thirteenth-century cloister; the soaring abbey; the underground labyrinth of crypts and chapels; the Salle des Chevaliers, with its pointed vaulting supported by a triple row of columns. It was such an extraordinary building that Monuments Man Bancel LaFarge told him it had inspired him to become an architect. The Mount had withstood a thousand years of attacks and sieges, due in no small part to the protection afforded by the surrounding water and its rapid tide, but the power of modern warfare could bring it all down with a single bombing run.

He didn't have to worry long. Mont Saint-Michel, he could see from a mile away, was still standing. At the entrance to the causeway, three "Off Limits" signs had already been posted by Captain Posey, the Monuments Man for Patton's Third Army. Unfortunately, they hadn't kept the island from being overrun. Troops were everywhere, fighting, shouting, and most of all drinking. Mont Saint-Michel, Rorimer soon realized, "was the one place on the continent which was unguarded, undamaged and open for business-as-usual....Each day more than a thousand soldiers came [on junket leave], drank as hard and as fast as they could, and, feeling the effects, became boisterous beyond the power of local control."[10] The restaurants were running low on food and, even worse, booze. The souvenir shops were empty. And despite the fact that a British brigadier general was supposedly shacked up at the local hotel with a female companion, James Rorimer couldn't find a single officer to take charge of the situation.

That night, after searching the monastery and ancient building, rousting troops from historic areas and padlocking the doors, Rorimer had dinner with the mayor, whose souvenir shop had been stripped clean days before. The men decided that, although arguments to the contrary were abundant, Mont Saint-Michel should stay open for business. It had been a long three months, and more than 200,000 Allied soldiers were wounded, dead, or missing. The stench of death—civilians, soldiers, farm animals, horses—had saturated the air, the water, the food, and the clothes. But it was over, at least for now. The battle of Normandy was a brutal, decisive, hard-fought, hard-won Allied victory, and there wasn't much one Monuments officer could do to keep the troops from celebrating. So when the weary mayor headed off to his wife, Rorimer went to a bar, propped his boots on a table, and considered the future between sips of beer.

Normandy was behind them, but the real work lay ahead. He thought of the German soldiers hauling away artwork in Red Cross ambulances. The Nazis had committed horrible crimes, he was sure of that, and if he was going to truly be a part of putting the art world right, he would need to find a way to get transferred from Comm Zone to the front. The evidence lay out there somewhere, waiting to be discovered. And he was the man to do it. The first step, though, was getting to Paris.

The next morning, Rorimer was approached by an air force military policeman. The officer demanded to see his papers. The papers seemed to confirm his suspicions, because the soldier smiled, nodded, and placed the Monuments Man under arrest. "No officer of such low rank would have the responsibilities you claim," he said. "And no officer, of any rank, would travel without his own transportation." Even at the local headquarters, the officers were convinced they had stumbled on a German spy. The MP was jubilant, no doubt envisioning promotions and commendations. The young man escorted the "spy" all the way back to Rorimer's headquarters before receiving the crushing news: there really was an MFAA, and Second Lieutenant James Rorimer really was a member of it. The Monuments Men may have considered their first months in Europe a success, but clearly the mission had a long way to go.

Dear Margie:

I found an air mail envelope and so can spread myself a little. It's been a week since I've got to my headquarters and had a chance at any mail. With a break of luck I may reach it tomorrow and have some new word from you, darling.

Work has been pretty consuming this week but not at all depressing. For two days I've billeted in a city, quite a decent-sized city, and have enjoyed a good room with a nice family.... A charming household of people like many we know and I am impressed with the slightness of difference between nations, at least between civilized nations.

As the front rolls along and the evidence piles up, the score against the Germans grows heavier. They have behaved very badly, and in the last days of their occupation, savagely. From here, now, they do not look like a simple innocent people with criminal leaders. They look like criminals. And I wonder how long it will take to get them to live fairly with the rest of the world.

Being in a city I feel very slouchy and ill-kempt in my field clothes—a steel hat, no necktie, generally dirty from the dust of the road, and carrying a gun. Keeping clean is always a problem.

Lately, I've not had time to do my own washing and, with short jumps, I can't farm it out.

There is no end to the friendliness of the welcome we get. In another town today, I saw a jeep roll in covered with flowers. The corporal driving said, "Jeez, you'd think we'd won the war." Yesterday in a village hardly damaged by war a girl brought up a little sister, about two, to give me an apple. She wouldn't take it back, nor would a little boy in another village, who gave me a tomato. They all want to shake hands all around, at least twice....

Do take care of yourself. By the time this reaches you, summer will be about over and you'll be looking grimly at teachers' meetings. Don't try to carry anything else after school starts. I'll try to get my pay straight one of these days and send you some money.

I suppose you hear much talk of fatalities. We hear none at all and seem not the worse.

I love you and think of you much.

Yours,
George

CHAPTER 12

Michelangelo's Madonna

Bruges, Belgium
September 1944

By the last week of August 1944, the northern European campaign had turned into a rout. The Germans had thrown almost all their reserves into preserving the "Ring of Steel" around Normandy, and once the ring was broken a wide open field of advance lay before the Western Allies. Racing forward with almost no resistance, they found millions of pounds of abandoned food, hundreds of carloads of coal, countless abandoned vehicles and wounded German soldiers, and even traincars full of looted lingerie and perfume. The villages were decorated with flowers, the townspeople openly cheering and handing out food and wine to their liberators. The surviving Germans had essentially thrown down their arms and were racing for home.

By August 28, the front lines had advanced more than one hundred miles, liberating Paris and pushing past its eastern outskirts. By September 2, the Allies had reached Belgium, and a day later cut through more than half the country and liberated Brussels, Belgium's capital and largest city. Four days later, very late in the night of September 7 or possibly in the early-morning hours of September 8, the sacristan of the Cathedral of Notre Dame in the Belgian city of Bruges was roused from sleep by a knock on his door. When the sacristan, tying on a robe, was slow to answer, the knock became louder and more urgent. By the time he reached the door, someone was pounding. "Patience, patience," he muttered under his breath.

Two German officers were standing outside, one dressed in the blue uniform of the German navy, and one in field gray. Behind them, in the dark street, the sacristan could see armed German sailors from the local barracks, at least twenty but possibly more. They had come in two trucks marked with the insignia of the Red Cross.

"Open the cathedral," one of the officers demanded.

The sacristan took the Germans to see the dean.

"We have orders," the German said, holding up a piece of paper. "We're taking the Michelangelo. To protect it from the Americans."

"The Americans?" The dean laughed at the audacity. "The British are said to be outside the city. I haven't heard anything about the Americans."

"We have orders," the German commander repeated, pushing into the doorway. A few sailors with guns stepped forward, too. There was no mistaking the message. The dean and sacristan accompanied the soldiers back to the cathedral, unlocking the massive doors with the old iron keys. Behind them, the street was quiet. Under the German occupation, nobody but partisans moved about at two in the morning, and they, of course, kept to the alleys. The blackout may have hindered Allied night bombings, but it was a great help to the Resistance as well.

"You'll never get her out of Bruges," the dean told the commander as he pushed open the ancient doors. "The British are already in Antwerp."

"Don't believe everything you hear," the German countered. "There is still a way."

Once inside, the Germans moved quickly. Guards were posted on the door. Soldiers circled the sanctuary, shading the windows, while two more stood watch over the dean and sacristan. The rest proceeded directly to the north aisle of the church, where the sculpture sat in a sealed room specially constructed by Belgian authorities in 1940. The Germans tore open the doors. In the light of their pocket lamps, the only light, it seemed, in all of Bruges, the *Madonna* glowed. She was life-sized and radiant, the gentle face and robes of a young woman carved by the young master, Michelangelo, from the richest, whitest marble in Italy. In the glow of her enemy's lamps, the *Madonna* seemed to look down with an almost serene look of sadness; the Christ Child, looking nothing like a helpless baby, seemed to step defiantly out of the alcove into the light.

"Get the mattresses," the commander ordered. Four days before, Dr. Rosemann, the head of the Belgian section of the Kunstschutz, the German arts and monuments protection organization, had visited the cathedral. He needed to see the *Madonna* one last time, he said, before he left Belgium. "I have kept a picture of her on my desk all these years," he told the dean. After viewing the sculpture, Dr. Rosemann ordered his men to place several mattresses in the room. "For protection," he said, "from Allied bombs. The Americans are not like us; they are savages. How can they appreciate this?" The mattresses were protection, the dean realized now, but not from bombs. They were the quickest and safest way to carry the statue to the trucks.

"What about the paintings?" a sailor asked. Near the *Madonna* hung many of the cathedral's most magnificent works.

The commander considered them for a moment. "You there," he said to one of the soldiers near the door. "Go bring another truck."

The dean held his breath as the men climbed onto the base of the precious statue. He couldn't look away, for fear any moment might be her last. Beside him, the sacristan crossed himself and muttered prayers, not daring to look as the statue started to teeter off its pedestal. The sailors were holding the mattress as the four-foot-tall sculpture slid forward, the weight of the marble pushing them all to the floor. But she was safe, at least as far as the dean could tell. She was lying face-down on a mattress, but at least she was safe.

As a dozen sailors moved the *Madonna* slowly toward a side door, others set up a ladder. The soldiers started removing paintings as the commanding officer paced and flicked spent cigarette butts onto the floor around him. Back and forth, back and forth.

"This one is too high," a sailor shouted. "We need a taller ladder."

"Keep your voice down," the commander ordered. It was still pitch-black outside; there was plenty of time. "Try again."

The *Madonna* was nearing the door. The sailors took the second mattress, as they had clearly been instructed beforehand, and placed it over the sculpture. It wouldn't offer much protection, but it might conceal the theft from prying eyes.

"No good, Commander," said one of the men on the ladder.

"Just leave it," the commander said, suddenly irritated by the whole operation. It was five in the morning; he hadn't slept all night. All for a statue. "Leave the painting; it's not important. Load the rest."

It took another half hour to heave the statue onto the back of one of the Red Cross trucks. The soldiers piled into the second truck. The paintings went into the third, the one the sailor had gone out an hour before to find. The first soft strip of daylight was just touching the horizon as the dean and the sacristan, standing in the side doorway in their night clothes, watched the *Bruges Madonna*, the only sculpture by Michelangelo to leave Italy during his lifetime, disappear.

The dean stopped his story and took a sip of his tea. His hand still shook, slightly but noticeably. "It is believed she left Bruges by sea," he concluded sadly, "although it is possible by air. Regardless, she is no longer here."

Across from him, Monuments Man Ronald Balfour, George Stout's roommate from Shrivenham, adjusted his scholar's glasses and recorded the information in his field journal. The dean's study, with its rows of books, reminded him of his own library back at Cambridge.

"Any idea when she left Belgium?"

"No more than a few days ago, I would think," the

dean replied sadly. "Possibly yesterday, who knows?" It was September 16, eight days since the theft and just days after the British had triumphantly entered the town.

Balfour closed his notebook. He had been so close. The *Bruges Madonna* had slipped through their grasp, through his grasp, somewhere between Bruges and the open sea.

"Would you like a photograph?"

"I don't need a photograph," Balfour said, preoccupied with his thoughts. He had been in the British army since 1940. Three years he spent recruiting infantrymen in rural England. Eight months training as a Monuments Man. He had thought he was ready. He was only three weeks on the continent, attached to First Canadian Army in the northernmost flank of the advance, and already the job seemed to be exploding out of his grasp. It was one thing to enter Rouen, France, and find the Palais de Justice destroyed. An errant Allied bomb had inadvertently started the destruction in April; the Germans completed it when they accidentally set the whole district on fire while trying to burn down the telephone exchange on August 26. Balfour had missed saving the Palais by less than a week.

But this was different. This wasn't war damage or an unfortunate decision made during a hasty retreat. The world had long known the Germans had looted artwork. The fact that they were *still* looting artwork, even in the face of a massive Allied advance, was beyond anything Balfour had imagined.

"Take them," the dean said, holding out a stack of

postcards. "Distribute them. Please. You know the *Madonna*. But many of the soldiers do not. What if they find her in a barn? Or in some German officer's home? Or"—he paused—"at the bottom of the harbor. Take these, so they will recognize her and know she is one of the wonders of the world."

The older man was right. Balfour took the cards. "We'll find her," he said.

CHAPTER 13

The Cathedral and the Masterpiece

Northern France
Late September 1944

*

Southern Belgium
Early October

In mid-September 1944, the last of the original MFAA field officer corps to arrive on the continent, the good-natured sculptor Captain Walker Hancock, flew directly from London to Paris. The plane was forced to fly low because of cloud cover, but the Luftwaffe had all but disappeared from the skies of France and there was little danger. Out the window Hancock could see Rouen, where a week or two before Ronald Balfour had discovered the burned-out hulk of the Palais de Justice. Even from the sky the destruction in the city was obvious, but beyond Rouen the countryside was quiet, the farmhouses, cows, and sheep clearly visible in their timeless array. The richly cultivated fields, with their craggy lines of hedgerows, made lovely patterns. The little villages, with their quiet lanes, seemed peaceful and prosperous—until you looked closer and saw the pockmarks of destruction. Every bridge, Hancock noticed, was smashed.

Paris was battle-scarred, but to Walker Hancock more beautiful than ever. The Eiffel Tower dominated the horizon, of course, but it was the smaller boulevards that held the wonder of liberation. Thousands of French, British, and American flags flew from the windows, and except for the occasional convoy of military trucks the streets were empty of motorized traffic. "Everybody gets about on bicycles," he wrote his wife, Saima, "the result being an abundance of handsome legs. It didn't seem possible to imagine Paris without its taxis—but I've *seen* it. Lights are turned on at 10 p.m.—after a long evening in the dark—and of course there are no street lights. But the Metro is running and more crowded than the NY subways. Allied soldiers walk in without paying. The Germans demanded the privilege, so the French have extended the courtesy to the 'Liberators.' . . . The first demonstrations of joy are over and so seem at first hardly to be noticed. But one soon finds what a friendly attitude is there. Very often a little boy with neat white gloves will come up and solemnly shake hands without saying a word. The poorer children all insist on giving us souvenirs—simple little things that they have collected, like pictures that (used to) come with chocolate bars or cigarette wrappers. . . . Today I bought some postcards in a village near the camp. The storekeeper refused to let me pay for them. 'We owe everything to you'—he said—'we can't repay the American soldiers.' "

Fall was in the air, and yet to Hancock the world seemed as fresh and bright as a Parisian summer. "I have been in Paris," he continued, "and will never cease to be thankful that I got there a month after its liberation."[1]

He stayed a night with James Rorimer, "Jimsie," his fellow officers called him, who had gotten the assignment he most desired: Monuments Man for Seine Section, which meant, essentially, Paris. Rorimer was staying in his sister and brother-in-law's apartment, which had not been used since before the war. For breakfast he served fresh eggs, the first Hancock had eaten in months, and the men talked about their experiences. Rorimer had arrived in the convoy of General Pleas B. Rogers, the first U.S. convoy to enter the City of Light. He had seen columns of smoke hovering over the city, framed by the Eiffel Tower. Bullets snapped from rooftops; the Chamber of Deputies smoldered. German prisoners were being led to the Comptoir National d'Escompte on the Place de l'Opera. In the Tuileries Garden, the muzzles of the abandoned German guns were still hot from firing. "I didn't rest, between my nerves and my excitement," Rorimer told Hancock, "until I was lying on my bed at the Hotel de Louvre. It was absurd, but here in the midst of destruction was this comfortable hotel with hot and cold running water and big, high-ceilinged rooms, each with French doors, drapes and a balcony. Just for a moment, it was like pre-war Paris."[2]

Walker Hancock wasn't staying. In fact, he was eager to leave Paris. He had a duty, one he believed in so strongly that he had left behind a life of contentment to perform it. Unlike some of his fellow officers, who felt the pull of war at least partially for personal reasons, Hancock could have gone on with his life in America exactly as it was. He was a well-known sculptor of monumental works, including the great winged horse known as *Sacrifice* on the World War I soldiers' memorial in his hometown of St. Louis. He owned two art studios, and although he was in debt (another reason not to pursue a low-paying army job), he had accumulated enough commissions and goodwill to sustain him for a lifetime. And a month before sailing to the continent at forty-two years old, he had married Saima Natti, the love of his life.

And yet no soldier had a better attitude about his service in the war than Walker Hancock. Filled with a sense of duty, but almost forty, he had applied for Army Air Forces Intelligence soon after Pearl Harbor. He failed his physical. So he joined Naval Intelligence, passing his physical with flying colors, only to be drafted by the army and sent to basic training. Not long after, the drill sergeant pulled him out of morning lineup and informed him he was being transferred. Hancock thought he was returning to Naval Intelligence; in actuality, he had won a competition to design the Air Medal, one of the army's highest awards for bravery. After striking the medal, Hancock entered the Italian section of the War Department. Finally, he was recruited by the MFAA.

"Doesn't life do strange things to us mortals!" he wrote his fiancée Saima in October 1943. "Here, in the midst of all my happiness about *you*, I suddenly get news that I'm going to be sent overseas to do the work I most want to do in the Army."[3] They were wed on December 4, 1943, in Washington, D.C. Two weeks later, Walker Hancock's duty orders came through. "I can still vividly remember that as the taxi sped away to begin the first leg of my journey, I looked back and saw Saima standing in the doorway, weeping.... I had never experienced such a dark moment."[4]

Hancock missed his battleship convoy in New York—again, they were unaware a Monuments Man was expected—so every day he was required to report for duty on the docks in case a ship had an open berth. He had to dress in his uniform and bring his bags, but there was nothing else for him to do. Sometimes it was positively depressing. "It's like prison—this having to be 'available' every day," he wrote Saima, "when I want only to be with you.... [But] in the meantime I'm walking on air—can't even remember to wind my watch. A fine officer I'm making!"[5]

But he couldn't contain his native enthusiasm and optimism. "Let's try to look at the happy side of matters," he wrote her, "the most wonderful thing of all—that we know how much we love each other, and that the joy of doing a useful service should be greater and not less because of that."[6]

Saima traveled to New York to stay with her new husband in a soldier's hotel, never knowing when he left in the morning whether her new husband would return from the docks. For two weeks, he came back to her, and then one evening, when he didn't return, she knew he was gone. The army hadn't even given him a chance to tell her goodbye.

"The sun and the wind and the inspiring site of shipping," he wrote Saima upon his arrival in England, "remind me of what a privilege it is to be a witness to some of the events of what will be the most dramatic year in many generations—instead of reading about them in the vaults of the Pentagon."[7] At forty-two, he assured her, he was old enough to have his eyes open to the wonders, and worried that "most of the boys will wake up later on and realize what they missed."[8]

Now, finally after eight months in England, he was in northern France. The breakout at Normandy had become a rout, and the Allies were racing toward the German border with almost no resistance from the retreating German army. General George C. Marshall, President Roosevelt's most trusted military advisor, confidently predicted the battle for Europe would end "between September 1 and November 1, 1944," and advised his officers to start considering transfers to the Pacific theater.[9] Almost as good, the bitterly wet summer of Normandy had finally faded to calm, clear weather, which made Walker Hancock's first official assignment as Monuments Man for the U.S. First Army—traveling by jeep with his fellow Monuments Man Captain Everett "Bill" Lesley to inspect protected monuments near the rear of First Army territory—seem almost a sightseeing tour. Hancock wrote Saima, in his usual buoyant manner, that "every hour of each day has been a pleasure."[10]

The damage he found was minimal. The Germans had steamrolled across northeastern France in 1940. Four years later, the Allies had quickly taken it back, leaving large swathes of country untouched by war. Most of the problems stemmed from the Nazi occupation force: local museums casually looted; fields strewn with mines or otherwise rendered unworkable; small objects like candlesticks and brass window handles stolen for souvenirs. Some paintings were missing, but the worst destruction was to the priceless Louis XIV furniture so common in the old, grand homes of France. Much of it was burned as firewood to make way for the overstuffed modern pieces German officers found more to their tastes. Every wine cellar, of course, had been emptied, with many of the most expensive vintages traded bottle-for-bottle for cheap apple wine, which the German soldiers preferred. The work proved idyllic, especially since most of the major sites had already been visited by the dapper conservator George Stout, who had covered an awful lot of ground for one man serving near the front.

Sometimes it was nothing short of spectacular. Chartres Cathedral rose, as always, like a mountain from the fields of wheat. But the usually bustling town of Chartres was quiet, the famous cathedral standing defiantly alone. Hancock found himself, even more than he had on previous visits as an art student at the American Academy in Rome, inspired by its enormity and complexity, its extraordinary ambition. The great walls and towers, with their rich ornamentation, had taken centuries to build; there was no way, he thought, that four years of war could destroy such beauty.

Would he have loved it more if he had known that wasn't true, that the Wehrmacht had almost destroyed in an afternoon what had taken four generations to build? When the Allies arrived at Chartres, they found the cathedral at risk of being damaged and possibly destroyed by twenty-two sets of explosives placed on nearby bridges and other structures. Demolitions expert Stewart Leonard, who after the end of active hostilities would himself become a Monuments Man, helped defuse the bombs and save the cathedral. As he later explained to Monuments Man Bernie Taper over drinks in a Berlin apartment, "There's one good thing about being in the bomb disposal unit: No superior officer is ever looking over your shoulder."

But was art worth a life, Taper wanted to know. Like all Monuments Men, it was a question that haunted him. "I had that choice," Leonard said. "I chose to remove the bombs. It was worth the reward."

"What reward?"

"When I finished, I got to sit in Chartres Cathedral, the cathedral I had helped save, for almost an hour. Alone."[11]

Would future generations, Walker Hancock wondered, understand the power of witnessing this cathedral under the threat of war? Would they appreciate its wonder more if they could see it now, with its windows removed, sandbags piled seemingly thirty feet high, and artillery holes peppering the towers? On the floor lay the twisting path that pilgrims had for centuries traveled on their knees to salvation. Above him, the torn plastic coverings of the window openings fluttered defiantly in the breeze.

"Here was an unexpected beauty," Hancock wrote. "The windows were open to the sky...so that we saw simultaneously the interior and exterior of that wonderful building. To follow the great flying buttresses as they entered the roof and turned into the ribs of the vaults was a graphic lesson in Gothic engineering. But it was more. Seen from within, there was something invigorating in the appearance of those mighty wheel-like arches, so characteristic of Chartres, seeming almost to turn in their pressure against the walls of the apse....One could stand within the enclosure and see in a new, overhead light the figures of the kings and queens of Judah and the Christ of the Apocalypse."[12] For a moment, the cathedral seemed both a monument to the Allied triumph and a structure out of time, beyond the war, something that would stand forever, even when the world was gone.

But it was not to last. The sun was setting, its beams slipping through the great open window arches and rising up the walls. The battle lines lay in the opposite direction, in the east. His help, Hancock knew, was required there. He shouldered his kit and turned back to the war.

———

A few weeks later, Walker Hancock was shaken awake from a too-brief sleep. Over his cot stood his fellow Monuments Man for U.S. First Army, George Stout, looking as well-groomed as ever despite the early-morning hour. "We've got work," he said, snapping his driving goggles.

Outside it was pouring rain. The mist was so fierce and the sky so overcast that Hancock could make out only the dark shape of the enormous army barracks where First Army was headquartered. He remembered with dejection that Stout's vehicle—the dilapidated German Volkswagen he had been driving since Normandy—had no top, and therefore offered no shelter. He pulled his coat closer. It was October 10, 1944, and he could feel winter approaching.

He ate breakfast with Stout in the mess hall. Hancock had arrived at First Army headquarters in Verviers, an eastern Belgian town about twenty miles from the German border, only a week before, and he was still unused to the routine of army life. He had parted with both Bill Lesley and the jeep outside Paris, and spent a week hitchhiking as best he could across northern France. Moving east toward southern Belgium, he had entered an area ransacked by the occupying Germans. Families were returning to find their homes destroyed or looted. Pillboxes and abandoned equipment dotted yards and gardens. The villagers, many short on food since the fields had gone untended, offered onions and tomatoes as thank-yous, and despite their circumstances asked for little in return. All told the same story: The Germans "were wonderfully disciplined and 'correct' while they had the upper hand—and went berserk when it was obvious that their visit was at an end."[13]

"I can see that letters are going to be few and far between from this end," Hancock wrote Saima. "My life is suddenly one of very great activity. It makes my head swim even to think of where I have been and what I've done in the last two days. But I'm so happy and interested in what I'm doing that it makes the months of waiting, planning, theorizing, and lecturing others very dull by comparison."[14]

Now he was passing through another region, the hilly, wooded areas of eastern Belgium. In the rain the hills looked dull, and he passed through them without the wonder of his early tour. Stout drove steadily, his eyes glued to the road. At least they were out of the rain, for Stout had sent his captured Volkswagen for repairs and been loaned a better vehicle, a situation that would prove far too temporary. Still, Hancock thanked his good fortune on this of all days as the rain hissed down so hard he could barely see the road. He wasn't even aware they'd crossed the border into Holland, in fact, until they stopped at the foot of yet another of the steep, scrub-covered hills. There were concrete walls at its base, holding back the mountain. At first Hancock thought it was a train tunnel, but the opening was locked tight by two enormous, bolted metal doors.

"What is this place?"

"Art repository," Stout said, as the doors opened and he drove the jeep inside.

The cavern, created in the 1600s to protect Dutch treasures from French invaders, had all the modern conveniences. The storerooms were well lit, the temperature and humidity controlled. And yet, as he passed deeper into the eerie silence of the mountain, Hancock felt it an unworldly place. The two civilians in charge of the repository led them back past walls of chiseled stone illuminated by long rows of buzzing lights. Near the back were several revolving screens that turned on swivels, like display racks of postcards in tourist shops. But instead of two-cent postcards these screens held paintings from the Netherlands' greatest museum, the Rijksmuseum in Amsterdam. As a curator turned the crank, the masterpieces by Dutch painters—still lifes of food on tables, exquisite landscapes full of rich skies dotted with sweeping grayish clouds, portraits of smiling, black-clad burghers—passed slowly by, the squeaking of the axle echoing in the empty vault.

"Amazing," Hancock muttered. He wished he could

write Saima about it, but the censors would never let through information this specific because of the ever-present fear of interception or spies.

Turning away, he noticed a large painting rolled on a spindle like a carpet. There was a metal crank on the end, and a wooden case had been built around it. The packing material rolled up with the painting stuck out like the torn, ragged ends of butcher paper.

"*The Night Watch*," one of the curators commented, tapping the wooden housing. Hancock's mouth dropped. He was looking at the rolled end of one of Rembrandt's most famous paintings, the great, wall-sized masterpiece of the militia company of Captain Frans Banning Cocq, painted in 1642.

Stout pulled back the ragged packing material, examined the edge of the painting, and frowned. It was never a good idea to store oil works in prolonged darkness. Parasitic microorganisms tended to grow on the surfaces of the oils. And the resins used to varnish the paintings would yellow in the darkness, muting the colors and obscuring the contrasts. As early as March 1941, Stout had heard from Dutch experts that *The Night Watch* appeared to be yellowing; Stout could see now, as he had feared, the intervening three and a half years had not been kind. If it sat here too long, the painting might have to be stripped and revarnished, a potentially harsh procedure for a centuries-old work. But he was most concerned with the fact that the painting was off its stretcher and had been rolled for an extended period of time, making it vulnerable to crack-ing, or even flaking or tearing…types of structural damage that were irreversible. Great masterworks were not made to be rolled up and buried inside mountain hideaways. But at the moment, there was nothing that could be done. In a world at war, *The Night Watch* was getting the best treatment possible. He wondered how other masterpieces—like Jan Vermeer's *The Astronomer*, which had been stolen off the walls of the Rothschilds' Paris mansion by the Nazis in 1940 and hadn't been seen since—were faring.

"Where are the guards?" Stout asked.

One of the curators pointed across the room at two policemen.

"Is that all?"

The curator nodded. These were lean years, and only a few guards were available, even for a nation's treasure. Besides, there hadn't been a need. The Germans had long known about this repository at St. Pietersberg, near Maastricht, and others like it. In fact, Nazi officials and soldiers had supervised a previous move of *The Night Watch*, which had been "hidden" in several locations before arriving in Maastricht, conveniently close to the German border, in 1942. Perhaps because of this, the Dutch curators seemed surprisingly unconcerned with the lack of protection. Cut off from the rest of the world in their hillside lair, they hadn't heard about the recent theft of Michelangelo's *Bruges Madonna*. They didn't understand, as George Stout had grasped, that the greatest danger wasn't when the Germans were in complete control, but now, when they were losing control and realizing this was their last opportunity to act. What had Dr. Rosemann told the dean of the church in Bruges? *I have kept a picture of her on my desk all these years.* What had the French peasants told Hancock?

The Germans were wonderfully disciplined and "correct" while they had the upper hand—and went berserk when it was obvious that their visit was at an end.

"We'll get more guards," Stout said. "At least ten until normal conditions are restored to the area."

The phone lines were broken; the request for guards would have to wait until they arrived back at headquarters. Stout was clearly displeased by the inefficiency and lack of planning, not to mention the danger inherent in a delay, but only for a moment. Then he was, once again, practical and unflappable. "The additional guards may be here tomorrow," he said, heading for the borrowed car. "But this is the army. I can offer no guarantees. Thank you, my friends, for a most unusual tour."

My God, Hancock thought, as he climbed in beside the conservator and took one last glance backward at Rembrandt's masterpiece, looking for all the world like a carpet about to be installed on a living room floor. *War is strange.*

CHAPTER 14

Van Eyck's Mystic Lamb

Eastern France
Late September 1944

Captain Robert Posey, Alabama farmboy and Monuments Man for General George Patton's U.S. Third Army, hung his towel on the peg and headed back to his pup tent. It was September 23, 1944, and he had just taken his first hot shower since landing at Normandy more than two months before. He ran his hand over his warm, freshly shaved face. For years he had worn a mustache, and he still wasn't used to its absence. Without hair on his lip, he looked like a kid, not a forty-year-old architect, husband, father, and soldier. And besides, the mustache was a statement. When called to active duty, he had shaved both ends, imitating Hitler's well-known style. It was his little jab at the Third Reich, but it hadn't gone over too well with the general.

"Dammit, Bobby, shave that dirt off your lip," Patton exploded upon seeing the patch of hair.[1]

Not that Posey minded his commander's occasional explosions. It was an honor to serve in Patton's Third, the finest fighting force on the European continent. The truth is that Robert Posey felt much closer to the men of the Third than he ever had to his fellow Monuments

Men, and he had quickly adopted their pride, brotherhood, and private exasperation that the other Allied armies had yet to admit their obvious superiority. They were the army that broke the "Ring of Steel" in Normandy. They were the army that had closed the Falaise Pocket, cutting off the last German retreat from western France. They were the army leading the charge on the southern flank, while the other armies straggled somewhere behind them to the north. If Eisenhower had just turned Third Army loose sooner, when Patton first suggested turning east to head off the Germans, they might have already ended the war. There wasn't a man in Third Army who doubted that. They were confident, and it was all because of the man in the big tent, General George S. Patton Jr. Sure, he was belligerent, arrogant, and at times damn near crazy, but Posey would do anything for the man. It was the general's dog, Willie, a bull terrier named after William the Conqueror, that Posey couldn't stand.

He sat down hard on his cot, slipped on his shirt, and picked up the recent letter from his wife, Alice. He read it again, for the fourth or fifth time, and felt once more the instant softening of the hard shell of the soldier. It was that old familiar pull of home. Alice was in South Carolina living with relatives for the duration of the war, but Posey thought of the home they had shared together. The little patch of yard. The "zoo," as he always called the scene inside. The crooked smile of his young son; the elegant confusion of his softspoken wife. He suddenly wanted to hold her, but since the censors had recently lifted the ban on specific details in letters home—at least for the territory already conquered—he wrote her a letter about his travels instead.

"Now that the campaign in France is about over," he wrote, "we are allowed to tell of the cities we have seen. I have visited the great cathedrals of Coutances, Dol, Rennes, Laval, Le Mans, Orleans, Paris, Reims, Chalons-Sur-Marne, Chartres, and Troyes. Chartres is the greatest of all. I have also seen many fine churches in villages and many chateaux. The famous Mont-Saint-Michel and Fontainebleau are also included. The little village whose description I gave [in a previous letter] is Les Iffs, about halfway between Rennes and Saint Malo on the Brittany peninsula. I have lots of souvenir cards with autographs."[2]

He shuffled through the cards, all intended for his five-year-old son Dennis, whom he called "Woogie." He loved to send the boy trinkets—postcards, buttons, and recently a swastika belt buckle and a towel with "*Kriegsmarine*" stitched on it that he had found at a German submarine base. They were soldiers' souvenirs, much like those sent back by the enlisted men of Third Army with whom he felt such kinship. They were his way of staying connected with his son, and of documenting his journey through Europe, which he was keenly aware could be ended by a mine or a bullet any day.

Thinking back on the journey now, fresh from his shower, he couldn't believe how far he had come. He had grown up in love with the military, having spent his school years in army ROTC. He had become an architect, but he was still enlisted in the Army Reserve when the Japanese bombed Pearl Harbor. He wanted to leave for the Pacific the next day, but in the confusion of that terrible time it was almost six months before he was called to active duty. He was sent to base camp in Louisiana in the middle of the summer, the hottest, most humid place he had ever been—and he had grown up in central Alabama. From there, he was flown straight to Churchill, Manitoba, Canada's only major port on the Arctic Ocean, and by far the coldest experience of his life. He spent most of his time designing and building runways against a possible German invasion via the North Pole.

The North Pole! What general had looked at a globe and suddenly broken out in the hot sweats thinking about that? Posey never met any Germans in the frozen tundra, but he did have regular contact with another enemy: polar bears. As the poor Alabama boy discovered, Churchill, Manitoba, was the polar bear capital of the world.

Now here he was outside a captured German barracks in eastern France. Within a few weeks, maybe even days at the rate Third Army was moving, he would be in Germany, and not long after Berlin...at least if Papa Patton had anything to say about it.

He finished the letter to Alice—adding a PS about the luxury of a hot shower—and then picked up the packet that had arrived a few days before from SHAEF. Inside were photographs, descriptions, and background information on missing Belgian cultural treasures. Two of them were clearly the most important. One was Michelangelo's *Bruges Madonna*, whose theft had been documented by Ronald Balfour exactly one week ago. The other was the Ghent Altarpiece.

The *Adoration of the Mystic Lamb*, more commonly

referred to as the Ghent Altarpiece, was Belgium's most important and beloved artistic treasure. Almost twelve feet high and sixteen feet wide, it consisted of two rows of hinged wood panels: four in the center, and four on each wing, with the wings painted on both sides. The twenty-four individual but thematically linked works were arranged to show a different view when the altarpiece was opened or closed. The central panel, and the one from which the piece derived its name, depicted the Lamb of God on an altar, with the Holy Spirit in the form of a dove shining above it and crowds gathered around. The altarpiece was commissioned from Hubert van Eyck, known as *maior quo nemo repertus* ("greater than anyone"), but upon his death in 1426 was taken over by his younger brother Jan van Eyck, the self-described *arte secondus* ("second best in art") and completed in 1432.

The altarpiece, when unveiled at St. Bavo's Cathedral in the city of Ghent, shocked the Dutch world. It was painted in a realistic manner based on direct observation, not the idealized forms of antiquity or the flattened images of the Middle Ages. The images on each panel, even the minor ones, were rendered with extraordinary attention to every detail, from the faces of the human figures, which were based on real fifteenth-century Flemish people, to the buildings, landscape, vegetation, fabrics, jewels, robes, and materials as well. This detailed realism, based on the skilled use of oil paint, was like nothing the art world had ever seen. It would transform painting and usher in the Northern Renaissance, a golden age of Dutch culture that rivaled the Italian Renaissance farther south.

Five hundred and eight years later, in May 1940, the hills and meadows portrayed so vividly in the van Eyck masterpiece were blitzkrieged and captured by German forces. While half a million British and French troops retreated north, pursued by the Wehrmacht, three trucks headed south carrying the most important works of the Belgian state, including the Ghent Altarpiece. They were desperately trying to reach the Vatican and the protection of the pope, but only made it to the French border before Italy declared war on the countries of Western Europe. The trucks, buffeted by German Panzer divisions rushing north to stop the evacuation of British troops at Dunkirk, changed directions and eventually found their way to a château serving as an art repository in the southwestern French town of Pau, where the weary and terrified drivers entrusted the safety of the altarpiece to the French government.

Hitler knew it was impossible to steal renowned masterpieces on the scale of the Ghent Altarpiece without drawing the condemnation of the world. While he had the conqueror's mentality—he believed he was entitled to the spoils of war, and he was determined to have them—Hitler and the Nazis had gone to great lengths to establish new laws and procedures to "legalize" the looting activities that would follow. This included forcing the conquered countries to give him certain works as a term of their surrender. Eastern European countries like Poland were destined under Hitler's plan to become industrial and agricultural wastelands, where Slavic slaves would produce consumer goods for the master race. Most of their cultural icons were destroyed;

their great buildings leveled; their statues pulled down and melted into bullets and artillery shells. But the West was Germany's reward, a place for Aryans to enjoy the fruits of their conquest. There was no need to strip such countries of their artistic treasures—at least not right away. The Third Reich, after all, would last a thousand years. Hitler left works of comparable stature to the Ghent Altarpiece, such as the *Mona Lisa* and *The Night Watch*, untouched, even though he knew exactly where they were hidden. But he coveted the *Lamb*.

In 1940, Hitler (through Goebbels, his propaganda minister) had commissioned an inventory, later known as the Kümmel Report after its chief compiler, Dr. Otto Kümmel, general director of the Berlin State Museums. The inventory listed every work of art in the Western world—France, the Netherlands, Britain, and even the United States (which Kümmel said possessed nine such works)—that rightly belonged to Germany. Under Hitler's definition, this included every work taken from Germany since 1500, every work by any artist of German or Austrian descent, every work commissioned or completed in Germany, and every work deemed to have been executed in a Germanic style. The Ghent Altarpiece was clearly a touchstone and defining emblem of Belgian culture, but to the Nazis it was "Germanic" enough in style to belong to them.

Even more important, six of the side panels (painted on both sides, representing fourteen scenes) of the Ghent Altarpiece had been owned by the German state prior to 1919. The Germans had been forced, under the terms of the Treaty of Versailles that ended World War I, to give the panels to Belgium as war reparations.

Hitler had always hated the Treaty of Versailles, seeing it as a humiliation of the German people and a symbol of the weakness that had defined his country's past leaders. When Germany overran France in June 1940, Hitler was determined to exact a symbolic measure of revenge by ordering his troops to locate the railcar in which the humiliating armistice had been signed in 1918, ordered the walls of the building in which it was housed torn down, and had the railcar hauled to the precise spot in Compiègne, France, where it had been positioned twenty-two years before. Sitting in the exact same chair as Marshal Foch, the French hero of World War I who had been the victor that day, Hitler forced the French to sign an armistice. After the signing ceremony, Hitler ordered that the railcar be taken to Berlin where it was towed down the city's historic street, Unter den Linden, through the Brandenburg Gate, then put on display at the Lustgarten on the banks of the river Spree. The seizure of the Compiègne railcar was proof that Germany had overturned the disastrous "crime of Compiègne," and had crushed its hated neighbor. But it also proved something else: that nothing was too big, or too sacred, for the Nazis to steal.

The Ghent Altarpiece, that great masterpiece that had changed the course of painting forever, thus represented two of Hitler's enduring quests: to right the historic "wrongs" of the Treaty of Versailles, and to add an undisputed world treasure to his Führermuseum in Linz.

By 1942, Hitler was unable to resist the temptation any longer. In July, he sent a secret delegation, led by Dr. Ernst Buchner, general director of the Bavarian Museums, to the repository at Pau. This was not a mission of force—the delegation consisted of only one truck and one car—but of stealth. When the French superintendent at Pau refused to hand over the altarpiece, Buchner called the Reichschancellery. Within hours, a telegram arrived from Pierre Laval, the chief of government in Nazi-controlled Vichy France, ordering the altarpiece turned over to Buchner. By the time the proper French and Belgian art authorities learned of the order, the Ghent Altarpiece had disappeared into Germany. The Belgian government protested vigorously—even accusing the French of treason against its culture—but there was nothing that could be done. The Ghent Altarpiece was gone.

And now, more than two years later, Robert Posey sat on his cot in a pup tent in France, looking at a picture of this irreplaceable treasure. He knew the world was counting on him and his fellow Monuments Men to track it down, find it, force the surrender of those who guarded or coveted or wanted to destroy it, and return it to Belgium unharmed.

CHAPTER 15

James Rorimer Visits the Louvre

Paris, France
Early October 1944

While Posey found himself surprisingly pleased with his experience in U.S. Third Army, Second Lieutenant James Rorimer, the bulldog Metropolitan Museum curator, was having a similar experience in Paris. Over his beer at Mont Saint-Michel, Rorimer had wished fervently to be assigned to the City of Light; after returning to headquarters, he soon learned he had in fact received "the plum of all the jobs in Europe for one with my background."[1] The French authorities had embraced him with "open arms and hearts" and he was regularly being feted by the rich and powerful of Parisian society.[2] They wanted his help; he wanted their information. It was satisfying to be embraced wholeheartedly as a liberator and a friend.

And Paris, that wonderful sanctuary of a city, was in fantastic shape. It was almost hard to believe, looking at her buildings and monuments, that she had been occupied by the Nazis for four years. Several landmarks—including the Grand Palais, burned by the Nazis in an effort to root out the Resistance—had been destroyed, but a stroll down any of the wide avenues revealed a city virtually unmarked and bursting with life. There was almost no gasoline, but on every corner the bicycles crowded the lockups, especially the tandems with their little carts that during the occupation had been the city's primary taxis. In the parks, the old men were back to playing cards in their berets and fedoras. At the Luxembourg Gardens, the children floated their boats in the fountain, their innocent sails white against the water. "From the long and wonderfully empty avenues leading into the heart of the city," wrote Francis Henry Taylor, who visited the city as a representative of the Roberts Commission, "one felt the elation which comes only to those emerging after a deep sleep from illness. The will to live had conquered. Paris as the supreme creation of the mind of man had paralyzed the hand that tried to seize her."[3]

But Taylor was only in Paris a few days. A more detailed look at the city revealed that while there was ebullience on the surface of Parisian society, it was undercut by crosscurrents of fear and mistrust. The sudden retreat of the Germans and the collapse of the French collaboration government had left the city short of civil servants like police officers, and there was no way to control the simmering emotions of an angry population. A wave of revenge had gripped the populace as citizens took the law into their own hands. Women who had slept with Germans were taken into the streets and their heads publicly shaved in front of rowdy mobs; suspected collaborators were brought before tribunals and summarily executed. Anyone reading one of the city's newspapers, *Le Figaro*, would easily understand the gravity of the situation. *Le Figaro* had resumed printing on August 23, 1944, after a two-year hiatus. Inititally the paper was only two pages in length, but it had one recurring feature that appeared every day. The first part of the feature appeared under the heading "*Les Arrestations et L'Epuration*" (Arrests and Purges) and detailed the previous day's developments in the pursuit of collaborators. Underneath the article appeared two lists: "*les exécutions capitales*" (death sentences) and "*les exécutions summaires*" (summary executions). Even the more civilized death sentences, Rorimer knew, must have been meted out in trials lasting a few hours, or at most a couple of days.

In this void—no working civil institutions, no working safety apparatus, and no trust in one's fellow citizens—there was plenty of work for a Monuments Man. There were 165 Parisian monuments in the army's *Civil Affairs Handbook*, fifty-two of which were officially protected. There were hundreds if not thousands of victims of Nazi looting. Hundreds of public sculptures were missing, especially the city's famous bronzes, and even the nineteenth-century lights had been stolen from the Senate building. And then there was the general confusion of a city trying once again to find its feet. Finding basic information and supplies was often impossible. Procedural questions could wrap him in knots for hours. Even locating the right official for a particular area or task took an inordinate amount of energy.

Just after his arrival in August, Rorimer had been temporarily assigned to Lieutenant Colonel Hamilton's detachment, and even in late September Hamilton wouldn't give him up. "No one officer should be tied up with Monuments duty alone," Hamilton had told

Rorimer when he pleaded for his release, which meant Hamilton needed an aggressive, competent, energetic officer who spoke French, and he wasn't about to let James Rorimer go.[4]

And then, of course, he had to make sure the American military didn't do anything to damage the city. In August, when he arrived in the convoy of General Rogers, Paris had seemed deserted; now there were American troops everywhere. Not that they weren't enthusiastic to help. One detachment, assigned by Rorimer to assess damage to the Place de la Concorde, counted every bullet hole in the enormous complex. Rorimer caught them the next day counting war damage holes in the Louvre. "General assessment," he told them. "Only the big stuff." The Louvre was so massive that counting each bullet hole would have taken them a year.

The real problem, Rorimer felt, was that the American military didn't understand the French. The park through which he was walking, the Jardin des Tuileries, was a perfect example. It was the heart of Paris, a great formal garden laid out for Louis XIV and familiar to all who had ever strolled this great city. On his first morning in Paris, Rorimer had seen it as few Parisians ever had: almost empty in the morning light. The abandoned German guns lining the perimeter seemed to have scared people away, but bivouacked under one copse of trees was a single American tank unit with small cooking fires going for breakfast. Otherwise, the gardens had been his alone.

A few weeks later, Rorimer discovered the Jardin des Tuileries was slated for use as a massive Allied

encampment. The Germans had dug trenches throughout the park and strung them with barbed wire, but the
idea of the Allies digging slit-trench latrines into the
heart of Paris was too much. The Tuileries, he argued
in a series of interminable meetings, were no place for
Allied waste. The gardens were as vital to the health
and happiness of Parisians as Hyde Park to Londoners
and Central Park to New Yorkers.

The army relented. But what had Rorimer really
accomplished? The Tuileries' famous central bou-
levard, down which he now turned, was lined with
ten-ton trucks, troop carriers, and jeeps. Nobody had
declared the gardens off-limits to vehicles, not techni-
cally anyway, and they were now the largest parking lot
in Paris. Six statues had already been knocked off their
pedestals and the terra-cotta pipeworks, laid out in the
seventeenth century, were bursting under the weight of
vehicles. It had taken ten days of research and planning
to find an alternative, but Rorimer was convinced the
paved Esplanade des Invalides would accommodate the
army's needs. And the Esplanade, appropriately, was in
a district dedicated to military history. Now if he could
only convince the army it was worthwhile to move their
parking lot across town.

Rorimer passed the fountain known as the Grand
Bassin—even in the shadows of the military trucks
young boys were out floating their sailboats—crossed
the Terrasse des Tuileries, and, after showing his credentials to the armed guards, passed into the courtyard
of the Louvre. On one side, the American anti-aircraft
installation bristled with guns, and he could still see
the fenced yard where the Allies had kept German pris-

oners during their first week in the city. But inside, as always, the museum was a sanctuary. In here, he couldn't see a single gun or armed guard, much less the supplicants who came continually to his office to plead for individual care. Beneath the vaulted glass ceiling of the Grande Galerie, the museum was as still and quiet as a grave. A largely empty, hollow grave, for on these walls where millions had once come to view the world's masterpieces, there were nothing but scribbled words in white chalk, notes to remind the curators where each magnificent painting had hung.

The works weren't stolen or missing. In fact, the Germans hadn't touched them. They were even now secure in the repositories to which the French had moved them in 1939 and 1940, just before the German invasion. The evacuation had been an extraordinary operation, overseen by one of the great heroes of the French cause, Jacques Jaujard, director of the French National Museums.

Jaujard may have been a French government official, but he was also one of the most respected museum men in Western Europe. He was only forty-nine, but with his swept-back jet black hair and handsome chiseled face, he had the look of a youthful grandfather, the vibrant patriarch, perhaps, of some French wine-making clan. He was a bureaucrat—but a man not afraid to get his hands dirty with work. During the Spanish civil war, Jaujard had been instrumental in evacuating the contents of Madrid's world-class museum, the Prado. In 1939, he was promoted to director of the National Museums and immediately began to plan the evacuation of the French museums, at a time when few thought the Nazis would attack, much less conquer, a country like France. Under his watchful eye, thousands of the world's great master-pieces had been crated, loaded, driven, and stored. Even the Winged Victory of Samothrace, the massive ancient Greek statue that had stood at the head of the Louvre's main staircase, was removed by means of an ingenious pulley and inclined wooden track system. The almost eleven-foot-tall marble statue of the goddess Nike, her wings outstretched (but her head and arms lost over the centuries), appeared solid, but in fact consisted of thousands of shards of marble that had been painstak-ingly reassembled. Jaujard must have held his breath, Rorimer thought, as the statue slid down the staircase on its wooden track, her great wings trembling slightly in the air above her. If she crumbled to pieces, Jaujard would be held responsible. But he had always been a man who welcomed such challenges. Like Rorimer, Jaujard believed it was better to assume the burden of leadership than to drift along in the shadows.

Rorimer stopped and, turning, stared up and down the Louvre's long, empty Grande Galerie. So much irreplaceable art, all gone, he thought. So much dan-ger. He stepped toward a shallow alcove, framed by pil-lars, where two words had caught his eye. The words *La Joconde* seemed to float on the wall inside an empty frame. *La Joconde*, the French name for the *Mona Lisa*. Most of the works were transported en masse, some-times over bomb-blasted roads, but the *Mona Lisa*, the world's most famous painting, had been loaded by ambulance stretcher into the back of a truck in the dead of night. A curator climbed in the back as well;

the truck was sealed to provide a stable climate. Upon arriving at its destination, the painting was fine but the curator nearly unconscious. There hadn't been enough air for him to breathe.[5]

There were other stories. The great Géricault painting *The Raft of the Medusa* was so large it became tangled in the streetcar wires of Versailles. At least they learned their lesson. In the next city with low-hanging wires, the truck was accompanied by telephone repairmen walking before it and lifting all the wires with long, insulated poles. The image was amusing: the truck creeping along with its pole-wielding escorts, the evacuating citizens racing around it, perhaps staring in wonder at Géricault's painting of the dying faces of victims stranded on a sinking raft. But the situation wasn't amusing at all. These were masterworks, not parade floats. And under Jaujard's careful guidance, there was no major damage.

But even Jaujard had not foreseen the lightning strike of the German blitzkrieg or the humiliating collapse of the French army. The placement of art in temporary repositories, mostly country châteaux and remote castles, was intended to prevent war damage, primarily from aerial bombardment. At the Château de Sourches near Le Mans, the curators had even spelled out on the lawn in huge white letters the words "Musée du Louvre" so that pilots flying overhead would know artistic treasures were housed inside and avoid bombing it. As the French army melted, Jaujard ordered the artwork moved to repositories farther west and south. The advancing Germans found him at the repository at Chambord southwest of Paris, directing the evacuation. "You are, sir," they told him, "the first top French civil servant we find present on duty."[6]

Nothing was harmed, thank goodness, by bombs and artillery, but there was not much that could be done about the Nazi occupiers. They knew almost every work of art comprising France's patrimony, and they acted quickly to seize it. Paris was occupied on June 14, 1940. On June 30, Hitler ordered his representatives in Paris to safeguard works of art from the French National collections, and also artwork and historical documents belonging to individuals, in particular Jews. These cultural objects were to be used as collateral for the peace negotiations. France had signed only an armistice; Hitler was planning to use the formal peace treaty to "legally" seize the country's cultural assets, much as Napoleon had used one-sided treaties to seize the cultural treasures of Prussia almost 150 years before. It was widely acknowledged, and with only slight exaggeration, that without the spoils of the Napoleonic campaigns the Louvre would be a mere shadow of what it had become.

The powerful Nazi ambassador to Paris, Otto Abetz, sprang into action, declaring that the Nazi-controlled occupation government would provide "custody" for the cultural assets. Three days after Hitler's order, Abetz ordered the confiscation of the holdings of the top fifteen art dealers in Paris, most of whom were Jewish. Within weeks, the embassy was overflowing with "safeguarded" artwork. And that, Jaujard told James Rorimer during one of their frequent chats, was when a true hero emerged: the art official Count Franz von Wolff-Metternich.

"A German?" Rorimer had asked in surprise.

Jaujard had nodded, a twinkle in his patrician eyes. "Not just a German," he said. "A Nazi."

In May 1940, Count Wolff-Metternich had been appointed head of the Kunstschutz, the German cultural conservation program. The Kunstschutz had originally been created as an army-based protection unit during World War I—the only true precursor to the Western Allies' MFAA—but had been reconstituted in 1940 as a branch of the Nazi occupation government, operating primarily in conquered Belgium and France. Wolff-Metternich, an expert on Renaissance architecture, especially that of the Rhineland of northwest Germany where he was born and raised, was plucked from a professorship at the University of Bonn for the top job.

Wolff-Metternich was chosen because he was a respected scholar whose credibility brought a sense of professionalism and legitimacy to the Kunstschutz program. He was not an avid member of the Nazi Party, but in instances such as this the Nazis were often more concerned with selecting qualified professionals than with their political associations. That the Wolff-Metternichs were a prominent German family, with a title dating back hundreds of years to the Prussian empire, was also an appealing factor.

Wolff-Metternich was given no instructions, but he had a clear idea what his Kunstschutz should do. "At all times," he would write, "we took as our legal determinant the relevant paragraphs of the Hague Convention."[7] His definition of cultural responsibility, therefore, was the internationally recognized one, not the Nazi version. "The protection of cultural material," Wolff-Metternich wrote, "is an undisputed obligation which is equally binding on any European nation at war. I could imagine no better way of serving my own country than by making myself responsible for the proper observance of this principle."[8]

"Count Metternich stood up to the ambassador," Jaujard had told Rorimer. "He went over his head to the military authorities. It was really a tug-of-war then to see who would control France, the Nazi military or the Nazi occupation government. Within days, the military forbade the embassy to seize any further cultural objects. At my suggestion, transmitted through Wolff-Metternich, most of the objects in their possession were transferred to the Louvre. When they arrived, many were already crated for shipment to Germany."

Jaujard took little credit for this success. He was a man who believed in discretion; that those who do not speak of their actions are the ones who actually perform them. But Rorimer knew the stories of his bravery; he had heard many times and from many different sources the awed reverence for the director's opposition to the Nazi threat. Defeating the ambassador merely meant the battle wasn't lost in the first days; it certainly didn't win the cultural war. Jaujard had worked closely with Count Wolff-Metternich on the ambassador affair— much closer than he had acknowledged—and he would continue to work with him through a long string of Nazi attempts to seize the patrimony of France. An official charged with confiscating French government documents also tried to confiscate its movable artwork. Other Nazis claimed the artwork was stored improperly at the repositories, and therefore needed to be moved to Germany for its own safety. Wolff-Metternich refuted that claim with personal inspections. Dr. Joseph Goebbels demanded almost one thousand "Germanic" objects held in the French state collections. Wolff-Metternich actually agreed with Goebbels that many of these objects rightly belonged to Germany; he did not agree with the propaganda minister that they should be sent immediately to the Fatherland. "I never hid my idea that this delicate problem," he wrote, "which touches the sense of honor of all people so deeply, could only be solved at the Peace Conference by a full agreement between peoples with equal rights."

"He risked his position, maybe even his life," Jaujard had told Rorimer during a previous meeting praising the Kunstschutz official. "He opposed Goebbels the only way possible, through a strict interpretation of the Führer's order of July 15, 1940, which prohibited the movement of artwork in France until the signing of a peace treaty. The order was meant to keep us French patriots from hiding artwork before the Nazis could claim it, but Wolff-Metternich quite cleverly applied the order to his fellow Germans as well. Without that principled stand, there would have been no hope."

"Not that we told them 'no' exactly. A straightforward 'no' would have only brought down Goebbels's wrath. We always told them 'yes,'" Jaujard told Rorimer, "but... there was always a detail that needed clarifying. The Nazis were—what is that delightful English language phrase?—paper-hangers. They were very bureaucratic. They couldn't make a decision without sending five or six letters to Berlin."

That's all Jaujard would say, that he and Wolff-Metternich killed the Nazi threat against the French state collections with a thousand paper cuts. He wouldn't acknowledge the difficulty of that task: the long years of guarding against forced entry; the threats of violence; the secret code Jaujard established with a friend to secret himself from Paris if the Nazis ever came to arrest him. The many calls to Wolff-Metternich in the middle of the night, urging him to come at once to throw paperwork in some Nazi looter's face, a call Wolff-Metternich always answered despite being seriously ill with kidney problems. His illness would have forced his retirement, in fact, but he stayed on "primarily because of confidence placed in me by persons of the French Art Administration."[9]

And Rorimer could not know, because Jacques Jaujard never spoke of it, that the museum director's influence went in other directions than into the Nazi hierarchy. That he had a network of museum personnel who worked as his eyes and ears; that he had contacts within the French bureaucracy; that one of his closest associates, the art patron Albert Henraux, was an active member of the French Resistance. Jaujard gave Henraux travel passes and museum authorization as a cover for his work in the Resistance; Henraux took Jaujard's information, gathered by his museum spies, and passed it through to the guerrilla fighters. And Wolff-Metternich almost surely knew of the whole thing. *He risked his career, maybe even his life*, Jaujard had said of him. The statement was true for both men.

The "good Nazi," as Rorimer liked to think of him, was relieved of his position in June 1942, but not before besting Goebbels, who gave up his attempts to seize the thousand "Germanic" objects at the end of 1941. The stated reason for the dismissal was Wolff-Metternich's public opposition to the most brazen theft of the Occupation: the seizure of the Ghent Altarpiece, under Hitler's direct order, from the repository at Pau. In reality, certain Nazis, most under the influence of Reichsmarschall Hermann Göring, the Nazi Party's second in command, had been undermining Wolff-Metternich for months. Their reasons ranged from claims his work was "exclusively in French interest,"[10] to complaints that he was too Catholic. The real problem was that Wolff-Metternich was not the man they wanted him to be. The Kunstschutz was supposed to provide a veneer of legality. They wanted a man who would bend the rules for the benefits of the Fatherland, but Count Wolff-Metternich would not. In the end, he was a "lost soul in the wasp nest of the Hitlerian gang."[11]

Soon after, Jaujard's violent denunciation of the theft of the Ghent Altarpiece cost him his position, too. In protest, the staffs of all the French museums quit en masse. That's how important Jacques Jaujard was to the French cultural community. The Germans were stunned; Jaujard was reinstated. Thereafter, his position was nearly inviolate. In the end, the Nazis secured only two objects from the national collections, both of German origin and of middling importance.

And yet it wasn't a total victory. The French state collections were safe, but the private collections of French citizens had been unprotected prey for the Nazi vultures. Himmler and his Waffen-SS. Rosenberg and his Einsatzstab Reichsleiter Rosenberg (ERR). And worst of all, Reichsmarschall Göring. Hanging over everything, always, was the threat of Hermann Göring.

Standing now before the empty wall of *La Joconde*, Rorimer remembered Jaujard's opinion of Reichsmarschall Göring: rapacious, insatiable, a man of appetites. A man who brooked no opposition and possessed no moral or ethical boundaries in pursuit of personal power and wealth. The man who could look on the cultural treasures of a nation like France and see nothing but plunder, ripe for the taking.

"James!" The word, echoing off the empty walls of the Grande Galerie, startled Rorimer from his thoughts. He turned from the alcove that had once held the *Mona Lisa* to see, coming toward him, none other than Jacques Jaujard, the guardian of the Louvre. Rorimer had known Jaujard before the war. He was always surprised to see how good the French patriarch looked after all those treacherous years.

"So glad you received my call," Jaujard said, clamping the Monuments Man on the shoulder.

"Good to see you again, Jacques," Rorimer said, taking the older man's hand. "And I have good news this time. The paperwork is straightened out. The tapestry is yours. At least for a few weeks."

"Bureaucrats." Jaujard laughed, turning and motioning down the hallway toward his office. *The man hasn't lost a step*, Rorimer thought. Jaujard not only had an office in the Louvre, but his apartment was inside the museum too. Rorimer wondered if he had left the building even once during the entire four years of the German occupation.

Or the month since liberation. In the first fevered days of emancipation, a mob had descended on the German prisoners being held in a camp outside the Louvre. Convinced they were about to be lynched, the Germans had broken the windows of the Louvre and leapt inside. A search found them scattered amid the artwork not evacuated, including several hiding in the pink granite funereal vase of the ancient Egyptian emperor Ramses III. The mob also found a curator helping a wounded German to the infirmary; all the proof it needed to condemn the whole staff as traitors and collaborators. How else to explain their survival, and that of the artwork they protected? No other institution had been so successful.

Jaujard and his loyal retainers—including his secretary, Jacqueline Bouchot-Saupique, who had been a primary conduit for reports to the Resistance at risk of her own life—were marched to the town hall while the mob yelled, "Collaborators! Traitors! Put them to death!"[12] There had been a very real chance they would be shot before reaching the government building. Only the timely testimony of several of Jaujard's contacts, including members of the French Resistance, had narrowly saved their hides.

Now, finally safe, he took no vacation. Instead, he was working endless hours to organize an art exhibition to lift the spirits of the wounded city. The centerpiece was the Bayeux Tapestry. Just more than a foot and a half high by 224 feet long and dating to the 1070s, the tapestry was without equal as a surviving relic of the early medieval period. There was no precedent: The lettering was unique, the figures more dynamic than any depicted before or for a hundred years thereafter. The unknown artist, whoever he or she was, had created no other surviving works. The Bayeux Tapestry, treated as a minor church relic for six hundred years and only rediscovered by the world in the 1700s, was a keystone in the cultural history of France.

It was also an important historical document, a nearly contemporaneous account of the French nobleman William the Conqueror's invasion of England in 1066. Stitched with narrative passages and depicting more than fifteen hundred objects—people, animals, clothing, arms, military formations, churches, towers, cities, banners, tools, carts, reliquaries, and funeral biers—it was by far the most detailed extant description of life in the early medieval period. With its focus on politics and military campaigns, culminating with the death of the Anglo-Saxon king Harold II in the battle of Hastings in 1066, it was also one of history's great depictions of conquest and empire. As such, it had long been coveted by the Nazis, and particularly the rapacious Reichsmarschall Göring, who had a special fondness for tapestries.

In 1940, fearful of its safety, the French moved the tapestry from Bayeux, one of the major cities in Normandy (William the Conqueror was a Norman duke), to the Louvre repository at Sourches. After their conquest of France, the Nazis made its possession a top priority, offering a steady barrage of monetary and artistic exchanges. Jaujard, as always, delayed and obfuscated. Then on June 27, 1944, with the Allies securely on the Normandy beaches and the tapestry on the verge of slipping out of their grasp, the Nazis transported it to the Louvre under German military escort. On August 15, with Paris on the edge of rebellion, the German military governor in France, General Dietrich von Choltitz, arrived at the Louvre to confirm the presence of the tapestry. After seeing it with Jaujard, he dutifully reported its location to Berlin.

On August 21, two SS officers arrived from the Reichschancellery to transport the tapestry to the Fatherland. General von Choltitz took them to his balcony and pointed to the roof of the Louvre. It was bristling with Resistance fighters; a machine gun was firing a burst of shots toward the Seine.

"The tapestry is over there," von Choltitz told the SS men, "in the basement of the Louvre."

"But Herr General, the enemy is occupying the Louvre!"

"Of course it is occupied, and rather well. The Louvre is now the headquarters of the Prefecture, sheltering the leaders of the Resistance."

"But under such conditions, Herr General, how can we get ahold of the tapestry?"

"Gentlemen," General von Choltitz replied, "you are the leaders of the best soldiers in the world. I will give you five or six of my own men; we will cover your back with sustained barrage fire to protect you while you cross the rue de Rivoli. All you need do is force open a door to fight your way to the tapestry."[13]

When the liberators arrived in Paris a few days later, on August 25, 1944, the Bayeux Tapestry was still safely ensconced in the Louvre sub-basement in its lead traveling box.

"What about the approval from Bayeux?" Jaujard

asked Rorimer over his shoulder. The tapestry was the pride of Normandy, and though it was still in the Louvre basement, gaining approval for public display had been a bureaucratic nightmare. Rorimer had cut through red tape in the American military and French government, but there was still the matter of officials in Bayeux, who usually did not allow the tapestry to be displayed outside the city.

"A young government official is off to ask permission. On a bicycle, if you can believe it. It's a 165-mile trip."

"At least there are some dedicated public servants left," Jaujard said, but not bitterly. Dealing with the overworked government was a fact of life in newly liberated France. "Speaking of which," he said, entering the reception areas of his office, "I'd like you to meet Mademoiselle Rose Valland."

"A pleasure," Rorimer said as the woman stood to greet them. She was generously proportioned, not heavy but solidly built, and at five foot five taller than many of her female contemporaries. She was not particularly attractive, Rorimer couldn't help but notice, a fact not helped by her drab, unfashionable outfit. Her hair was in a bun, like a kindly aunt, but her mouth was drawn. Matronly. That was the word that came to mind. And yet there was unexpected determination in her sharp brown eyes as she stared down the American Monuments Man, something that couldn't be missed, even behind her delicate wire-rimmed glasses.

"James Rorimer, from the Metropolitan," Rorimer said, extending his hand. "And the United States Army."

"I know who you are, Monsieur Rorimer," Valland said. "I am glad I have the chance to thank you for the special attention you paid the Jeu de Paume. It is unusual for an American to be so sensitive to the concerns of the French."

He realized suddenly that he had met her before, at the small Louvre outpost known as the Jeu de Paume, located at a far corner of the Jardin des Tuileries. The building had been constructed by Napoléon III for an indoor tennis court—or *jeu de paume*, as the sport was then known—but had been converted into an exhibition space for foreign contemporary art. The U.S. Army had planned to use the building as a post office; Rorimer had successfully argued, in tense meetings over a series of days, that it was part of the Louvre and therefore protected.

"Mademoiselle Valland has been managing the museum," Jaujard explained. "She stayed on as a servant of the French government, at my urging, during the Nazi occupation."

"No doubt a bitter duty," Rorimer said. He thought of the descriptions of the occupation he had heard so often since his arrival in Paris: no meat; no coffee; no heating oil; hardly a cigarette to be found. Desperate people tearing chestnuts from the trees in the public squares to keep from starving, then leaves and branches to fuel their furnaces. Women forced to stitch new handbags out of four or five old ones. Wooden soles carved into high heels. A paste that made it seem you were wearing silk stockings, since the stockings themselves were unavailable. Some women even traced a dark line down the back of their legs to imitate a seam, then complained about the leers and advances of the German troops. "Why couldn't they just go to Montmartre?" one woman had scoffed over a black-market dinner, now available to those with money and connections. Because of the nightly blackouts and frequent electrical outages, the bawdy theaters of the red-light district had taken off their roofs and let the sun shine in. The prostitutes had done a brisk business, but Rorimer suspected even they had their complaints about the Germans.

But not Rose Valland. She simply smiled and said, "We all had our jobs to do."

She must have simply been dropping off paperwork, because a minute later she was excusing herself to return to the Jeu de Paume. Rorimer, watching her disappear down the hall, had only one clear thought: Rose Valland had never drawn a dark line down the back of her legs to imitate silk stockings. She was clearly not that kind of woman. But otherwise, he found her completely inscrutable. So he put her out of his mind.

"She's a hero, James," Jaujard said, preparing to turn back to the tapestry and other matters at hand.

"You all are, Jacques," Rorimer replied. "I won't forget."

Letter from James Rorimer
To special friends, including his family and his
patron at the Cloisters, John D. Rockefeller Jr.
September 25, 1944

Dear Ones:

One month ago today I arrived in Paris. I
suppose that by now it is old news that that
was the day that the Americans arrived here.
Our section came here at the same time as the
combat troops. Shortly after the Germans had
surrendered in their last stronghold we were
working our way in and out of barricaded streets
and going to the agreed meeting place. The
Germans were still spending their last night
in the Senate buildings and fire had just been
set to the Chamber of Deputies. We slept in
beds in a hotel where the Germans had been less
than twenty-four hours previously. The following
day I paid my respects to M. Jaujard, Director
of National Museums, at the Louvre and began
thinking of the work I would have in Paris as the
G-5 Monuments, Fine Arts and Archives Officer for
Seine Section which includes Seine-et-Marne and
Seine-et-Oise as it did with the Germans.

As one of the first officers to arrive in
Paris I came to know the authorities—perhaps
it is still too early to mention names even
if they do appear in the local newspapers—
and I was commanded to do special work not in
any way related to Fine Arts. After helping
establish our headquarters I was asked to take

charge of the information section, and ran the
Information Desk for eight days rather than for
the forty-eight hours originally anticipated.
I met everyone in Paris who had to do with the
Franco-American relations. There were many
generals, officers of all kinds, hotel people
and business representatives of every sort and
description, old friends, civil authorities and
national ones, locksmiths, bomb disposal squads
and intelligence people. . . . I gave orders and saw
that they were carried out. I snapped the whip at
a point where military necessity demanded that
I leave Fine Arts alone and sort out the French
from the Germans, the true from the false,
the weak from the strong and the lazy from the
willing. There were hundreds of taxi drivers
to be employed and interpreters galore. Often I
had a queue of fifty or more and I would stand
up at my centrally located desk and help grease
the wheel of progress. Yes, I really helped in
winning the war during those hectic, exciting,
unbelievable days. . . .

Here I am in the greatest art center in the
world. There are the museums, the libraries, the
archives, the chateaux, the public buildings of
all kinds and descriptions which come under my
scrutiny. Help is to be given and our directives
are to be carried out by decisions which must be
clear and have no reverberations. So far they
have not and I have urged action that would make
your hair stand on end. When the war is over I

shall be able to tell many exciting adventures where a second lieutenant dared stand his ground. If I am relieved of my present position it will not be said that I didn't try to do all I could to save the treasures which the ages have produced. . . . I am determined to do my job—sometimes I wonder if it isn't all just another pipe dream like The Cloisters. Those good old days of activity and accomplishment seem to be here again after long months of teaching motor maintenance and languages. . . .

There are so many other things to write about. The suffering through the years of the French, one and all, except for a very few who profited handsomely by the occupation—one doesn't see these people at all—is not forgotten, but the joys of a freedom not known is exciting to all. . . . The Lord knows what actually happened. It wasn't pretty, I can assure you.

This must suffice for tonight. I have not received word from any of you for a month and am trying hard to trace the letters. What APO do you write to? Please check the new address and don't fail me.

Love,

James

CHAPTER 16

Entering Germany

Aachen, Germany
October–November 1944

For two weeks, Walker Hancock watched the bombs fall on Aachen, the westernmost major city in Germany. It was mid-October 1944, but already cold. He huddled into his jacket and stared at the horizon. Where had the sun of September gone? Smoke curled into a gray sky. The city was on fire. Behind him, the radio crackled as information passed back and forth from the front line.

Hancock had met his colleague George Stout at Verviers, U.S. First Army's advanced headquarters, just as the Western Allied war machine ran low on fuel and ammunition. The armies had raced hundreds of miles in two months, almost unopposed, to the German border. They found there not an enemy in retreat, as they had expected, but a line of pillboxes, barbed wire, minefields, and antitank barriers known as the Siegfried Line. The pillboxes were rusty with age, and most of the 700,000 troops that manned them were green recruits plucked from the decimated German population, many too young or too old to have fought in previous campaigns. Nonetheless, the Siegfried Line was a defensive bulwark the overstretched Allies couldn't charge through. At Normandy, the Allies had crashed into the German lines in overpowering waves; at the Siegfried Line, they rolled to a stop in staggered units, their supplies and momentum spent. General Bernard Montgomery's Twenty-first Army Group (which included the First Canadian Army in which Monuments Man Ronald Balfour served), was turned back in the Netherlands attempting to cross the Rhine. Patton's U.S. Third Army was halted near Metz, France. Hancock and First Army met their first stiff resistance since Normandy at Aachen.

The plan was to bypass Aachen altogether, surging by to the north and south and reuniting on the ridge east of town. Aachen, a city of nearly 165,000 whose population had dropped to six thousand as the Allies advanced, promised the kind of protracted fight the Allies wanted to avoid, especially since the city had little heavy industry or tactical value. What it possessed instead was history. Aachen was the seat of power of the Holy Roman Empire, which Hitler referred to as the First Reich. It was at Aachen that Charlemagne consolidated his power and united central Europe under his rule. While it was in Rome, in the year 800, that Pope Leo III crowned him Holy Roman Emperor, the first such ruler in Europe since the collapse of the Roman Empire, it was at Aachen that Charlemagne ruled. Aachen Cathedral was his St. Peter's Basilica. Beginning in 936, Charlemagne's prayer hall, the Palatine Chapel, was the coronation hall of the German kings and queens. It would serve in that capacity for the next six hundred years. Aachen Cathedral and the surrounding old quarter were undisputed historic treasures. The Allies had every reason to leave the city untouched.

Unfortunately, Aachen held major symbolic value for Adolf Hitler, not just as the birthplace of the First German Reich (and perhaps one of the inspirations for his Führermuseum at Linz) but as the first German city threatened by Allied troops. As retreating German soldiers mustered in the city, the local citizens cheered. But when the Allies appeared on the horizon, the local Nazi officials commandeered the last train out of town, loaded it with personal possessions, and abandoned the citizens to their fate. Hitler didn't care about the citizens—to give your life for Germany, after all, was considered a high honor by those not yet asked to do so—but he was so irate that the local Nazi officials had abandoned a major German city that he ordered them to the Eastern front as privates, a virtual death sentence. He then sent in a five-thousand-man division with orders to fight until Aachen lay about them in ruins and the last man was dead.

The Allies faltered. Having flanked the city and conquered the high ground beyond, the commanders decided that leaving five thousand soldiers behind the front near their supply lines was too risky. On October 10, 1944, they demanded a German surrender. The Germans refused. On October 13, First Army attacked. It was fairly easy to justify the need to spare the monuments of conquered countries like France and Belgium. But what about Germany? To Hancock, the aerial bombardment already seemed more intense. The men, he knew, were not entering with mercy on their minds. The motto of one battalion said it all: "Knock 'em all down." The Allies seemed eager to level Aachen.

The battle raged for eight days. The Allies had superior forces, but the Germans were hidden everywhere, including the sewer system, and the struggle quickly devolved into a chaotic, building-to-building fight. Bombers called in by spotters on the ridge dropped long-fuse bombs that detonated not on roofs but several floors into buildings, blowing them to smithereens. Artillery and tank fire knocked the city down block by block. The ancient stone buildings in the city center proved too well-built for tanks, so the Americans wheeled in their largest artillery piece and aimed it point-blank into walls. A bulldozer cleared the rubble for the advancing troops, who took a savage joy in the destruction. A few miles back the Allies had crossed an invisible line. This wasn't France; it was Germany. From Hancock's perspective, it seemed the prevailing attitude was that Aachen deserved everything the Allies could throw at her and more.

On October 21, despite Hitler's order to die for the Reich, the surviving Germans surrendered. As soldiers and civilians were rounded up and marched out, Walker Hancock and his colleagues headed into Germany. They passed through the minefields of the Siegfried Line, marked with white tape by army engineers. Behind the minefields were the dragon's teeth, staggered concrete pylons lined up row after row like the white military tombstones at Arlington National Cemetery, but too thick and heavy for a tank to drive over or through. Then barbed wire, followed by more minefields, gun pits, and the heavy concrete pillboxes that had proved impervious to aerial assault.

Before them, Aachen was smoldering. Two weeks earlier, Hancock had thought the Dutch repository at Maastricht unworldly, but here was a true alternate universe, the "weirdest and most fantastic" sight of his life.[1] Windows were blown into the streets; trolley tracks reared up from the pavement like wicked metal fingers; piles of debris were all that remained of many homes. At a point where the destruction widened out, leaving a vast field of broken lintels and cornerstones, some GIs had posted a sign with a quote from Hitler: "*Gebt mir fünf Jahre und Ihr werdet Deutschland nicht wiedererkennen.*" Below was the English translation: "Give me five years & you will not recognize Germany again."[2]

Hancock turned away from the main line of advance, where tanks rolled and patrols still scrambled back and forth with supplies and orders, and walked toward the city center. Around the first corner, the world closed in on him and he was utterly alone. "One can read all kinds of descriptions of the destruction caused by air raids, and see any number of pictures, but the sensation of being in one of these dead cities just can't be imagined."[3] The rubble was twenty feet high, the side streets long claustrophobic corridors of broken, gap-toothed facades. Occasional phantoms flashed by—a group of marauding Belgians, an American soldier on horseback wearing a full Native American headdress taken from the city opera company. *Did I really see that?* Hancock wondered, as the smoky world swallowed the rider. The city disintegrated, great chunks of concrete fall-

ing down around him. He looked through the face
of a building, roofless and empty, showing in broken
concrete frames little pieces of the sky. The windows
were shattered, the floors inside collapsed. "A skeleton
city," he would later comment, "is more terrible than
one the bombs have completely flattened. Aachen was
a skeleton."[4]

Near the city center, Hancock was forced to scramble over a succession of putrid rubble. Occasionally
he would glimpse the cathedral dome, miraculously
untouched, rising above the flattened buildings. Then
he would turn a corner and it would be gone. The only
sound was the whistle of artillery shells, still being
lobbed by both sides. The bombardment intensified.
For twenty blocks, down the narrow winding streets
of the ancient city, Hancock had to scramble for cover
from doorway to rubble pile, rushing forward each
time a shell exploded.

The doors of the cathedral were open. He crossed
the courtyard on a dead run and entered the Palatine
Chapel. The octagonal structure had for hundreds of
years swallowed each entrant, be they worshipper or
pilgrim, cutting them off from the outside world and
delivering them into the hands of God. It was no different for Walker Hancock. Inside, he felt safe. All
the windows were blasted to bits, but even that did
not disturb the profound sense of peace and security.
Around him, the great choir hall was filled with shards
of glass and chunks of masonry. Beneath the rubble,
he could see mattresses and dirty blankets. He walked
slowly down the central aisle, glass crunching under-
foot. Unfinished meals sat on chairs, coffee still in the

cups. A makeshift altar had been placed at the far end of the hall against a temporary screen. As he moved into the Gothic Choir Hall, he saw that an Allied bomb had pierced the apse and demolished the high altar. Hancock could see its smooth gray fins cradled in the shattered wood. Amazingly, it hadn't exploded, saving hundreds of lives and a thousand years of history.

Hancock turned back to the ghost city of blankets and cups. He stared up through the holes where the stained glass had once been. The delicate stone window frames crisscrossed the sky. It reminded him of the sight of the great empty windows of Chartres Cathedral. Then several shells exploded in rapid succession; smoke blew across the sky, dropping the cathedral into shadow. He looked down at the blasted refugee camp around him; a broken statue caught his eye, staring at him from the gloom. This was nothing like Chartres.

"For more than eleven hundred years," Hancock mused, "these massive walls have stood. That I should have arrived just in time to be the sole witness to their destruction is inconceivable but, somehow, reassuring."[5]

He was back in the Palatine Chapel, examining the damage more closely, when a figure stepped out of the darkness. It was less frightening, Hancock realized with surprise, than extraordinary. He had felt alone in another world. "*Hier*," the figure said, motioning Hancock toward him.[6] It was the vicar of Aachen Cathedral, slight and worn, a lantern trembling in his hand. He led Hancock silently up a narrow staircase, stepping carefully around the debris. The passage at the top was tight, hardly more than a shoulder width, and Hancock realized they were inside one of the great stone walls. The vicar had set up a few chairs in a small den, and he motioned Hancock into one of them. Only then did Hancock notice how badly the man was shaking.

"Six boys," the vicar said in trembling, broken English. "Age fifteen to twenty. Our fire brigade. Eight times they put out fires on the roof and saved the dome. They have been taken by your soldiers to the camp at Brand. There is no one for the pumps and hoses. One shell, and the cathedral could be lost."

The feeble lantern threw shadows across the man's tired face. In a corner, Hancock noticed the old mattress and the remnants of the food on which the vicar had lived since the bombardment began more than six weeks before. "They are good boys," the vicar said. "Yes, they belonged to the Hitler Youth, but"—he motioned to his heart—"they did not feel it here. You must bring them back before it is too late."[7]

Hancock didn't know whether he meant too late for the boys or for the cathedral, but either way the vicar was right. He took down their names: Helmuth, Hans, Georg, Willi, Carl, Niklaus, Germans all.[8] But Hancock was smart enough to know the Germans weren't all Nazis or all bad.

"How will you care for them?" he asked. The city was without food, electricity, running water, or basic supplies.

"They will sleep here. We have water and basic supplies. As for food..."

"I might be able to get you some," Hancock said.

"We have a cellar that will keep it fresh."

The mention of the cellar brought another thought

to Hancock's mind. Aachen Cathedral was famed for its relics—the gold and silver-gilt bust of Charlemagne, containing a piece of his skull; the tenth-century, jewel-encrusted processional cross of Lothar II, set with the ancient cameo of Augustus Caesar; and other Gothic reliquaries. He hadn't seen any of them.

"Where are the treasures, Vicar? Are they in the crypts?"

The vicar shook his head. "The Nazis took them. For safe-guarding."

Hancock had heard enough about Nazi "safeguarding" to shudder at those words. "Where?" he asked.

The vicar shrugged. "East."

CHAPTER 17

A Field Trip

East of Aachen, Germany
Late November 1944

The enclosed staff car bounced over a muddy, cratered road, Monuments Man Walker Hancock at the wheel. It was late November 1944, almost a month since Hancock had entered Aachen and discovered the condition of its cathedral. At their former rate of advance, U.S. First Army would have been halfway to Berlin by now, but they had bogged down in the dense, foggy forests east of Aachen. They were making yards per day now, not miles, against a hidden, entrenched enemy. And if that wasn't bad enough, the chill of what would be forever remembered as the coldest winter in the recent history of northern Europe had settled in. Even on the best of roads, and this certainly wasn't one of them, ice filled the ruts and clung dangerously to the edges of the curves.

"Careful," the colonel said from the passenger seat. "If I'm going to die out here, I want it to be from German shells, not a damned car accident." In the backseat, Hancock noticed, George Stout hadn't even blinked.

The danger of shells was real. The hole at the command center at Kornelimünster, made only two or three days before, proved that. Next to the hole, a poster read, "When you have entered these halls you may say you have been to the front."[1] And as they arrived at Büsbach, Hancock calculated that Kornelimünster was three miles behind them. This was truly the front. Yesterday, on his first visit to the isolated command post, Hancock had found soldiers digging through smoldering rubble. The rubble was a little house they had turned into sleeping quarters; it had been destroyed less than half an hour before his arrival.

The damage reminded Hancock of the Suermondt Museum in Aachen, where he had spent a considerable portion of the last month. Except for minor provincial works, all the paintings in the museum had been evacuated before the fighting. As a Monuments Man, his job was to find out where they had gone. So he had pulled a dusty chair and begun searching through the battered files still standing in the bomb-cratered offices. There was no electricity, and the hulking piles of debris threw odd shadows in the beam of his flashlight. His lips were constantly blackened, the result of the dust still hanging in the stagnant air, and the water in his canteen never lasted long enough. But he hardly noticed his discomfort. His large sculptures took years to complete, sometimes decades; he had learned to be a patient, meticulous man. And despite the occasional glamour of the Dutch art repository at Maastricht or Chartres Cathedral, this was the real work of a Monuments Man: the careful sifting of information, the patient study, the watchful eye.

Hancock's persistence paid off. First, he found a list of rural schools, houses, cafés, and churches where paintings and sculptures had been stored. He had checked several of the sites, yielding an impressive cache of paintings, but nothing world-class. Then, near the end of his searching, he had found the Suermondt's Rosetta Stone buried in a stack of debris. It was a dusty catalogue of the museum's collection, with each item marked in red or blue. A handwritten note on the cover explained that the items in red, which Hancock recognized immediately as the museum's most important works, had been moved to Siegen, a city about one hundred miles east behind enemy lines.

Hancock thought about it now, as he eased the enclosed staff car—such luxury after all those days of hitching and nights without food!—along the road to the front. There must be a large repository in Siegen, a storehouse of some sort. Possibly located in a concrete tower or a church or, like the repository he had visited with George Stout in Holland, at the base of a hill. And if the best works of the Suermondt Museum were there, why not the treasures of Aachen Cathedral? The bust of Charlemagne; the cross of Lothar decorated with Caesar's cameo; the shrine holding the robe of Mary. Were they in Siegen, too?

But if they were in Siegen...what then? Siegen was an entire city. There were hundreds of possible hiding places. And there was no guarantee the repository was even in the city itself. It could easily be five, ten, even twenty miles outside of town.

He had begun to search for human intelligence. Somebody knew more. He was sure of that. But who? With the help of an MFAA archivist, he had combed the rolls of the Allied detention centers, where most of the citizens of Aachen were being held, cross-checking them against lists of the city's cultural leaders. No matches. Eventually, he found an elderly painter, who led him to a museum caretaker, who suggested some architects, but nobody knew anything about Siegen.

"They're all gone," the young caretaker told him. "Only trusted Nazis knew the details of the operation, and they all went east with the troops."

But the search for the treasures of Aachen Cathedral, and information on the mysterious repository at Siegen, was only part of his duties. Since hitting the combat zone, he had spent most of his time on errands like this one, examining liberated monuments and answering calls from combat commanders. It seemed the Americans couldn't enter a house without finding a "Michelangelo" amid the paintings of forest nymphs and flowers.

But this call, this might be the one. That's why he had brought George Stout back with him. If anyone could identify the proverbial needle in the haystack, it was Stout. Not that he didn't trust his own judgment; it just seemed a little convenient. After all, the painting had turned up just when he had begun to wonder if the haystack even contained needles at all.

He thought back twenty-four hours, to his first sight of the painting. He had recognized the style immediately. Flemish. Sixteenth century. Was it by Pieter Bruegel the Elder, the great Belgian master, or someone who worked closely with him? He had seen works of comparable quality at Maastricht, but none had taken his breath away like this one. To see a painting of this quality leaning against the wall of a command post amid the bullets and the grime was to understand that great works of art were part of the world. They were objects. They were fragile. They were lonely, small, unprotected. A child on a playground looks strong, but a child wandering alone down Madison Avenue in New York City—that's terrifying.

"Where did you find it, sir?" he had asked the commanding officer.

"Peasant cottage," the CO had replied.

"Anything with it?"

"That's all."

Hancock's mind had slipped through the facts. This was no peasant painting, but a museum-quality work. It was clearly stolen, then left behind as the Germans retreated. But it was only one painting, casually cast aside. Probably the result of individual looting, found by a passing officer in some country estate and abandoned when it became a life-threatening burden. It wasn't the key to anything. But that didn't make it any less valuable as a work of art.

He had stared at the painting, thinking about the muddy road back to Verviers, open for miles to German shelling. The uncovered jeep was protection enough for his own life, but he didn't feel comfortable trusting it with a cultural treasure.

"Congratulations, Commander," Hancock had said. "This is a real find." An artillery shell detonated outside, shaking splinters from the roof. Hancock had jumped; the CO seemed not to even notice.

"I knew it," he said. "I knew it."

"Unfortunately, sir, I don't have a truck. I'll have to leave it here for now, but I'll be back tomorrow."

"Are you going back to headquarters?"

"Yes sir, I am."

"For God's sake," the officer said, "get them to send out a lamp. We haven't got anything that will give light here—not even a candle—and this is a hell of a place to be after dark."[2]

At headquarters the following day, Hancock had picked up not only the lamps but the colonel, who had just arrived from SHAEF and was eager to witness actual combat, and George Stout, who had just returned from the field. The American presence in Western Europe had grown to more than a million soldiers, so Eisenhower had created an administrative division under the command of Lt. Gen. Omar Bradley. Bradley's U.S. Twelfth Army Group had jurisdiction over First Army, Third Army, Ninth Army, and the newly arrived Fifteenth Army. George Stout had just been assigned to the Twelfth as their Monuments Man. In short, his worst fear had come true: He'd been kicked upstairs to management. Hancock had noticed Stout was in no hurry to head back to Paris to assume that command.

The man was a true professional, a real working fellow, and the one qualified conservator in a world of curators, artists, and architects. *An expert and a precisionist first makes his analysis*, Hancock thought as he drove, recalling Stout's advice on one of their first trips together, *then his decision*.[3] Hancock was glad to have him along because George Stout always knew what to do. He would make the decisions and accept the responsibility. The colonel he could take or leave. He was nothing but back-office blowhard, the kind that infuriated the grunts, but at least agreeing to bring him along for a sightseeing tour of the front meant an enclosed staff car instead of a hazardous one-ton truck. After months in the field, Hancock felt like a chauffeur in a limousine.

"There she is," the colonel said. "It's about damn time."

The command post looked precarious, a rickety wooden cottage in a muddy yard. Allied aircraft roared overhead as Hancock hit the brakes. The air was thick with smoke and dust. The fighting, Hancock noticed, seemed closer than it had been the previous day. *Maybe the fire's just hotter*, he thought, as the big guns recoiled. He could hear shells exploding, but he couldn't tell whether they were coming or going. This was clearly no place for artwork—or a Monuments Man. Hancock's plan was simple: Grab the painting and go.

Stout had other ideas.

"You take the notes," he told Hancock, kneeling before the painting after a wave of introductions all around.[4] Gently, he ran his fingers over the surface like a blind man greeting an old friend. "Kermess," he said firmly. "Sixteenth-century Flemish, workshop of Pieter Bruegel the Elder."[5]

I knew it, Hancock thought. "Workshop" meant the master had advised on it, at least, if not worked on some of it himself.

Stout turned the painting over. "Support: oak panel." He pulled out his tape measure. "0.84 meters by...1.2 meters by...0.004 meters. Three members of equal width, joined on the horizontal."

The concussion of shells rattled the ceiling beams,

knocking loose plaster dust and debris. Outside the window, Hancock noticed the colonel standing atop a pile of rubble, watching the battle through his binoculars.

"Cradle: low, seven longitudinal, oak, ten sliding transverse, pine. Multiple warp. Slightly worm-eaten. Broken lower corners, planed down at the time the cradle was applied."

Stout again turned the frame over to examine the painting. *Analysis first*, Hancock thought, *then decision*. Stout never hurried. He never guessed. He never acted out of fear or ignorance, even if just this one time Walker Hancock wished he would.

"Ground: white, very thin. Broken and flaked, sparse, buckled: lower moderate, extensive upper."

Hancock noticed men gathering out of the shadows. These were infantrymen, young soldiers drafted right out of school, the first into the fight. For months they had been shot at, mined, counterattacked, and shelled. They bathed out of their helmets, or not at all, and ate out of ration tins, wiping their spoons on their pants. Their billet had been destroyed, so they threw themselves down wherever they could find a comfortable spot. As always, Hancock wanted to say something to them, to thank them somehow, but Stout spoke first.

"Paint: oil, rich, and generally thin with translucent film in dark areas and monochrome drawing sparsely visible underneath."

Outside, the colonel was cheering, delighted by his first encounter with warfare. Inside, two Monuments Men bent over a four-hundred-year-old painting in the faint light of a newly arrived lamp. The first was kneel-

ing on the ground, studying its surface like an archeologist in an Egyptian tomb or a medic with a wounded
man. The second hunched behind him, concentrating
on his notes. The soldiers, tired and dirty, huddled
around them like the shepherds at the manger, staring
silently at a painting of expressive faces and peasant villagers and at the two adult men in soldiers' garb fussing
over every square centimeter of its surface.

Letter from George Stout
To his colleague Langdon Warner
October 4, 1944

Dear Langdon:

  The news about our directors' resignation
[from the Fogg Art Museum] did not come from
them first or in fact at all. Margie told
me.... I suppose I should write them but I'm
mildly troubled as to what I should say. Hall's
"Social and Business Forms," a sure guide to
propriety in such matters and one that stood
on my father's bookshelf, had no example of
a letter addressed to co-directors of an art
museum in which the writer has worked, upon
being indirectly apprised of their retirement
from office....

  Koehler is quite right. The job ought to fall
to somebody who will make the museum a working
part—one working part—of the department.... I
don't believe I've ever been more certain than
I am now that the development and understanding
of man's workmanship is the fundamental need
of man's spirit; or that we can never look for
a healthy social body until that need, among
others, is fed. I hope to put in the rest of my
life really working at that job.

  From my point of view, this [being a
Monuments Man] is not a bad job. During the
last three weeks I've been in harness with an

Englishman who's gone horribly sour and says we're wasting our time. I don't know what he expected. Some strange romantic adventure, personal glory, or great authority, perhaps. He doesn't convince me. We can't count the result but I'm satisfied, not with what I've done but with what the job stands for. One little thing that is neither here nor there and won't stand on any record pleases me. That is the attitude of the men I run across. They don't really care what's been damaged but they seem to figure it's part of the game and they want to know more about it. Men and officers, all down the line. Yesterday, a fellow I'd seen before, a sergeant I'd known back a ways and a fellow who couldn't get out two consecutive words that would print in the Monitor, wanted to know if the monuments were much shot up around there. And I remember back in France, some weeks ago, a rough old colonel I had to make some parlay with. I told him what my office was. His eyes looked incredulous in a face that seemed to have been worked over with one of these hammers they use to pound steaks. He said, "What the hell's that?" So we went into it a little. It was past lunch time. He stuck around with his executive while I ate some K rations off the fender of my jallopy and they kept on talking about it until I had a hard time to get away. These fellows are just naturally interested in a good piece of work and have no unnatural restrictions in looking it over. Perhaps, and may the sahibs of the Fogg forgive me for thinking it, this simple, curious outlook of healthy men is more important than some of the monuments themselves.

    Yours,
    George

CHAPTER 18

Tapestry

Paris, France
November 26, 1944

More than 250 miles away in Paris, a more traditional art museum—the Louvre—was finally alive with artwork. The pieces were mostly the classical sculpture collections, and not nearly as much as James Rorimer would have preferred, but Rorimer knew what an extraordinary accomplishment even this much was. The French government was finally closing the void in leadership that had developed after the Nazi departure, but the bureaucracy was a nightmare. And everyone, at every level, seemed to be pushing their own agenda. Rorimer had been pushing everywhere as hard as he could; he was, as one observer would later note, "not by talent much of a diplomat."[1] The staid French were often mystified by his bravado and more than one had complained of his "cowboy tactics."[2] But even with his bulldog tenacity and take-no-prisoners attitude, Rorimer hadn't been able to make much headway.

He was convinced it had something to do with his rank. He wouldn't trade his infantry training if he could, but coming in as a private put him at a tremendous disadvantage. He was a second lieutenant, and he was never going to be promoted, even though many of those around him felt he deserved a rank of major for the work he was doing. It chafed him. He couldn't help it. And it wasn't just personal pride, although that was part of it. His lowly rank was interfering with his work.

He thought of the day, back in September, when he learned that General Eisenhower's office in Versailles was being furnished with items from the palace and the Louvre. Jaujard, the patrician director of the French museums and hero of the Louvre, knew of the "loans," but had acquiesced in the interest of Allied cooperation. Rorimer did not. He raced to Versailles—Eisenhower's office was in a house in the surrounding town, not the palace—and found soldiers moving furniture. A beautiful Regency desk sat on top of an ancient Persian rug from the Mobilier National. A terra-cotta statue was in the corner, while paintings and etchings from the Museum of the Palace of Versailles leaned against the wall.

The captain in charge, the delightfully named O. K. Todd, had personally selected the items, and he was not taking the opportunity to ingratiate himself with the Supreme Commander lightly. When Rorimer began to argue with him, Todd simply stepped out of the room and called Colonel Brown, Eisenhower's headquarters commandant. Rorimer had argued with him, too: impractical, expensive, unguarded. Was it necessary? Was it wise? "General Eisenhower would be personally embarrassed," Rorimer had said, "if it should leak out that he was using protected works of art for military purposes contrary to his explicit orders. And wouldn't the German propaganda office have a holiday if it could report that General Eisenhower had appropriated art objects from Versailles for his personal use?"[3]

He had gone too far. "Let's see what your General Rogers has to say about this," Brown thundered, seizing the phone and dialing Rorimer's commanding officer.[4]

As luck would have it, General Rogers was out. Colonel Brown was in no mood to wait. The next morning, the cultural objects were returned. O. K. Todd received a commendation from the city of Versailles for this selfless act. Eisenhower, arriving a few days later, found even the stripped-down office too large and grand, so he ordered a dividing wall installed and gave half the space to his secretaries. In the end, it was a small event, a piece of trivia perhaps, but except for a lucky break it might have cost Rorimer his commission. And that was the problem: too many toes to step on, too many egos to stroke, too much time wasted. It was almost as frustrating as museum work!

Rorimer banished the thought. He had spent much of the last month in the Île-de-France region, at a series of ancestral estates that ringed Paris. The great rooms of many châteaux had been blackened because neither the Germans nor the Americans knew how to use the old fireplaces. Four lovestruck American soldiers had given important paintings to young women from a local village. At Dampierre, the Germans had installed a cocktail bar in front of *Golden Age*, one of France's most celebrated murals. But all in all, it had been a good trip. Damage was minimal; spirits still high. Another story from Dampierre seemed to epitomize the situation. The Germans had used the library's renowned Bossuet letters for toilet paper, but after they left, the caretaker found the letters in the woods, cleaned them off, and returned them to the library. Now that was dedication. That was service!

Besides, this was no time to be negative. It was November 26, 1944—the Sunday after Thanksgiving in America—and James Rorimer had much to be thankful for. After weeks of demands, arguments, and supplication, the military trucks had been moved from the Jardin des Tuileries, and the garden was officially opened to the public. And now the Louvre was open, too. Voices were echoing where, two months ago, Rorimer's footsteps had been the only sound. The Bayeux Tapestry, which he had discussed with Louvre director Jacques Jaujard so many weeks before, was on display in Paris for the first time in almost 150 years. He had accompanied General Rogers to the opening two weeks before; he was back now to walk the halls. The heart of Paris was coming to life, and Rorimer couldn't help but think of his contribution.

He needed that encouragement because the rest of his work was slow. On the surface, the city of Paris looked majestic and indestructible, but underneath the Nazis had hollowed out catacombs of theft and destruction. The French national collections had been preserved through the cunning of Jacques Jaujard and the "good" Nazi Count Franz von Wolff-Metternich, but the collections of private citizens had been ransacked. Before the war, much of the artistic wealth of Paris had rested in the hands of its prominent citizens and art dealers—the Rothschilds, David-Weill, Rosenberg, Wildenstein, Seligman, Kann—all of them

Jewish. Under Nazi law, Jews weren't allowed to hold property, so the collections had been "appropriated" by the German state. When the looters had exhausted those collections, the confiscations trickled down to the lower-level Jewish aristocracy, and then to the Jewish middle class, and finally to anyone who even had a Jewish-sounding name—or possessed something the Gestapo wanted. In the end, it had been a mass pillage, as Gestapo officers broke down doorways and hauled valuables away—artwork, desks, even mattresses. Jaujard estimated that 22,000 pieces of important artwork had been stolen.

So far, Rorimer had been able to find information on approximately none of it. The Nazis had taken or destroyed almost all their records. The victims were usually absent, having fled the country or disappeared into the Nazi work camps. Witnesses were reluctant to speak. The wave of terror had subsided—no more forced public haircuts of young women or summary executions of suspected collaborators—but confidence in the new order was still dangerously low. There was too much risk and not enough reward, at least for the time being, in speaking out. It was best, most ordinary Parisians believed, to sip the champagne of celebration and keep your mouth shut.

The French museum establishment wasn't faring much better. The first meeting of a group calling itself the Commission de Récupération Artistique (Commission for the Recovery of Works of Art) had occurred on September 29, 1944. The commission's leader was Albert Henraux, the art patron and one of Jacques Jaujard's key contacts in the French Resistance. The secretary was Mademoiselle Rose Valland, the assistant in charge of the Jeu de Paume museum. This was enough to prove to Rorimer that, no matter who took the lead, considerable power would always lie in the hands of his friend Jaujard. And yet, with all of Jaujard's influence, the commission had only been formally recognized by the government two days ago, on November 24. As far as Rorimer knew, they had not made much headway in the recovery of artwork either.

So at the end of his tour of the Louvre—perhaps his first afternoon of sightseeing, he realized, since his arrival in Paris three months before—Rorimer stopped by his old friend's office. It was almost time for closing, the last patrons being hustled swiftly out of the museum, but Jaujard, as always, was still at his desk. The man was indefatigable.

"Quite a success," Rorimer said, referring to the opening. The crowds had been lining up and waiting hours to see the Bayeux Tapestry despite a ten-franc charge (about 20 cents U.S.); only the military was being allowed free entry.

"The public is happy to have an exhibition again," Jaujard replied. "It is an important step."

"And yet no one understands, outside the museum community, how much work went into making this exhibition possible."

"It's like that all over, James. I'm sure the dairy farmers complain about how little we understand the difficulty of getting milk to the market."

"And the American soldiers complain about how difficult it is to chase Parisian women and buy perfume. Some merchants have even started charging for it!"

Jaujard laughed. "Only you Americans could joke about your presence here. We Parisians...we complain, but our memories of the occupation are too fresh not to appreciate you. Even if we no longer give everything away for free."

They chatted a few minutes more about the exhibition and the city. They were friends now, bonded by circumstance and mutual admiration. Eventually, when he sensed an opportunity, Rorimer brought up the commission.

"I'm glad you asked," Jaujard said. "There's a matter you might be able to assist us with." He paused, as if trying to find the right way to explain the situation. "You know about the Nazi looting of the private collections, of course."

"Twenty-two thousand works of art. Who could forget?"

"Oh, it might be even more than that. They stole from all over Paris and the surrounding area. To track down every source, as you know, is next to impossible. So why not start instead at the end? Before leaving Paris, the looted artwork was all brought to one spot for cataloguing and crating: the nearby Jeu de Paume. And we had a spy inside."

Rorimer felt himself edging toward Jaujard. A spy? Was this the break he had been hoping for?

"Who?" he asked.

"Rose Valland."

Rorimer thought of the Jeu de Paume administrator he had met almost two months before in Jaujard's office. He had seen her several times since then, and yet he found it hard to remember much about her besides her drab outfits, small wire-rimmed glasses, and ever-present grandmotherly bun of hair. Matronly. It was still the word that came to mind. She left the impression of a harmless spinster.

And yet...he had always believed there was more to her. And it wasn't just the fire and intelligence in her eyes. Or that he had begun to suspect the depth of her involvement in Jaujard's world. Because he hadn't, not until now. She had, over the weeks of their occasional acquaintance, remained as inscrutable as at their first meeting. She rarely spoke, and almost never revealed anything of interest. She wasn't afraid to challenge his assumptions, often with a dry sarcasm, but never in a way that left him dwelling on it later. He could never, in fact, remember much of what she said at all, which in itself, he now realized, should have made him suspicious. She wasn't just a frumpy, anonymous museum employee. Or perhaps because she was a frumpy, anonymous museum employee, she was also something else. She was the ideal spy.

Jaujard smiled. "I told you she was a hero, but you didn't understand. No one ever does. Rose Valland is not young or particularly attractive, but both qualities served her well in her duties. She is middle-aged. Simple in her manner. Imminently forgettable. What are you doing, James?"

"Middle aged. Simplicity in her manners..." Rorimer repeated, taking quick notes on a few torn-out sheets of paper.[5]

"Self-reliant. Independent," Jaujard continued. "Not reliant on her feminine charms, but as inscrutable as the cat in a game of cat and mouse...if the cat could make you think she was the mouse. But a playful sense of humor when you know her. A way of sighing before speaking, almost a womanly affectation, but never anything but cheerful. And yet she never values her feminine wiles over her strong will. She always wanted to carry her own suitcase, you know, no matter how heavy. Let's see. Sensitive. Indefatigable. Painstaking... Is that enough?"[6]

Rorimer looked up from his notes. "More than enough," he said. "Especially since I don't know why I'm writing it down."

"Because we want you to talk to her, James."

"Why?"

"You've been in Paris for three months and in that short time you've seen what's going on... the absence of trust, the difficulties of restarting government, the bureaucratic delays with which we must contend. It's not surprising that after spending four long years inside the Jeu de Paume with the Nazis, Mademoiselle Valland is reluctant to turn over all her records and information."

Rorimer took his pieces of paper and stuck them into the Louvre's exhibition pamphlet on the Bayeux Tapestry, which he had picked up at the door. "Maybe she doesn't know anything," he said.

"That's what your British colleague Monuments officer McDonnell thinks. He's been investigating the matter, and he thinks there's nothing there. But he's wrong."

Rorimer thought for a moment. "It doesn't make sense. If she had information, why wouldn't she share it?"

Jaujard leaned back in his chair. "She has shared it... at least some of it... but only with me. You must consider the experience of living with the problem of collaborators during the four years of Nazi occupation. Even today it is a very real concern for all of us. That well-known fact makes trusting your fellow countrymen very difficult. You don't know who you can trust—even now."

"But surely she can trust you."

"Trust is only part of it, James. I am a creature of the French bureaucracy. When she has given me information in the past—and believe me, the information has been invaluable—I have done my duty and passed it to the proper government authorities. Unfortunately, the intended action was not always taken, or at least not taken as urgently as needed. It took the government two months—two months, James—to track down 112 cases of looted artwork Mademoiselle Valland had informed me about. During that time, the cases were lightedly guarded. By the time they were retrieved, several had been rifled." Jaujard looked at Rorimer, but the Monuments Man didn't respond. "It has to be an outsider, James," he said. "Someone who can get things done. There's no one else she will trust."

"But she doesn't even know me."

"You may not know her, but she certainly knows you. She's been watching. And she's impressed with what you've done for France. She told you that herself, when you met her in my office."

Jaujard held up his hand. "Don't protest. You've done more than you think. And when you've had obstacles placed in your path…well, at least you've bashed your head against the bureaucratic wall. That counts for something."

Jaujard rose from behind his desk. "But let's not spend all evening talking about Rose Valland. Talk to my friend Albert Henraux. He heads the commission, and he is of the same mind. He will tell you everything." He picked his hat off the stand by the door and started down the corridor. "I never tire of looking at the Bayeux Tapestry. Can you believe it is finally here, in the Louvre? Do you know the last time it was in Paris? 1804. Napoleon seized it from Bayeux and brought it here. He was planning to invade Britain, and he wanted to inspire his generals."

Rorimer glanced at the walls, still empty in this part of the museum. Only a small portion of the collection had been returned; much less than the number of works stolen from the citizens of France. But it was still a hopeful sight.

"I hate to ask, Jacques, but . . . how do you know she wasn't one of them? I mean, how do you know Rose Valland wasn't working for the Nazis?"

"Because she spied for me. I ordered her to stay at the Jeu de Paume, and she did, willingly, despite the danger. She brought me information almost every week. Valuable information. Because of her, the Resistance managed to delay indefinitely the departure of the last German trains transporting priceless art stolen from France's greatest private collections."

Jaujard stopped. "I know her, James. Her loyalty to France and to the artwork is beyond question. When you get to know her, you will understand that, too." He started walking again. "If you doubt her," he said with a smile, "ask her about the details of the art train. Rose Valland probably saved more important paintings,"

Jaujard added absently, "than most conservators will work with in a lifetime. Especially the ones who didn't have to live through this damn war. Ah, here we are."

They were entering the room where the Bayeux Tapestry was spread along the length of two walls. Rorimer walked slowly along its length, absorbed in the artistry. The effusion of detail, the extraordinary range of the storytelling and the scenes of medieval life flashed before his eyes in all their glory, a novel in picture form.

"I've been wondering about this since my visit two weeks ago," Rorimer said from the far end of the room. One of the last scenes, which if he recalled correctly featured scattered soldiers, their arms and weapons held high in the air, was covered by a temporary wall. "Surely it wasn't damaged? Not after all these centuries."

Jaujard shook his head. "It wasn't the condition of the tapestry," he said. "It was the inscription: *In fuga verterunt Agli*—The English Turned in Flight."

Rorimer remembered suddenly what the scattered soldiers represented: the English army retreating before the might of the French. He couldn't help but laugh. "A little sensitive, aren't we?"

Jaujard shrugged. "We are at war."

CHAPTER 19

Christmas Wishes

Metz, France
December 1944

The winter of 1944 was perhaps the most brutal period of the war on the Western front. General Montgomery's combined British and Canadian Twenty-first Army Group, pushed back at the Rhine by entrenched German forces, spent weeks slogging through the river's hazardous delta to open the important port city of Antwerp, Belgium, for delivery of much-needed supplies.

U.S. First Army had entered the Hürtgen Forest, a perilous corridor of steep wooded valleys shot through with German fortifications, dug-in troops, and mines. By December, the snow was thick in the trees and in places the ground was frozen too hard to dig foxholes. Advancing was arduous. In one deeply forested section, the army gained only 3,000 yards in a month, and lost 4,500 men in the process. The Battle of Hürtgen Forest, destined to be the longest in U.S. military history, would last from September 1944 to February 1945. When it ended, First Army had conquered less than fifty square miles.

Farther south, General Patton and U.S. Third Army

barreled into the heavily fortified city of Metz, on the eastern border of France. The city, surrounded by forts and observation posts connected by trenches and tunnels, had been a citadel since the time of the Romans, and was the last city in the region to surrender to the Germanic tribes. Since then, it had been a crucible of west-central Europe, a city fought over by everyone from the first Crusaders, who slaughtered Jews there in 1096, to Bourbon kings and English bandits. In 1870, during the Franco-Prussian War, it withstood a massive assault but fell to a Prussian siege and temporarily became part of the German state. The French won it back, but with diplomacy, not direct attack. In November 1944, Third Army became the next in a long line of armies to try to conquer Metz.

When aerial bombardment failed, Patton sent in the troops. The fighting lasted almost a month, with soldiers climbing sheer stone fortification walls and battling in underground tunnels laced with razor wire and iron bars. In the end, every German position fell but Fort Driant, their defensive pivot, which surrendered without being conquered. The advance from the Moselle River had cost more than 47,000 American casualties and gained less than thirty miles. General Patton, exasperated with both the German defenses and the seven inches of rain that had fallen during the advance, wrote the secretary of war, "I hope that in the final settlement of the war, you insist that the Germans retain Lorraine, because I can imagine no greater burden than to be the owner of this nasty country where it rains every day and where the whole wealth of the people consists in assorted manure piles."[1]

December proved worse. On December 8, the day the last Germans officially surrendered at Metz, General Patton sent his troops a Christmas greeting containing the following prayer: "Almighty and most merciful Father, we humbly beseech Thee, of Thy great goodness, to restrain these immoderate rains with which we have had to contend. Grant us fair weather for Battle. Graciously hearken to us as soldiers who call Thee that, armed with Thy power, we may advance from victory to victory, and crush the oppression and wickedness of our enemies, and establish Thy justice among men and nations. Amen."[2]

The Weather Prayer didn't work. The skies remained cloudy; the temperatures plunged. Snow piled up shoulder-high in wooded ravines and tumbled off branches in dangerous, icy clumps. The dense fog would roll in, plunging the world into shadow, only to suddenly roll out again and leave the dark-clad soldiers easy marks against the white snow. In the Ardennes Forest, the ground froze so hard the soldiers' folding shovels and pickaxes could not break its surface. A few fortunate units were given dynamite sticks to create foxholes; others made do with line-strung pup tents and shared blankets. The stinging cold took off fingers, even through gloves. Trenchfoot, a rotting of the foot caused by prolonged exposure to dampness and subfreezing temperatures, was epidemic among weary soldiers too cold or swollen to remove their combat boots. Frostbite and hypothermia became an enemy to rival the German artillery positions, which seemed entrenched on every square inch of ground from the North Sea to the Swiss border. The Western armies, so recently racing forward, had entered a brutal war of attrition along both sides of the German border, one that would be measured in yards, not miles.

Monuments Man Robert Posey, the architect from Alabama, must have thought of his first posting, in the bleak reaches of northern Canada, and thanked his stars he was billeted in the French city of Nancy instead of his tent. In Metz, where he traveled frequently for inspection tours, the cultural damage was immense. The city's famous collection of medieval manuscripts had been destroyed by fire. He had found most of the valuable artwork in repositories, but the city's relics, including its most precious possession, the cloak of Charlemagne, had been shipped to Germany for "safe-keeping" along with the cathedral treasury. But Nancy had suffered little damage, and since Third Army would be headquartered there for most of the winter, Posey decided to write a short letter of historical notes on its architectural and artistic history. After his experiences in the field, he had embraced the idea of an educated, interested army.

The letter would prove immensely popular with the men, giving some context to the ground they were fighting over, but that didn't make it easy to write. Nancy was a commercial and artistic hub, but the history Posey kept thinking back to on those cold December days was that of the military. The troops were out there fighting and dying in the cold, and he could never for a moment forget it. He was as much a military man, he had begun to realize, as an architect; he had written his wife, Alice, that "the army is better than college for meeting people you enjoy knowing. There seems to be a closer common bond."[3] And he hadn't been referring to his fellow Monuments Men.

Posey wasn't a privileged man. He had been raised on a dirt farm outside the small town of Morris, Alabama, where architecture meant slapping new pieces of plywood on the side of the house and art was only the reflection of the sky in a muddy puddle after the rain. But what the Posey family lacked in social standing and material comfort, they compensated for with history. Every member of the family—every male member, at least—could recite the roll call of honor from which he was descended: Frances Posey, who fought in the colonial wars against French and Indian troops; Hezekiah Posey, a minuteman in the South Carolina militia during the Revolutionary War, wounded by Tories in 1780; Joseph Harrison Posey, who fought the Creek Indians in the War of 1812; Carnot Posey— Robert's son Dennis's first name was Carnot after this ancestor—who survived Gettysburg but died from a battle wound four months later; Carnot's brother, John Wesley Posey, who fought with the 15th Mounted Mississippi Infantry—they would ride horses to the battle, then fight on foot—and was the only one of the eight fighting Posey brothers to survive the Civil War.

In the eastern French provinces of Alsace and Lorraine, a similar history of honor and sacrifice was all around him. As the cemeteries attested, hardly a generation had lived here in peace since Attila plunged the Roman Empire into darkness. Earlier, he had passed near the French city of Verdun, the site of the bloodiest battle of World War I, where a million men had been wounded and 250,000 had died. He had inspected the military cemeteries at Meuse-Argonne and Romagne-sous-Montfaucon, filled with the dead of that war. "The Great War," they called it. "The War to End All Wars." But at Montsec the memorial to the fallen heroes of World War I had been chipped to hell by the bullets of this war. And at St. Mihiel, an American military cemetery, German soldiers had destroyed all the headstones featuring the Star of David.

He thought about Christmas. Would Woogie miss him? Would they have presents and stockings, turkey and stuffing, or was that lost to rationing, too? Over here, there would be little celebration. Christmas was just another workday, just as it had been growing up in Alabama. In a good year back then, little Robert got a handkerchief and an orange. One year his father fashioned a little cart—although come to think of it that was in the spring, not at Christmastime—and the children took turns being pulled around the yard by the family goat. Then he died. His father and the goat. And eleven-year-old Robert, having seen his little sister given away to his aunt because she simply couldn't be fed, had started working two jobs, one at the grocery store and the other at the soda fountain.

The military rescued him. He had joined army ROTC as soon as he was old enough. It provided him with food, money, a future. It paid his way to Auburn University. He was supposed to go one year, then switch with his younger brother, since even with ROTC funding the family couldn't afford two tuitions. Robert proved such a good student that his brother insisted he go straight through. That's when Robert discovered his second love: architecture. And that's the way it had been ever since: the army and architecture, mingled together in his mind and his heart.

He put down his pencil and reached for his preserved figs and peanuts, a Christmas present from Alice. Figs and peanuts: It was more than he could ever have imagined as a child. And there were still several boxes of presents to open, some even wrapped with paper. He was saving those for Christmas morning.

He thought of the moment he had realized there was a world out there. He was eight years old, and he saw a picture of a mountain. There was snow on top, but in the valley below there were flowers. He didn't have a way to find out why that was, so he started trying to figure it all out in his mind. The more he thought, the more complicated and wonderful life became. There were so many questions, he realized, that he would be busy trying to answer them for the rest of his life.[4]

He wondered what that boy would think if he could see himself now. He had seen actual mountains. He had seen ice a thousand feet thick in the Arctic. He had designed runways on that ice, in case American pilots needed to fly there. He had designed a pontoon bridge, only to see it fail and plunge a tank into the muddy waters of a Pennsylvania river. He had been in London. He had not only visited but worked in New York City.

Now he was in Europe. He could walk outside into an ancient city and see snow in piles along the streets and rows of buildings wrapping behind them. No, he wasn't just here. He was an expert; it was his job to preserve this city. And he was a soldier. He had met with General George S. Patton Jr., the greatest fighting man in the U.S. Army. A man who when you called him a bastard—and every man in Third Army sometimes did—you did so with admiration.

Posey remembered a story he had heard other soldiers telling about Patton's days commanding U.S. Seventh Army in Sicily in 1943. General Patton, upon seeing the Roman ruins at Agrigento, remarked to a local expert, "Seventh Army didn't cause that destruction, did it, sir?"

The man replied, "No sir, that happened in the last war."

"What war was that?"

"The Second Punic War."[5]

The story got a laugh, but hid a serious message: That history was long; that legacy was important; that Third Army must strive in all ways to be the greatest fighting force since Hannibal took his elephants across the Alps in that Punic War and almost crushed the fledgling Roman Empire. Robert Posey wasn't an infantryman. He didn't fire a gun. But his job was important, and he was determined to put his heart and muscle into it. Weather and danger be damned. There was no place in the world Robert Posey would rather be than in Third Army.

Except maybe home.

Once again, he put down his pencil. He looked at the other boxes from Alice and Woogie. It was December 10, two weeks until Christmas, but he didn't want to wait any longer.

The first box contained little presents for French children. He had told Alice not to send them, that he was always moving and didn't know any children, but she sent them anyway. He went out with the presents the next day and, to his surprise, found children in the streets gathering handfuls of tinfoil to decorate Christmas trees. German airplanes had dropped the tinfoil to break up Allied radar transmissions; it was the only thing in abundance that year. It reminded him of his own deprived youth, and he wondered at Alice's understanding. He found a group of French girls. He offered them Alice's presents, but under one condition: that they write letters in French to his son.

Dear Dennis:

I am sure you would like to have this Third Army Christmas card all for yourself. I hope you received the Third Army shoulder patch I sent you about two months ago in a letter.

The card shows our tanks breaking through the German lines in Normandy, crashing through into Brittany, racing across France and now headed for Berlin. I have been here to see it all and we are so very strong that I am sure it will not be too very long until we are in Berlin.

All of this is very spectacular and dramatic but it is also bad for it causes great suffering to people who live where the actual fighting is going on. It also takes soldiers away from their homes and causes them to become tough and sometimes bitter.

Germany started this war by invading one small country after another until finally France and England had to declare war on her. We helped France and England but didn't start fighting. Then suddenly Japan attacked us and Germany declared war on us at the same time. And so we had to fight, painfully at first for we were unprepared. Now we are strong; England is strong; Russia, who was attacked by Germany is strong;

Italy who fought with Germany has been defeated
by us and has swung over to our side; France
who was defeated by Germany but liberated by us
is building a powerful army. Greece, Belgium,
and part of Holland have been liberated and are
helping us; China is painfully shaking off the
treacherous Japanese yoke.

And so, these are the reasons that I think
we will soon defeat Germany and Japan and teach
them such a lesson that when you and other little
boys like you grow up you will not have to fight
them all over again. And I hope no other country
will start a fight to get its way for wars are
bad.

Realizing all of this helps me to be
satisfied with being away from you and Momie this
Christmas. I hope that you have a wonderful time
with lots of nice presents. Please take my place
and buy Momie nice presents for her birthday
anniversary and Christmas.

Good bye for now with love.

Bob

CHAPTER 20

The Madonna of La Gleize

La Gleize, Belgium
December 1944

While Robert Posey worked in eastern France, the sculptor Walker Hancock drove through the Belgian countryside, consolidating his work in the conquered territory just behind the front lines. Places like the Belgian village of La Gleize, one of the middle stops on his tour, didn't offer the awe of Aachen or the thrill of finding a possible Bruegel painting on the front lines, but it was peaceful here, nothing more than a small group of rough buildings sitting quietly atop a hill beneath a huge white winter sky. Hancock had come to inspect the cathedral, described on his list of protected monuments as dating to the eleventh century. Looking at it now, he was deeply disappointed. He could see immediately the building was beyond salvage. The tower was lopped off and the old stone walls destroyed. This wasn't the brutality of war, however, but of ill-conceived renovations. The monument was clearly unworthy of inclusion on the list.

He decided, especially given the cold, to go inside. Just beyond the door, on a pedestal in the middle of the nave, stood a small wooden statue of the Virgin Mary.

He stopped. The workmanship was crude, but the rough exterior heightened the figure's extraordinary grace. She was only a few feet tall and fragile in appearance, but somehow she seemed to dominate the interior of the church. She held one hand over her heart, the other open, and although the fingers of her raised hand looked impossibly delicate, the gesture would stop anyone in their tracks. It was a rough yet simple work of art, and it possessed a beauty that transcended its humble surroundings.

The *curé* of the cathedral was away, but a young woman in the tourism office agreed to give Hancock a tour of La Gleize. The view over sloping fields to the Ardennes Forest was sublimely beautiful, but the town, almost deserted, was little more than farmers' dwellings and small stores. Hancock found it charmless, but the young woman delightful. Her father ran the local inn, but since tourism was nonexistent he spent most of his time farming. The statue, known as the Madonna of La Gleize, was the envy of the neighboring parishes. It was carved in the 1300s, but had been found in the tower only fifty years prior during one of the ill-conceived renovations. She had stood in the nave only a few years.

The young woman gave Hancock a postcard of the Virgin, the only photograph available, and invited him to dinner. The house was a pleasant two-story stone structure, built by her father, Monsieur Geneen. The food was almost too good to be eaten after a month of living on K-rations, and the company lively and warm. The simple beauty of people who worked the land, and of the rural village that he had just that afternoon found so crude, came flooding in as Hancock sat at the rustic wooden table. The memories of that dinner and of the miraculous, unknown Madonna stayed with him in the months that followed, through the rain and the cold, the trenches, the bombardments, and the ruined towns. If ever a place seemed untouched by the war, it was La Gleize.

Precious Saima—

   This is the great day of our lives—the
anniversary of the happiest one in mine. And
if I loved you a year ago today, I do so many
times more this fourth of December. For even
though we have spent such a small part of this
year together, we have been together the whole
time in the best sense, and you have helped me
and nourished me through these interesting but
trying months in a way that you would hardly
have had the opportunity to do in a happy normal
life at home. That will come, and our joys will
be boundless, but what you have been to me
during these months of separation is something
that I never could have imagined without the
experience. Your letters have been my mainstay.
Just the simple account of what you do and think—
and between letters I think about *you*.

   Today has been rather a grind—and one of
those days when one seems to have just missed
accomplishing something all along the line. But
I hope I'll be able to make up for it during the
week. One just has to learn that things have
to be done a little bit at a time in the army—
and it doesn't pay to bite off more than can be
chewed.... There's a Polish soldier sitting on
the bunk beside me, saying that this will be

his sixth Christmas in the army and away from his people. He's pretty discouraged—but we are guaranteeing him this will be the last away from home.

Tomorrow or the next day I expect to see George Stout. I wonder if he will be coming back to the First Army. I hope so, for there is more work than I can keep up with at present. Worlds of love to you—you sweet creature—I *love* you—

Walker

CHAPTER 21

The Train

Paris, France
August 1944 and
Late December 1944

Rose Valland thought again of those last days at the Jeu de Paume. After the defeat of Ambassador Abetz by Jaujard and Wolff-Metternich, the Nazis had hit on a new scheme for "legally" transporting cultural objects out of France. On September 17, 1940, the Führer had given the ERR (Reich Leader Rosenberg's Special Task Force) the authorization to "search lodges, libraries and archives in the occupied territories of the west for material valuable to Germany, and to safeguard the latter through the Gestapo."[1] The official role of the ERR was to provide material for Alfred Rosenberg's "scholarly" institutes, whose prime objective was to scientifically prove Jewish racial inferiority. It didn't take long for the Nazis to realize the ERR was the perfect cover for moving valuable artwork and cultural treasures out of France. In late October, only weeks after the authorization of the ERR, an artwork cataloguing, crating, and transporting operation had been established at the Jeu de Paume.

For the next four years, the Nazis had used the

museum, *Valland's museum*, as their clearinghouse for
the spoils of France. For four years, the private collections of French citizens, especially Jews, moved through
its galleries like water flowing downhill to the Reich. For
four years, Gestapo guards assured that no one could
enter but the chosen, those bearing the mark of Colonel
Kurt von Behr, commandant of the Jeu de Paume and
the local leader of the ERR. The staff had never been disciplined; in fact, the Jeu de Paume had been a hothouse
of backstabbing, stealing, and intrigue since the moment
the Nazis occupied it, and that was just among its leaders. But the operation had always run with depressing
efficiency, moving load after load of stolen items through
its processing rooms and on to the Fatherland.

But in the summer of 1944, it was coming to an end.
The Allies were on the beaches at Normandy; everyone
believed their arrival in Paris was just a matter of time.
In June, Bruno Lohse, a slick, reptilian German art
dealer who had schemed his way through the hierarchy
of the ERR, returned from a ski vacation with a broken leg and kidney pain; both faked, the gossip said,
because the desperate Germans were throwing every
able-bodied man at the front lines. In late July, with
the fighting at a critical stage, Lohse left for Normandy
with a revolver stuck in his belt. His parting words were
"off to battle!" but when he returned two days later,
his truck was filled with chickens, butter, and a whole
roasting lamb. There was a big party at his Paris apartment, and even Colonel von Behr, his boss and rival at
the Jeu de Paume, was invited.[2]

And then, suddenly, they were finished. "*Ouf!*" Valland wrote in her notes. Relief, finally![3]

But it was relief mixed with trepidation. In her four years at the museum, she had developed a routine, an understanding that made her isolation in the lion's den almost...not pleasant, but acceptable. She knew what to expect. She had a good read on everyone. Dr. Borchers, the art historian charged with cataloguing and researching the looted goods, even trusted her with his confidences; she used him, without his knowledge, as one of her primary sources of information. Many a secret conveyed by Borchers had wound up in the hands of Jacques Jaujard and the French Resistance. She knew Borchers would never betray her; he considered her his only...non-enemy. Hermann Bunjes, a corrupt art scholar who had been lured from Wolff-Metternich's noble Kunstschutz to the service of Reichsmarschall Göring and the ERR, found her beneath contempt. The wily, cowardly Lohse wanted her dead. She was sure of that. He was tall and handsome and very popular with the women of Paris, but Valland found him slick and cold-blooded. If a high official was going to have her killed, she felt it would be Lohse. He had said as much in February 1944, when he discovered her trying to decipher an address on some shipping documents.

"You could be shot for any indiscretion," he told her, looking her straight in the eye.

"No one here is stupid enough to ignore the risk," she replied calmly, without backing down from his stare.[4]

That was the way to handle Lohse. Never show fear; never back down. If the Nazis discovered they could push you, they would push you to your death. You had to be too much trouble to make it easy, but not so much they grew tired of you. A delicate balance, but one she had perfected. She had been thrown out of the museum many times on charges of spying, stealing, sabotage, or informing the enemy. She always vehemently denied involvement, and recriminations would fly for days. In the end, they always took her back. The more "suspicious" she became, in fact, the more valuable she was to her Nazi overlords because they could use her as an excuse for every problem. Especially Lohse, whom everyone suspected of stealing items for his personal use and as gifts—for friends, for his mother. Valland knew he was stealing; she had seen him hiding four paintings in his car trunk as early as October 1942. She never said anything. Partly it was the bitter irony of the thieves stealing from the thieves. Partly it was that Lohse valued her silence and assertiveness. She was a great distraction. Her worst enemy, she suspected, was also her secret protector.

But that was when it was convenient to keep her; with the looting operation winding down and the Allies on their way to Paris, she was an inconvenience. In June, a French secretary working for the ERR had disappeared, and the Nazis were convinced she was a spy. Shortly after, a German secretary married to a Frenchman was arrested on charges of espionage. The Nazis weren't just clearing out the artwork; they were clearing out the staff. Rose Valland was fairly certain, ironically, that she was one of the few French workers above suspicion. But that didn't mean they wouldn't kill her. If the Nazis felt the cause was lost, they wouldn't be eliminating spies; they would be eliminating witnesses.

By August 1, the endgame had begun. The Germans were clearing the museum, rushing to get everything out before the Allies arrived. Rose Valland stayed to watch and to listen. Lohse was nowhere to be found; Bunjes was sulking the corridors in a bad mood. But in the middle of the mad rush of activity stood the Jeu de Paume commandant, Colonel Kurt von Behr. She remembered the first time she had seen him, in October 1940. He was in his full uniform then, standing straight and stern with his arms behind him, like the well-known prints of a German warlord in a triumphant pose. Tall, handsome, a cap shading his eyes, which she would learn had the advantage of hiding his glass eye. He was quite charming, a worldly German baron, and spoke French well. Still celebrating his victory, the conqueror was friendly and clearly eager to persuade her that the Nazis were not total savages. In this magnanimous spirit, the warlord granted her permission to remain in her former museum, now his kingdom.

Four years later, he looked quite different: harried, stooped, lined, and balding. It didn't help his image that in the intervening years she had discovered he hailed from a broken, impoverished baronial line, and that in his youth he had been a dissipated failure. He wasn't even a soldier. He was, of all ironies, the Nazi-appointed head of the French Red Cross. He had no official rank, even though he called himself colonel. And he had his own Red Cross uniform: black, decorated with swastikas, and suspiciously similar to the original uniforms of the Waffen-SS.

He was pathetic, but also dangerous. For if there was one thing striking about him, as he watched his kingdom being hastily disassembled, it was the look in his eyes. Four years before, he had seemed worldly and relaxed, the perfect conqueror. Now there was anger there, an anger at the realization that everything would soon be lost.

"Careful," he hissed at the hapless German soldiers who were banging paintings together and shoving them into crates without packing material. There was panic in their eyes, their desire to flee. What had become of the vaunted German discipline?

Rose Valland remembered wanting to approach him, to say something to break him down. But the colonel was heavily guarded by men with machine guns. "*Dommage*," she had thought.[5] A pity. Then he had glanced at her, and she had seen anger edged with menace. A thought echoed in her head: *Liquidate the witness.*

"Colonel von Behr," a soldier had said, breaking his gaze. Von Behr had turned with a glare. "The trucks are almost full, sir."

"Get more, fool," he growled.

Before he could turn back to her, Rose Valland had slipped away. It wasn't her place to taunt von Behr, and she was certainly no assassin. Her role was to spy, to be the quiet mouse that slowly but surely chewed a hole in the foundation of the house. Four years of occupation was ending in a matter of days, if not hours. If ever there was a time to lie low, this was it.

But her persistence, as usual, had paid off. The trucks leaving the museum with the last of the looted French artwork weren't heading straight for Germany. In her trek through the museum, Valland had learned they were going to the Aubervilliers train station on the outskirts of Paris to be loaded onto railcars. Trucks would have been nearly impossible to track; a train was easier. Especially since she had discovered the railcar numbers.

The next day, August 2, 1944, five railcars containing 148 crates of stolen paintings were sealed at Aubervilliers. The ERR had rushed to pack the final shipment from the Jeu de Paume, but a few days later the railcars still hadn't left the station. The art train was scheduled to contain forty-six additional cars of looted objects obtained by another Nazi looting organization controlled by von Behr, "M-Aktion" (M stood for *Möbel*, German for furniture). Much to von Behr's disgust, those cars weren't yet loaded.

Train no. 40044 was still parked at the rail station a few days later when Rose Valland paid a visit to her boss, Monsieur Jaujard. She had copied the Nazi shipment order which contained the train and railcar numbers, destinations of the crates (Kogl castle, near Vöcklabruck, Austria, and Nikolsburg depository in Moravia), and their contents. Wouldn't it be wise to try and delay the train, she suggested. The Allies could arrive any day.

"Agreed," Jaujard said.

As von Behr huffed on the train station platform, berating the armed guards and the privates trying desperately to load the other cars, Jaujard's contacts in the French Resistance set out to stop the train using the information Rose Valland had obtained, and subsequently relayed to them by Jaujard. By August 10, the art train was packed, but by then a thousand French railroadmen had gone on strike, and there was no way to depart Aubervilliers. By August 12, the tracks were again open, but instead of departing for Germany the art train was shunted to a side track to make way for other trains carrying personal possessions and terrified German citizens. The German guards, exhausted after ten days, walked nervously back and forth, wishing they were already home. The French army, it was being whispered, was hours away. And yet small technical problems kept cropping up, pushing the train to the end of the priority line. The French army never showed. The young men sighed with relief. After almost three weeks, the train finally began its journey home to Germany.

But it only got to Le Bourget, a few miles down the track. The train, fifty-one cars packed full of loot, was so heavy that it caused a mechanical breakdown (or so went the excuse), necessitating a forty-eight-hour delay. By the time that problem was solved, it was too late. The French Resistance had derailed two engines at an important bottleneck in the rail system. The art train was trapped in Paris. "The freight cars with their 148 crates of art," Valland wrote to Jaujard, "are ours."[6]

But it hadn't been so simple. When the Second Armored Division of the Free French army arrived a few days later, the Resistance alerted them to the importance of the train. The detachment sent by General Leclerc found several crates broken open, two crates pillaged, and an entire collection of silver missing. They decided to send thirty-six of the 148 crates filled with important works by Renoir, Degas, Picasso, Gauguin, and other masters to the Louvre. It was the bulk of the collection of Paul Rosenberg, the famous Parisian art dealer, whose son by coincidence was the division commander of the Free French troops who inspected the train. But much to Rose Valland's regret and frustration, almost two more months would pass before the rest of the crates were removed from the train and returned to the museum. Even in the cold snow of December, waiting for the stationmaster to show her the last contents of the train, it was an oversight that gnawed at the corner of her mind.

———

"We'd like to see the stationmaster, please," James Rorimer told the attendant at the Gare de Pantin, blowing on his hands against the winter chill. Behind him, Rose Valland took a long drag on her cigarette, deep in her own thoughts. "I know it's a vice," she had told him during one of their first conversations, "but if I can smoke, nothing else but my work matters."[7]

She was mysterious like that, always saying sly, inscrutable things. He could never, for the life of him, understand exactly where he stood with her. They had a good relationship, he was confident of that. It wasn't just that Henraux, who like Jaujard had urged Rorimer to learn what he could from Valland, agreed that she had been watching and admiring him. It was what Valland said to him the week before, on December 16, when he turned over to the commission several minor paintings and engravings found in an American military installation. "Thank you," she had said. "Too often, your fellow liberators give us the painful impression they have landed in a country whose inhabitants no longer matter."[8] It was about as personal as Rose Valland ever got.

But how good was their relationship? And how much did Valland really trust him? He thought of the story Jaujard had told him: Rose Valland alone, holding her ground against the French crowds that stormed the Jeu de Paume in celebration on the day General Leclerc liberated Paris. She wouldn't allow the mob into the basement, where the museum's collections had been stored during the occupation.

"She's sheltering Germans!" someone shouted.

"*Collaborateur*!" The cry rang through the building. "*Collabo-rateur*!"

Calmly, despite the gun at her back, Valland had showed her fellow Frenchmen that the basement was indeed empty of everything but boilers, pipes, and artwork. And then, despite their protests, she kicked them out. She was no pushover, that was for sure. She was strong, opinionated, easy to underestimate and misunderstand. She had her own ideas about duty and honor, and she kept to her principles even with a gun in her back. Rorimer wasn't sure if Jaujard had told him the story to explain her secretiveness and determination, or to draw a subtle line between the two of them. Jaujard, after all, had been threatened by his own countrymen, too.

But he had made progress. While he was delivering the recovered objects to Valland at the Jeu de Paume on December 16, Rorimer had visited Albert Henraux, director of the Commission de Récupération Artistique. He informed Rorimer of the locations of nine ERR storehouses and also told him about the unopened traincars. Henraux encouraged him to work with Valland to investigate the locations. "She knows more than she has revealed to us, James. Perhaps you can find out what it is."

Rorimer had heard the story of the nine locations from Rose Valland as they traveled together to inspect them. While working as a spy at the Jeu de Paume, she had compiled the addresses of all the important Nazi storehouses in Paris, as well as the home addresses of all the important Nazi looters. She had provided the information to Jaujard in early August. He, in turn, had given the addresses to the new French government to investigate. Although a few objects had been returned to the Louvre, nothing further had been heard. This was her first visit to the Nazi storehouses she had worked so hard to uncover.

They didn't find much. One site contained thousands of rare books; a few others held minor pieces of art left behind during the French government sweep of the building. In some ways, it was simply another dead end, another setback. And while he still professed in his letters home to love his job, Rorimer's satisfaction was being undercut by crosscurrents of doubt and frustration.

For one thing, he was homesick. In England, he had agreed not to send sentimental letters home because they would "only cause the writer and the recipients unnecessary emotional disturbances."[9] For six months he had dutifully obeyed this rule. But in late October, he had broken down, writing his wife that "I think of your problems often, perhaps even constantly. It is not that I do not want to help you lead your life with you these days, but rather that I know how foolish it would be to do anything but plan for our happy future years together. I do not ask about our child, nor tell you how I long to see Anne. That would not be fair. It's for this same reason as I have told you before that I do not write very personal, sloppy letters about wasted emotions. When I see the concierge's child at our apartment I realize how deprived I am of these moments which we should be having together."[10] Anne was eight months old, and her father had never seen her. And he had no hope of doing so anytime in the near future.

He was worn out, absolutely dead worn out. And the difficulties of the job—the ceaseless dead ends, the brutal bureacracy, the endless small disturbances, the isolation from family and friends—were building up. What finally pushed him over the line in late November was small: His beloved typewriter, which he had purchased on his crossing to France, was stolen. Seemingly minor, maybe, but there were no other typewriters available, and he couldn't find one to buy, and he had to write home to ask his mother to send him one, which required special army permission. His mother wanted letters, letters, letters, and how was he to compose them without his typewriter?

Looking back on it weeks later (but still without a typewriter), he didn't understand why he had exploded. He didn't know it was a deeper, more fundamental issue. Despite the dinners with society figures, Paris' glorious monuments, and his belief in the work, he had slowly come to realize that Paris wasn't central to the monuments effort. The important work was not here, but in Germany, and Rorimer hated to be too far away from the important work. He would not have acknowledged it, because he probably did not yet know it himself, but he viewed the war as an opportunity to perform "what is called a service to humanity," and he was eager to make his mark.[11]

That's why the lack of material in the ERR storehouses didn't faze him. As he stood there, looking at those empty rooms, he could see that they were merely entry points into another world. For the first time in months, he felt himself being drawn into something larger. Just seeing the warehouses the Nazis had filled with "confiscated" items brought home to him the size and complexity of their looting operation. This wasn't accidental damage or angry retaliation, but an enormous web of deliberate deceit that stretched all over Paris and down all the roads back to the Fatherland and all the way to Hitler's office in Berlin. Jaujard had pushed him into this web. He was the orchestra conductor, the man at the center of his own circle of intrigue, the one person who had the connections and foresight to effectively counter, as much as possible, the Nazi will to possess. He had protected the museums and state-owned collections, but by comparison he could do little to save the private artistic wealth of France—the invaluable cultural objects held by her citizens. Jaujard had opened a door into that lost world, but Rose Valland, James Rorimer realized, was going to be his guide.

The first nine locations Valland had identified were buildings. The tenth, and clearly the most important to her, was the art train. Thirty-six of the cases she had identified during the last harrowing days of the Nazi occupation had been returned to the Louvre for safekeeping in August, but by early October the other 112 cases were still believed to be on the train...somewhere. And despite Jaujard's freqent requests, no one would tell the art community their status. Someone, somewhere, knew down which track the remaining cars of the art train had been shunted, but the information wasn't being communicated through the bureaucracy. The mystery was finally solved on October 9, when the municipal police in Pantin contacted the Louvre. They had made frequent requests to the government, but nobody had done anything about the train parked near the Pantin railyard under the Edouard-Vaillant Bridge. The municipal police didn't have enough men to guard the valuable art; and besides, the train was parked dangerously close to freight cars filled with ammunition. The museum community once again sprang into action.

On October 21, Rose Valland sent a memo to Jacques Jaujard telling him that, between October 17 and 19, the last 112 cases of "recovered paintings" had finally been transferred to the Jeu de Paume. Several had been opened and pillaged, she noted, and she feared that "most of the freight cars in this convoy transporting the expropriated goods of Jews have been similarly looted."[12] It was these forty-six railcar loads that she and James Rorimer were back to investigate.

"I'm Monsieur Malherbaud," an older man said, stepping out of the door of the station. "I am the stationmaster."

"Are you the man who routed the art train, the one carrying the Cézannes and Monets?"

The man looked warily at Rorimer's uniform, then at the commonplace woman smoking a cigarette behind

him. There were still plenty of German spies and saboteurs in Paris, and most were specialists in retaliation. It
was wise to be cautious.

"Why do you ask?"

"I'm Second Lieutenant Rorimer of United States
Army, Seine Section. This is Mademoiselle Valland,
from the Musées Nationaux. She informed the Resistance of the shipment."

"I'm sorry," he said. "The artwork was cleared.
There was nothing left."

"We're looking for the rest of the train."

The man looked surprised. "Then follow me."

The railcars had been unloaded into a nondescript
warehouse. "Here goes nothing," Rorimer said to Valland as the stationmaster pulled open the warehouse
door. The previous nine Nazi storehouses Valland had
identified had been mostly cleared by the time the two
of them arrived; this one promised to be full. Rorimer
was excited by the prospect of what they would find.

The sight that greeted him in the cold warehouse
was not at all what he had expected. He didn't know
exactly what he had expected, but it certainly hadn't
been an enormous, jumbled pile of ordinary household
items. For there before him, at least twice as tall as he
was, rose an endless pile of sofas, chairs, mirrors, tables,
pots, pans, picture frames, and children's toys. The
amount was staggering, although in reality it was nothing, only forty-six railcars full. M-Aktion, it was determined after the war, had shipped 29,436 railroad cars
full of such ordinary household objects to Germany.

They delayed the art train for this? Rorimer thought,
his heart sinking inside him. *It's all worthless. It's all*

just junk. Then he stopped himself. It wasn't worthless; these objects were people's belongings—the detritus that had made up their lives. The Nazis had gone into people's homes and simply cleared them out, all the way down to the family photographs.

"It's not what you were expecting, is it?" Valland said, shoving her hands into her pockets.

The hidden message in her simple statement struck him like a thunderbolt. She had known the boxcar numbers where the valuables were hidden; Rose Valland had known, or at least strongly suspected, there wasn't anything else important on that train. But she had wanted to see for herself. Stopping the art train was a great personal triumph for her, but she had never been allowed to see it for herself. She was nothing more than a minor government bureaucrat, a woman. Valland had the information, but as a U.S. Army officer Rorimer had the access. He was her entry into places she had never been allowed before—places she had risked her life to discover.

He thought of the information she might possess. She was the key to understanding the whole Nazi looting operation; her cooperation provided the only real possibility of finding what had been stolen and bringing it back. But she was stuck at the bottom of an endless pyramid of functionaries, and she needed him as much as he needed her.

"You know where it is," he said. "The stolen artwork."

She turned and started to walk away.

"You know where it is, don't you, Rose?" He jogged to catch up to her. "What are you waiting for? Someone you can trust?"

"You know enough," she said with a smile.

Rorimer grabbed her by the arm. "Please share your information with me. You know I will use it only as you wish: for France."

She pulled out of his grip, no longer smiling. "I'll tell you where," she said, "when the time is right."[13]

CHAPTER 22

The Bulge

The Western Front
December 16–17, 1944

Robert Posey couldn't wait. He had intended to keep the last Christmas present in the shipment from his wife, Alice, the big one marked "With love from your family," until Christmas Day.[1] But he had waited six days, and it was only December 16. He simply couldn't wait any longer. So he ripped open the box and dug eagerly down into the packing material. Eventually, his fingertips touched cold plastic. He lifted the present out of the box. It was a phonograph record.

"The greatest surprise of all," he wrote Alice later that night, "was the record letter Christmas greeting. I immediately raced over to the Special Services company where the sergeant put on one of those radio-victrola hookups and I sat in another room and heard it come over the radio. It is the finest present one could have. Your voices were perfect; even the off-the-record instructions you gave Dennis to 'say anything you want' came over without a syllable dropped. It was the same as a re-broadcast over the radio with the two of you joining together in the program. By simply turning the knob I could make it louder or softer as the case required. The little song was delightful. It was very reassuring to hear the two of you together. I do not note any change. I had sort of expected to hear Dennis' voice older than when I saw him last; but from the sound of it now he is still a little boy and the Kitten [Alice] is still a bit shy."[2]

Later that night, he got another surprise. The Germans had launched an offensive, the interservice radio reported, and the Allies were falling back.

Walker Hancock heard of the Ardennes Offensive, more commonly known as the Battle of the Bulge, the next day, when he was stopped by an advanced unit and told the village he was planning to inspect, Waimes, was now in German hands. He spent the next night heading west in a blacked-out convoy, following for hours the small green "cat's eye" light on the bumper of the jeep in front of him. They were strafed only once. He spent Christmas Eve in a cellar in Liège, Belgium; the next morning, Christmas Mass was interrupted by German bombs.

Ronald Balfour, the British scholar at the northern spear of the Allied trident in the First Canadian Army, spent the Bulge in the hospital. On November 29, four days after advancing into Holland, he had suffered a broken ankle in a serious truck accident. He would not report back to duty until mid-January.

George Stout, despite his best delaying tactics and Walker Hancock's sincere hope for his mentor's return to U.S. First Army, had been officially transferred to U.S. Twelfth Army Group in early December. This meant a prolonged assignment at headquarters in Versailles, outside Paris. He spent December 14, 1944, inspecting the palace's medieval collection with James Rorimer, and the next few weeks in an office, writing summaries of the Monuments Men's work for 1944 and reworking their official procedures. "Most of my time is spent indoors," he wrote his wife, Margie, "working at a table. I don't object, for the weather is severe."[3] It was the worst winter in modern history: icy, foggy, and so cold that diesel fuel was known to freeze. Even Paris was under a miserable blanket of snow.

With the infantry decimated by the sudden German advance, U.S. Third Army went looking for replacements. They found a ready volunteer in Robert Posey, the Alabama Monuments Man who, more than any of the others, wanted to be a soldier. Posey wasn't trained for combat and his eyesight was so bad he couldn't see an enemy soldier a hundred yards away, but his instructions were simple: "Keep firing until you can't fire anymore."[4] And that's what he did. He fired through the frosty, snow-covered Ardennes Forest until his ammunition was gone, then stopped to reload. Enemy bullets tore through the icy trees, but when his fellow soldiers began to fire and advance he followed, shooting across a clearing and into the foggy woods.

CHAPTER 23

Champagne

Paris, France
Just Before Christmas, 1944

In Paris, Rose Valland trudged her way through the snows that were blanketing Western Europe. A few days before, as the Germans swept down on Robert Posey and the faltering Western Allied lines in the Ardennes, she had sent James Rorimer a bottle of champagne. She feared she had been a bit abrupt at the art train, and she didn't want to leave him with the wrong impression. She had been pleased with his clear desire to share her information, and with all the days she had spent with him inspecting the Nazis' storerooms. They had the bond of museum professionals laboring out of a shared love for art, but she admired his personal qualities as well: diligent, opinionated, bullheaded, and insightful enough to grasp immediately the scope of the situation...and the potential. Above all, perhaps, he was respectful. He appreciated what she had achieved. She wanted him to know how much it meant to her that they were friends and peers. Thus the champagne. In return, he had invited her over to drink a toast. She couldn't help but think, as she struggled through the snow, that she was walking toward some sort of decision. She just wasn't sure what kind.

It had been a long road. She had come from a modest background, without the privilege of money or the arts. Having grown up in a small town, she studied fine arts in Lyon before making her way to Paris as a starving artist, a rather romantic notion until you discover just how hard the penniless existence can be. Reality drove her to obtain a degree in fine art from the Ecole des Beaux-Arts and art history degrees from the Ecole du Louvre and Sorbonne. Valland was determined to be successful in the art capital of Europe. Her first opportunity came at the Jeu de Paume, where she began work as an unpaid volunteer just to be near the art. This was not uncommon; art people were very passionate about their subject and many were willing to work at museums—especially ones as prestigious as the Louvre—for free. Most of these volunteers came from wealthy or aristocratic families; they didn't need the low salary the museum usually provided. Rose Valland, without money and not socially connected, was an exception. She supported herself as an independent teacher—a tutor. In her spare time, she made woodcuts, painted, and studied. She was never promoted at the Jeu de Paume. The French were very particular about the title of "curator"; it could only be used if it was officially bestowed. And Valland knew, after a decade in Paris, how difficult it would be for that honor to be granted her. Still, she was determined to contribute.

And then came the war.

In 1939, she had helped Jacques Jaujard, the patrician director of the National Museums, with the evacuation of France's state-owned artwork. She had fled Paris with the rest of the citizens as the Germans advanced in 1940, stuck in the terrible traffic outside the city as Luftwaffe bombers roared overhead and the cows lowed pitifully in the fields because there was no one left to milk them and relieve their pain. But she had returned as soon as the fighting was over, back to her unpaid position and the museum that had become her home.

And then, in October 1940, her life had changed. With the Nazi occupation only four months old, Jaujard had personally ordered her to stay in the Jeu de Paume to observe the Nazis' activities and report anything important back to him. It was quite a request, to ask a minor employee to remain, *unpaid*, in the hazardous position of spying on the Nazis, but Valland jumped at the chance. She had planned to stay anyway—she was one of the few French staff still coming to the museum every day—but Jaujard's trust lifted her mission to a higher level. It provided the opportunity to contribute in a way that was meaningful for both her and France.

Soon after, Jaujard approached her again with a special project. He and the "good" Nazi Count Wolff-Metternich had negotiated the transfer of looted objects from the German embassy to three rooms at the Louvre. Now those rooms were full. Colonel von Behr and Hermann Bunjes, the corrupted art scholar then in the employ of Wolff-Metternich's Kunstschutz (a convenient cover for a man not yet discovered to be a scoundrel), had come to Jaujard requesting additional storage for confiscated art. It was chaos in those early

days, just after the fall of the city, and every Nazi organization was grabbing what it could. Jaujard saw the
wisdom of consolidating it in one place, so he arranged
to place the Jeu de Paume at the disposal of the Nazi
officials. But with one condition: that the French be
allowed to inventory everything. He wanted Rose Valland to create that inventory.

Sometimes, Rose Valland thought as the snows of
December 1944 floated down around her, *your destiny
is thrust upon you.*

That assignment had not gone well. She was aware,
almost from the start, that something was terribly
wrong. On the first morning of the Nazi occupation
of the Jeu de Paume, November 1, 1940, she arrived
expecting bureaucrats. The Nazis came with an army.[1]
They had it all prepared. She could see that immediately. Truckload after truckload of artwork arrived,
unloaded and carried in by soldiers in uniform under
Colonel von Behr's command. It was stunning to hear,
in that formerly quiet museum, the sound of military
boots and the guttural bellowing of German orders.
Even more stunning to see soldiers with crates lined up
all the way to the front door, and trucks full of crates
lined up outside.

The soldiers returned the next morning. They tore
open the crates with crowbars and passed the paintings
hand-to-hand to the back galleries, where they were
stacked five or six deep against the wall. The activity
was violent, feverish. Paintings were dropped, canvases torn, only natural in such a storm. The officers
shouted only "*Schneller, schneller.*" Faster, faster. When
a room was full, the paintings were stacked in another.

Rose Valland walked the museum in a daze. She saw great works of art, many without frames, others damaged from the hasty moves, and witnessed them trampled beneath German boots. The officers yelled only, "*Schneller, schneller.*" By the end of the day, more than four hundred cases had been offloaded and placed in the museum, many bearing the names of their owners: Rothschild, Wildenstein, David-Weill.

The next day Valland, along with several assistants, set up a desk in a hallway. As the artwork passed by, they wrote down, as quickly as they could, the name, artist, and origin. Vermeer. Rembrandt. Tenier. Renoir. Boucher. Many of the paintings were so well known as to be instantly recognizable, but they passed so quickly she couldn't write them all down. She was deep into her work when suddenly she realized a uniformed man was standing over her, staring down at her list. It was Hermann Bunjes, the corrupt Kunstschutz official who had schemed with von Behr to requisition the museum. He was stern and unkind, very young but already stooped beneath the weight of his perpetual disgust. Bunjes, who had been a minor scholar so much like Rose Valland herself, had sold out everything he believed in for the illusion of Nazi power. He would work hand in hand over the next few years with Lohse and other ERR officials who schemed and stole and abused and threatened. But on that first day he simply looked down at what she was writing—the very inventory he and von Behr had told Jaujard they would accommodate only two days before—and slammed her notebook shut.

"That is enough," he said. Three words, and Jaujard's inventory was finished.

But they didn't throw her out. Colonel von Behr, with the generosity of the untouchable warlord, allowed her to stay as guardian of the museum's permanent collection, which with modern art, like *Whistler's Mother*, was detestable to the Nazis anyway. *Destiny is not one push*, she thought as she waited to cross a quiet street on that cold Paris evening years later, but a thousand small moments that through insight and hard work you line up in the right direction, like a magnet does with metal shavings.

She did not have to wait long for her destiny to arrive—only three days, in fact, after her assignment by Jaujard. On the first, the museum was empty. On the second, it was filled with artwork piled into every nook and cranny. On the third, it housed an exhibition fit for a king. Paintings and tapestries were hung tastefully on the walls, with complementary statuary between them. Couches for viewing were arranged in every gallery, with expensive rugs beneath them on the floor. Champagne on ice sat almost unnoticed in the corners. The guards stood at attention, red armbands and black swastikas against brown uniforms. Colonel von Behr, Hermann Bunjes, and the other leaders of the museum wore uniforms, too; some even wore helmets. Helmets, as if this was an army and they were going to battle. To see all those Nazis in their high polished boots, standing at attention, was an impressive and terrifying sight. They were waiting, Rose Valland knew, for their king.

The man who arrived was not Hitler. And it was not Alfred Rosenberg. The looting operation at the Jeu de Paume may have been run in the name of the Einsatzstab Reichsleiter Rosenberg—Reich Leader

Rosenberg's Special Task Force—but only in name. Rosenberg was a die-hard racist intent only on proving Jewish degeneracy. He had no interest in art. He couldn't see the potential of the blank check Hitler had given him: the right to transport to the Fatherland anything that would aid in his research into Jewish inferiority. Valland remembered one of Rosenberg's rare visits from Berlin to the Jeu de Paume. By that time, late 1942, he must have realized that he had lost control. He shuffled through the museum accompanied only by a few associates. The only accommodations made for his visit were pots of chrysanthemums in some of the rooms. It smelled like a funeral.

It was so different from the visits of the true kingpin who had risen up to exploit the ERR opportunity. For him, personal exhibitions were set up with exquisite care, selected to match his personal taste. Champagne bottles weren't just opened, they were "sabered," a dramatic and theatrical process in which the force of a saber, slid along the body of the bottle toward the neck, snaps the collar from the neck of the bottle, leaving the cork intact but the bottle open. The obsequious ERR officials toasted his tastes and his triumphs, then followed on his heels, hungering for his every compliment and laughing at his foolish jokes. And the kingpin adored the attention, for Hermann Göring, the Nazi Reichsmarschall and Hitler's second in command, was a vain and greedy man.

Rose Valland knew she would always remember his excesses. He had dozens of specially tailored uniforms, most with gold stitching and braided silk, each with more epaulettes, tassels, and medals than the last.

He carried emeralds in his pockets and jingled them with his fingers like other people jingle loose change. He drank only the finest champagne. When he came to rifle the Rothschild jewelry collection in March 1941, he took the two finest pieces and simply shoved them in his pocket, like he was shoplifting licorice whips. When he stole larger works of art, he simply added another railcar to the back of his private train and hauled it away, like Caesar hauling the spoils of war behind his imperial chariot.[2] On the way to Berlin, he would lounge in an enormous red silk kimono weighed down with heavy gold trim.[3] Every morning, he would luxuriate in his red marble bathtub, built extra wide to contain his girth. He hated the rocking of the train. It made his bathwater slop. When Reichsmarschall Göring was in his bath, his train stopped on the tracks. This, in turn, forced the stopping of every other train in the nearby rail system. Only after the Reichsmarschall had bathed could the shipments of armaments, equipment, and soldiers proceed to their various destinations.

But that would come later. On his first day in the Jeu de Paume, in the midst of all the glory set up by the ERR, the rotund Reichsmarschall slouched through the museum in a long brown overcoat, a battered fedora pulled low on his head, dressed in the suit of a dandy accented with a bright colorful scarf. She remembered her first thoughts upon seeing him that day: fat, flamboyant, pretentious, yet strangely mediocre in his tastes.[4]

She would find out why later. In addition to being Reichsmarschall, Göring was the head of the Luftwaffe, the German air force. He had staked his reputation with Hitler on the fact that the Luftwaffe would knock Britain out of the war. When he appeared at the Jeu de Paume on November 3, 1940, the Luftwaffe had been fighting the Battle of Britain for four months, and blitzing London for three. And they were losing. For the first time, the tyrants were losing. And Göring was responsible.

At the same time, Göring's personal battle for the plunder of Western Europe was not going well. For the rapacious Reichsmarschall, this was an equal or perhaps even greater setback than the battle over the English Channel. After the Nazi blitz, the art markets of the Netherlands and France burst open. They were hives of vermin, full of collaborators, opportunists, and shady middlemen with no qualms about stealing, pawning, swindling, and exchanging artwork for visas out of Europe. There were hundreds of Germans with their hands out, trying to take advantage of the upheaval of the century. Göring was ruthless, efficient, and powerful, but he was also conceited and easily duped. He was spending a vast amount of his time and energy dealing with art agents, and he still wasn't getting even half of what he wanted. He had come to Paris to banish his depression with a buying spree.

On this cold winter day at the Jeu de Paume, November 3, 1940, his representatives showed him not just the kind of artwork he coveted; they showed him a new world. That was their genius. They showed him a tiny speck of the riches of France, and how easy it was to attain the rest. Why buy it? Why negotiate and haggle and try to outmaneuver his fellow Nazis when Rosenberg had been given a loophole to steal? In

hindsight, Rose Valland could see that it was all a stage.
Colonel von Behr, Hermann Bunjes, and Göring's personal art curator Walter Andreas Hofer had set it up
for him. They knew what the Reichsmarschall wanted,
and they knew they could give it to him. All they had
to do was show him that now all things were possible.
In their own way, those vile Nazis had also seized their
moment. They had lined up the metal filings of their
own destinies like so many dastardly magnets. They
said to him: We are your men, your organization, and
this is what we can provide. All you have to do is ask.

When Göring returned to the Jeu de Paume two days
later, on November 5, 1940, he was a new man. Valland
could see the wolfish pleasure in his eyes, the triumph.
He discussed the works of art loudly and boastfully
with his experts, espoused the virtues of his favorite
pieces, took paintings off the wall so he could examine
them more closely. By then, in just two days, he had
worked it all out. He even had a proclamation already
drawn. From then on, by order of the Reichsmarschall
and approved by the Führer, Hitler would have first
choice of the ERR confiscations. Göring would have
second choice. Rosenberg was third. Rosenberg complained, of course, but Hitler sided with Göring. They
had no respect for Rosenberg at Nazi headquarters.
The whole world, Valland thought, hated that man.
And of course Hitler was happy with first choice. The
Reichsmarschall, far from alienating himself from the
Führer through his power grab, had ingratiated himself
with his patron. And at the same time, he had gotten
power over the patrimony of France.

After that, the pattern was set. The ERR operation

in Paris, for all intents and purposes, was Göring's personal looting organization. He came twenty-one times to the Jeu de Paume, always feted by personal servants: Colonel von Behr, Hermann Bunjes, and later the reptilian art dealer Bruno Lohse, Göring's personal representative to the ERR. They were drawn in because, in a Nazi world, the position of Reichsmarschall came with all the trappings of power. Real power, the kind where you can make a fortune, take people's lives, and change the world. The men at the Jeu de Paume swallowed it all. They thought they were serving in the court of the king. The greedy Lohse tried to make money wherever possible. The social-climbing von Behr was elevated to the highest ranks of society in occupied Paris. The power-hungry Bunjes was given a position.

When Wolff-Metternich found out Bunjes was undermining the Kunstschutz mission, he fired him. Göring gave Bunjes an officer's commission in the Luftwaffe and named him director of the SS Kunsthistorisches Institut in Paris. Before, Bunjes was a minor functionary and scholar; now he ran a prominent institution. That was the power of the Reichsmarschall. And the corrupt young souls of the Jeu de Paume, Bunjes and Lohse especially, idolized that power.

The wind blew chill down the streets of Paris. Even with her heavy coat, it was so cold that Rose Valland stepped off the sidewalk into the shelter of a doorway. She was close to James Rorimer's apartment, just another block or two, and she really did feel like she was approaching a decision. She lit a cigarette. She lived an ascetic life: small apartment, bare furnishings, not many luxuries or friends. It was part of her protective shell. She had no attachments the Nazis could exploit. She had no close companions to discover her secrets, personal and professional. She was safe. Her closest personal contact, she realized, may very well have been her boss, Jacques Jaujard. She admired him immensely, and would be forever grateful for the opportunity he had given her.

But was Jaujard now pushing her toward Rorimer? It was a question she had puzzled over for a week. The American Monuments Man definitely had Jaujard's trust and admiration. He had pushed them to work together several times, which in turn had led not only to progress in the recovery of Parisian property but to a growing friendship between them.

But could she confide in him? She had spent four years gathering her information. Four years of deprivation. For the first months, it had been nothing but fear. But she had grown into her position. In July 1941, the French curator at the Jeu de Paume fell ill, and Jaujard placed her in charge of the museum in the *paid* position of attaché—and later "Assistante du Jeu de Paume," after all those years as a volunteer! By then, she was running the maintenance staffs for the Nazis, a task that made her indispensable and allowed her free movement throughout the museum. She was also passing information regularly to Jaujard, oftentimes through his loyal secretary Jacqueline Bouchot-Saupique. Sometimes her reports were written on Louvre stationery, most often they were scribbled on whatever slip of paper was available. On occasion they were oral reports conveyed during a brief visit to Jaujard's office. As attaché for the Jeu de Paume, Valland had the right of passage into the Louvre. She knew her homely looks, carefully cultivated during those years, allowed her to slip past the guards without being searched.

In later years, as her fear subsided, she began to accept the risk. The shipping manifests, train numbers, and addresses were too hard to memorize, so she began to take notes. Then she began to take them home at night so she could copy them down, always returning them to their files before the Nazis arrived the next morning. She trolled for information from packers, secretaries, and Nazi officers. She memorized overheard conversations, the Nazis never suspecting that she understood German. The Nazis were fastidious about documentation; they reported and photographed everything. She filched and then developed negatives at night, so she had photographs of them all: Hofer, von Behr, Lohse, and Göring studying looted art. She even had the watchman's logbook. She had information on everyone who had come and gone through those closed halls. And she had lists: of artworks, of traincars, of destinations.

It had cost her so much. Years of sleepless nights. Weeks of terror, subsiding to the dull knowledge that she might never make it out of the occupation alive. Could she really share everything she had learned and gathered with an officer of the U.S. Army?

She stared across the street at a nondescript doorway, watched a bundled woman go trudging by. Instead of the answer to her question, what came was the elation, after all those years, at her ability to make the decision as a free French woman. She recalled that moment of hope when the first shots of resistance rang out on August 19, 1944. Who could forget that date? The Metro workers had gone on strike; then the police; finally the postal service. Everyone expected the uprising any day, but when they heard the first shots...the skies of Paris lifted like the lid off a frying pan. The city resounded with the enthusiasm and joy of its inhabitants. She was at the Louvre with the other curators. They wanted to raise the French flag over the museum. Jaujard said no. Their duty was to protect the collections. They could not risk a German reaction.[5]

She left the Louvre and went to the Jeu de Paume, determined to stay with the art to the end. On the corner outside was a German observation tower. On the steps, the German machine-gun barrels were still hot from firing. All night, German units descended on the Jardin des Tuileries to prepare their defenses. Across the garden from the museum, partisans cut down trees and tore up paving stones to form barricades. From a window on the top floor, she could see Citroën sedans painted with the emblems of the Free French (FFI). But nothing happened; for days, Paris simmered.

The tension broke on the night of August 24. Lightning split the sky; the police rose up. Artillery shells whistled down the Seine. The barrels of the German guns shone red-hot in the thunderstorm. The next day, German soldiers were crouched behind statues in the courtyard of the museum, surrounded by sandbags. She saw them shot dead, one by one. A terrified young soldier became separated from his unit and was gunned down on the museum steps. The rest surrendered. Within two hours, General Leclerc's tanks were lined up on Rue de Rivoli. His troops stacked captured German ammunition and helmets inside the Jeu de Paume while Parisians crowded the terrace, cheering the soldiers down the street.

And then the sound of gunfire, screaming, the crowd tumbling through the doors and windows of the Jeu de Paume. A museum attendant, foolish enough to climb on the roof to watch the arrival of Leclerc, was accused of being a German spotter. She had to plead with several of Leclerc's officers before one finally intervened. When she wouldn't let the mob into the basement, where the Jeu de Paume's permanent collection was stored, they accused her of harboring Germans. Collaborator! Collaborator! A French soldier pressed a gun to her back. As she descended the staircase into the basement, she thought of the young German soldier she had discovered earlier in the day, huddled in one of the sentry boxes. What if they found another? She had wondered, after all she had been through, if this was the way it was going to end. *My duty*, she thought then, as she did now, *is to the art*.

She thought of the near disaster with the art train: priceless artwork sitting on a side track for two months because of a bureaucratic muddle. She was concerned that some members of the art establishment might think that she was selfish. That she was withholding her information to make herself more important. Some were already whispering that she had made it all up, that she didn't have anything worthwhile to share. After all, she was a mere assistant, not even a curator. They suspected she was just trying to make a name for herself.

Maybe they had a point. She had been incensed

when *Le Figaro* ran a story about the art train on October 25 because it gave the French rail system credit for the recovery. She had written Jaujard, reminding him that the article "deprived the National Museums of the merit that they deserve." But her real frustration had been evident in an earlier paragraph. "At a personal level," she had written, "I would deem myself happy if this clarification reestablishes the facts as they are, for without the information I was able to provide, it would have been impossible to report and pinpoint this shipment of stolen paintings among the numerous convoys headed to Germany."[6]

She threw down her cigarette and stared out at the snowy Parisian street. Yes, she wanted credit for the work she had done. Destiny might have placed her in the right place at the right time, but she had seized it. Others had run or hid; some had even turned to the Nazi side. She had risked her life for her principles and her country. It wasn't for personal glory. It never was. She had protected the art. She had stood up for what was right. And the best thing for the artwork, she knew, was to cut through the bureaucracy and the infighting of the French government and go straight to James Rorimer. There simply wasn't time for anything else. The American military would be the first to reach the Nazi repositories in Germany and Austria. Rorimer was the only man she could trust. And Jaujard trusted him, too. She felt sure Jaujard wanted her to go to Rorimer, even if he'd never said so out loud.

She started walking. A few minutes later, she arrived at the American's apartment. Inside, the room was lit by candles because of the nightly blackouts, still a fact of Parisian life. There was a small fire in the hearth; the room was warm. He took her coat and offered her a seat. It was a world away from the frozen reality of the front lines, but intimately connected to it. Sometimes the parameters of a mission are decided in a little back room over a glass of champagne.

In later years, James Rorimer would write that this Christmas meeting was a turning point. Perhaps for him it was, because for the first time Rose Valland gave him a hint of the breadth and scope of the information she possessed: in short, everything the right person would need to find the stolen patrimony of France.

But for Valland, what happened that night was merely another confirmation that James Rorimer was her man. His trust, his insight, his respect and intelligence and bulldog intensity were all on display, as always. It would be difficult for him to understand her sacrifice, she realized sadly, but that was a meaningless personal consideration. She could see that he shared something more important: her sense of purpose. Like Valland, Rorimer believed that his destiny was bound up in the information she possessed.

"Please give me the information," Rorimer said. "Share it with me."

She knew she would. She had of course given her reports and some of her hastily prepared notes to Jacques Jaujard, because that was her obligation. But she was so suspicious of the bureaucracy, because one careless or stubborn person, anywhere in the chain of command, could bring the flow of information to a halt. And that's exactly what happened. Months later, long after the end of the war, photographs provided to

SHAEF by Valland were found shoved in a file drawer in some out-of-the-way office with a bunch of other "useless" documents.

Fortunately, she had another copy of the documents for Rorimer. But she didn't give them to him, at least not in December 1944. She had one more condition. She didn't want Rorimer passing her information to someone else. She didn't know about the good, capable men of the MFAA already on the front lines: Stout, Hancock, Posey, Balfour. But even if she had known about them, it wouldn't have mattered. Valland didn't want Rorimer sharing information, she wanted him using it. And that meant he needed to be at the front.

She had been hinting for weeks, but she tried again. "You're wasted here, James. We need men like you in Germany, not Paris."

"Your information," he said.

She knew he was going to the front. He couldn't resist the challenge . . . and the opportunity. It was only a matter of time. But time was not a luxury they could afford. She had only one trump card to play: her information. Her mind turned. She would have more leverage if she held back; it was safer to wait until she was sure he was going to Germany. Or maybe, she thought, she really did like the attention and respect her secrets brought.

"Rose," he said, grasping her hand lightly.

She turned away. "*Je suis désolée, James,*" she whispered. "*Je ne peux pas.*"

I'm sorry. I can't.

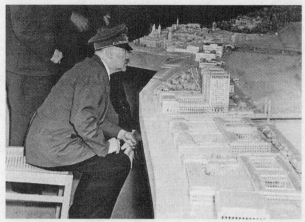

BERLIN, MARCH 1945: Only weeks away from committing suicide, Adolf Hitler periodically escaped the depressing reality of Germany's hopeless military situation by entering the dream world embodied in this scale model of his hometown of Linz, including the Führermuseum. *(Ullstein Bild, Frentz)*

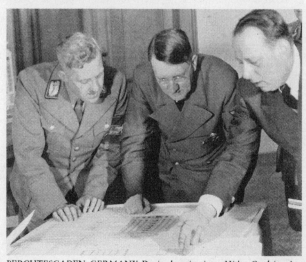

BERCHTESGADEN, GERMANY: During happier times, Hitler, Gauleiter August Eigruber (left), and architect professor Hermann Giesler studied plans for the redesign of Linz. This photo was taken at Hitler's home in Berchtesgaden, known as the "Berghof." *(Walter Frentz Collection, Berlin)*

WESTERN UNION

The filing time shown in the date line on telegrams and day letters is STANDARD TIME at point of origin. Time of receipt is STANDARD TIME at point of destination

```
NA341 70 NT 1 EXTRA=NEWYORK NY 11

DAVID E FINLEY=

    DIRECTOR NATIONAL GALLERY OF ART WASHDC=

AFTER CONSULTATION WITH FINLEY AND OTHERS WE BELIEVE IT
NECESSARY CALL EMERGENCY MEETING ART MUSEUM DIRECTORS AT
METROPOLITAN MUSEUM SATURDAY AND SUNDAY DECEMBER 20 AND 21.
HOPE VERY MUCH YOU CAN COME DISCUSSION WILL BE LIMITED TO
CONCRETE PROPOSALS FOR EMERGENCY. SUGGEST THAT YOU CONSULT
WITH YOUR COMMITTEES BEFORE COMING SO THAT WE WILL KNOW HOW
FAR YOUR TRUSTEES ARE WILLING COOPERATE NATIONAL EMERGENCIES.
SESSIONS OPEN PROMPTLY 10 A.M.=

        FRANCIS HENRY TAYLOR    PRESIDENT.

20 21 10 A.M.
```

THE COMPANY WILL APPRECIATE SUGGESTIONS FROM ITS PATRONS CONCERNING ITS SERVICE

This Western Union telegram alerted prominent museum leaders to the urgent meeting at the Metropolitan Museum of Art in New York City held on December 20, 1941, less than three weeks after the bombing of Pearl Harbor. (*National Gallery of Art, Gallery Archives*)

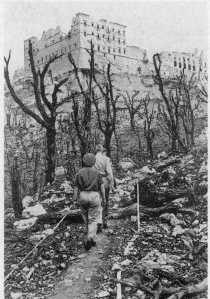

MONTE CASSINO, ITALY, MAY 27, 1944: Monuments Man Lt. Col. Ernest T. Dewald (center) makes his way up to the ruins of Monte Cassino, the Benedictine abbey destroyed by controversial Allied bombing in February 1944. (*National Archives and Records Administration, College Park, MD*)

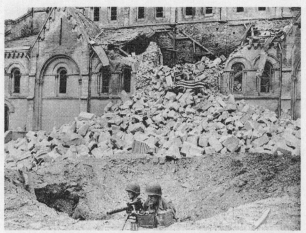

SAINT-LO, FRANCE, JULY 1944: "Covered with the American flag, the body of Maj. Thomas D. Howie (upper center), commander of the Third Battalion, 116th Infantry, rests amid the ruins of the Cathedral of Notre-Dame in Saint-Lô, France. Howie had been killed outside of the city on July 17, by mortar fire, and the task force that entered the city the next day carried his body by ambulance and jeep as a symbol of their comradeship and will to win." This scene of devastation was an all-too-common occurrence in many of the towns and villages of Normandy following the D-Day invasion. *(AP Images/ Harry Harris)*

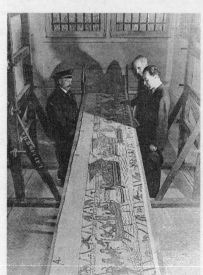

PARIS, AUTUMN 1944: Jacques Jaujard (far right, foreground), director of the National Museums of France, examines the world famous Bayeux Tapestry with W. Verrier, inspector general of French Historical Monuments and attaché of the Louvre (left) in conjunction with its exhibition at the Louvre in late 1944. *(Archives des Musées Nationaux)*

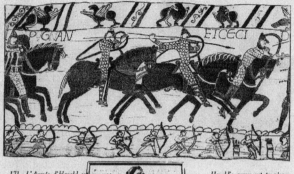

TAPISSERIE DE LA REINE MATHILDE — — THE QUEEN MATHILDA TAPESTRY

171 L'Armée d'Harold est taillée en pièces.   Harold's army cut to pieces. ND

1 JULY

CORRESPONDANCE

DEAR WALKER,
    YOU CAN SCARCELY
IMAGINE THE LIFE. IT'S
WORKING OUT MARVEL-
LOUSLY, BUT WOULD HAVE
BEEN COMPLETELY
RUDDERLESS WITHOUT
THOSE WEEKS WITH YOU.
GOT YOUR DEPOSITS
YESTERDAY. + ALSO
SHIPPED OFF THE FIRST
LONG REPORT. IT MUST
BE VERY HARD FOR YOU
TO GUESS WHERE I AM.
    YOURS, Bancel

ADRESSE
CAPT. L. B. LAFARGE
0-905778
1st CA UNIT ECAD
APO 658 % P.M., N.Y., N.Y.

CAPTAIN
WALKER HANCOCK
SHAEF, G-5
APO 757,
U.S. ARMY

A postcard sent July 1, 1944, from Monuments Man Capt. Bancel LaFarge to fellow Monuments officer Capt. Walker Hancock, advising him of LaFarge's arrival in Bayeux, France. (Walker Hancock Collection)

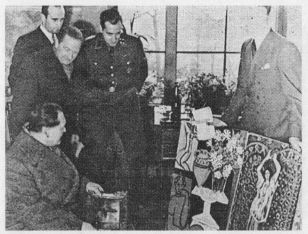

PARIS, DECEMBER 2, 1941: At the Jeu de Paume museum, Reichsmarschall Hermann Göring, painting in his left hand and cigar in his right, sits gazing at two paintings by Henri Matisse being supported by Bruno Lohse. Standing to Göring's left is his art advisor, Walter Andreas Hofer. Note the bottle of champagne on the table at center. Both paintings were stolen from the Paul Rosenberg collection by the Nazis and were recovered and returned after the war. The painting on the left, titled *Marguerites*, today hangs in the Art Institute of Chicago. The other, titled *Danseuse au Tambourin*, is at the Norton Simon Museum in Pasadena, California. *(Archives des Musées Nationaux)*

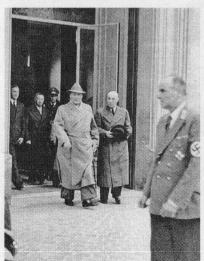

PARIS: Göring departs the Jeu de Paume in Paris after one of his twenty visits to select works of art stolen from French collectors to add to his vast collection. Col. von Behr is in the foreground; Bruno Lohse is standing in the doorway on the left, next to Walter Andreas Hofer. *(Library of Congress, Washington, D.C.)*

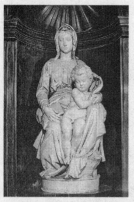

MICHELANGELO, *BRUGES MADONNA*, 1503-04. Marble, H. 121.9 cm (48 in). Notre Dame Cathedral, Bruges, Belgium. *(Scala/Art Resource, NY)*

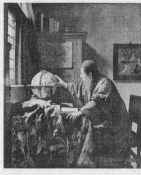

JAN VERMEER, *THE ASTRONOMER*, 1668. Oil on Canvas, 51 x 45 cm (20 x 17¾ in). Louvre, Paris, France. *(Réunion des Musées Nationaux/Art Resource, NY)*

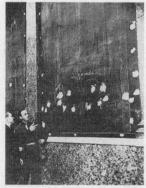

PARIS, SEPTEMBER 12, 1944: Monuments Man James Rorimer (right) and Ecole du Louvre director Robert Rey stand before the empty wall where the *Mona Lisa* (*La Joconde*) once hung before its precautionary evacuation from the Louvre in 1939. *(National Archives and Records Administration, College Park, MD)*

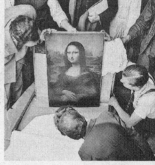

PARIS, 1945: The *Mona Lisa* was moved on six separate occasions from 1939 to 1945 before being uncrated upon its return home to the Louvre. *(Roger-Viollet)*

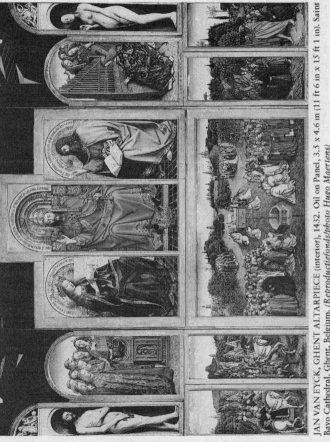

JAN VAN EYCK, GHENT ALTARPIECE (interior), 1432. Oil on Panel, 3.5 x 4.6 m (11 ft 6 in x 15 ft 1 in), Saint Bavo Cathedral, Ghent, Belgium. *(Reproductiefonds/photo Hugo Maertens)*

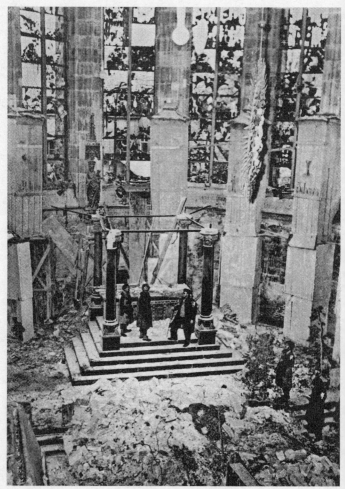

AACHEN, GERMANY, OCTOBER 1944: This was the scene of devastation that greeted Monuments Man Walker Hancock and other troops of U.S. First Army upon their arrival at the Aachen Cathedral on October 25, 1944. *(National Archives and Records Administration, College Park, MD)*

Germany

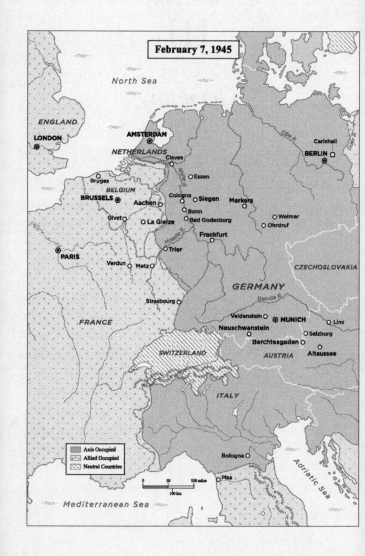

February 7, 1945

North Sea

ENGLAND

LONDON

AMSTERDAM

NETHERLANDS

Cleves

Bruges

BELGIUM

BRUSSELS

Aachen

Givet

La Gleize

Essen

Cologne   Siegen   Merkers

Bonn

Bad Godesburg   Welmar

Ohrdruf

Frankfurt

Carinhall

BERLIN

Elbe R.

Oder R.

Rhine R.

Ruhr R.

Moselle R.

PARIS

Verdun   Metz

Trier

FRANCE

Strasbourg

SWITZERLAND

GERMANY

CZECHOSLOVAKIA

Danube R.

Veldenstein   MUNICH   Linz

Neuschwanstein   Salzburg

Berchtesgaden   Altaussee

AUSTRIA

ITALY

Bologna

Pisa

Adriatic Sea

Mediterranean Sea

Axis Occupied
Allied Occupied
Neutral Countries

0   50   100 miles
100 km

CHAPTER 24

A German Jew in the U.S. Army

Givet, Belgium
January 1945

Every morning, Harry Ettlinger, the last boy to celebrate his bar mitzvah in Karlsruhe, Germany, took a commuter bus from his home in upper Newark, New Jersey, to his high school downtown. After three years in America, his father had finally secured his first job, as a nightwatchman in a luggage factory. The family was so poor that Harry barely noticed the war rationing. But along the bus route, the changes were clear. In the tiny front yards of urban New Jersey, everyone was growing beans, carrots, and cabbage, just as Eleanor Roosevelt was doing on the front lawn of the White House. "Victory gardens," they called them. Even the empty lots had been cleaned by schoolchildren and planted with beans. Those children and their parents now rode "victory bikes," made of reclaimed rubber and metals not needed for the war effort. The bus passed a poster taped to a lightpole: "When you ride alone, you ride with Hitler." It was a plea to use public transportation, or at least to carpool. Harry was glad his family didn't have a car. Nobody drove anymore;

it was almost a sin to consider it. He heard rumors you could be fined if you were caught pleasure-driving with no particular place to go.

The bus entered the industrial section of Newark, where the factories hummed through the night. The bus was always full, even though this route had been mostly empty before the war. At the factory stops it would become completely jammed, not even standing room, with workers coming off the midnight shift at the war factories. He could see them waiting patiently on the sidewalks, mostly older men or women, exhausted but proud. In order to save fabric for tents and uniforms, women wore shorter dresses, and he could see their well-turned legs as they walked home or waited for the next bus. For the same reason, men weren't allowed to wear pants cuffs. He wasn't as impressed with this change.

What he really noticed, though, were the flags. Every factory, and almost every house, flew an American flag. In the residential areas, almost every window also displayed a white banner featuring a blue star and a red border. The banner meant someone in the household was in the service. If the banner featured a gold star and a yellow border, someone in that household had been killed in action.

When he graduated from high school, Harry knew his parents would post one of those blue-and-red banners; probably two, since his brother Klaus planned to join the navy as soon as he turned seventeen. Already, boys had started to drift out of his high school, including the valedictorian, Casimir Cwiakala, who would be shot down over the Pacific. Only a third of the boys in Harry's class, in fact, were planning to attend their graduation ceremony. The rest were already in the army or the navy, training to be pilots, tankers, and infantrymen.

Harry had no desire to avoid the war, but he was also in no rush to enlist. The war wasn't going away; it would always have room for him. Deep inside, that didn't make him comfortable, but his duty to fight was never something he questioned. Like every other young man in the spring of 1944, Harry Ettlinger was going to join the army, be sent overseas, and become a proud, disciplined, terrified soldier. He couldn't imagine his life unfolding any other way. Until then, he had responsibilities. In the morning, he went to high school. After school, he worked in a factory to help support his family. Before the war, Shiman Manufacturing had made jewelry; now it churned out disposable chisels for army dentists.

The draft notice arrived, as expected, soon after graduation, and on August 11, 1944, Harry Ettlinger shipped to basic training. The Allies had broken out at Normandy, and no doubt his mother watched the daily map in the newspaper, the front lines spreading north and east across Europe. Harry and his fellow recruits didn't follow the army's progress. It didn't matter to them. They were going to Europe, they were going to fight, and some of them were going to die. Where exactly that happened wasn't of any consequence.

For now, they were stuck in a place called Macon, Georgia, and their life was rise early, wash and dress, bunks spick and span, breakfast, march here, march there, take an M1 rifle apart and put it back to together, yes sir, no sir, march, eat, march, clean, back to sleep, and rise early and do it all over again. They lived every minute of every day in a ten-man unit, lined up from tallest to shortest (Harry was number four), and that unit seemed their whole world.

In mid-November, near the end of training, Harry Ettlinger was called out of the morning roll-call line. "Are you a United States citizen, Private Ettlinger?" an officer asked him.

"No sir."

"You are a German, is that right, Private?"

"A German Jew, sir."

"How long have you been in this country?"

"Five years, sir."

"Then come with me."

A few hours later, in front of a local Georgia judge, Harry Ettlinger was sworn in as a U.S. citizen. Six weeks later, he was in Givet, Belgium, only a few miles from his native country, awaiting the orders that would send his unit to the front.

Givet was a replacement depot, known to the men as a "repple depple," a staging area for replacement troops being deployed to units that had suffered heavy casualties. At Givet, Harry Ettlinger and a thousand buddies lived in triple bunks in an enormous barn. It was the coldest January on record; the heat from the coal stoves fled straight up while the freezing wind blew freely through the gaps in the old wood facing of the barn. The snow was so thick that Harry never saw a single blade of Belgian grass. The sky didn't clear for two weeks, and when it finally did he stepped outside to see airplanes from horizon to horizon, his first sight of the magnificent Western Allied war machine. The Battle of the Bulge had turned. The Germans had been beaten back at Bastogne and the Ardennes, and the Allies were once again on the advance. But nobody had any illusions. The Germans weren't going to surrender, not until every one of their cities lay flattened and destroyed. Thousands of Allied soldiers were going to die fighting for every inch of soil, and thousands of German soldiers and civilians, too. Clear skies meant bombs, death, and, more important at the moment to the men at Givet, freezing temperatures. That night was one of the coldest of Harry's life.

A few nights later, the orders arrived. The replacement soldiers were moving out. The next morning, more than a hundred trucks were lined up in the snow outside the barn. The officers called out unit numbers, and the men climbed onto the trucks with their bags, guns, and other gear. They had no idea where they were going, only that it was to join the 99th Infantry Division somewhere at the front. Harry was in the fifth truck with the other eight men in his unit (one had mysteriously dropped out), the men he had lived with now for more than five months. They didn't say much to each other as the other trucks in the line were loaded, and they didn't say much when they heard the truck in front of them shift into gear and begin to move out. This was it, they were on their way, together, and they were both excited and afraid.

And then, suddenly, a sergeant was running alongside the convoy, waving his arms for the lead truck to stop. When the trucks ground to a halt, the sergeant walked up and down the line, calling out again and again so that the thousands of men in the trucks could hear: "The following three men get your gear and come with me." Harry was so shocked when he heard his name, he didn't get off the truck.

"That's you," someone said, nudging him.

Harry climbed down and placed his gear on the ground at his feet. Down the line, he saw two more men, out of more than twenty-five hundred, climb off their trucks and throw down their gear. He looked back one last time at the eight men left in his squad, his brothers in arms. Within a month, three of them would be dead. Four others would be seriously wounded. Only one man would make it out of the war unscathed.

"Private Ettlinger, sir." Harry saluted as the sergeant approached. The sergeant nodded, checked the name off his clipboard, then signaled for the convoy to move out. As the trucks rolled away, Harry hefted his bag and started back to the barn, unsure of where he was going or why, but sure that it wasn't to the front. It was January 28, 1945, his nineteenth birthday. Harry Ettlinger would always consider it the best birthday of his life.

CHAPTER 25

Coming Through the Battle

La Gleize, Belgium
February 1, 1945

Walker Hancock arrived in La Gleize, Belgium, on a deadly cold February afternoon. Before the Bulge, he had spent a delightful afternoon here in the company of a kindly hostess and a lovely, unknown sculpture of the Virgin Mary. During the Bulge, he had watched with dismay as the enemy lines advanced west across the map, engulfing Aachen, crossing the Siegfried Line, and finally bulging into Belgium, where they began to slow, then creep, and then finally grind to a halt in the Amblève Valley. Right at the point of stalemate, underneath the pin on the map, was the town of La Gleize. Every time he looked at that pin, he thought of the young woman and the extraordinary Madonna, only weeks earlier so far removed from the war. *Nothing is beyond this war*, he kept thinking, wondering if they had survived. *Nothing is immune.*

Now that the Bulge was over, and the Allies had pushed back the German advance, Walker Hancock was anxious to see what had become of the peaceful little village. Bill Lesley, the first Monuments Man to tour the valley after the Battle of the Bulge, had reported La

Gleize virtually destroyed, but nonetheless Hancock was surprised by the horrid conditions. The houses were all ruined, the stores burned out and abandoned, shattered equipment and spent bullet cartridges lined the streets. The cathedral, battered by heavy artillery, was little more than a shell. It appeared to teeter on the hillside, ready to fall and wipe out the last remnants of the town. Strangely, the door was locked; Hancock entered through a gaping hole in the wall. The roof had been blown apart, and the broken beams swayed in the vicious wind heavy with snow and ice. The pews had been turned over and piled up to form barricades, the chairs tossed. In the wreckage, he saw ammunition, bandages, ration cans, and shreds of uniforms. The Germans had used the cathedral as a fortress, then as a field hospital, and Hancock suspected bodies, perhaps both German and American, were frozen under the snow. *Nothing is beyond this war*, he thought again.

But one thing was: the Madonna. She stood just as he had seen her two months ago, in the middle of the nave, one hand on her heart, the other raised in benediction. She seemed hardly to notice her surroundings, focused as she was on the distant divine. But against that backdrop, she looked more miraculous and hopeful than ever, her beauty triumphant even in the midst of devastation and despair.

The town wasn't abandoned, at least not entirely. As Hancock walked down the icy main road, he noticed a few stragglers, shell-shocked and worn, peeking out from the ruins of their homes. The *curé* of the cathedral was again missing, but a man named Monsieur George, the perfect picture of a war survivor right down to the bloody bandage around his head, offered his assistance.

"I've come for the Madonna," Hancock said, sitting across the table from Monsieur George and his wife in their sparse kitchen. He produced a letter signed by the bishop of Liège, who held authority over this parish. "The bishop has offered the crypt in the seminary at Liège until the end of the war. The weather is bad, I know, but there's no time to lose. I have a truck and a good driver. We can take her today."

Monsieur George frowned. So did his wife. "The Madonna isn't leaving La Gleize. Not today, not ever." In fact, Monsieur George had no desire to even see her moved from the cathedral.

What about the snow, the cold, the wind, the unstable roof? Hancock argued as best he could, but the man would not be moved.

"I'll call a meeting," Monsieur George said eventually, ending the conversation. An hour later, a dozen frowning people—Hancock wondered if this was every living person in town—were crowded into Monsieur George's house, listening to Hancock hopelessly argue his case.

"This house has a good cellar," Monsieur George said finally. "The *curé* stayed with us here during the battle. Though some of us were wounded by bullets that came through the little window, that danger is now past. I propose we bring the Virgin to the cellar."[1]

Hancock wasn't happy, but it seemed the best possible compromise. At least the house wasn't in imminent danger of collapse. "She can't be moved," someone said. "The attachments between her irons and the stone pedestal are unbreakable. I should know. I cemented them together myself."

"Then surely," Hancock replied, "if you did such clever work to bond them, your cleverness can part them, too."

The mason shook his head. "No power under heaven can break that bond. Not even me."

"What about removing the pedestal from the floor?"

The mason thought for a moment. "It might be done."

"She will not be moved," another voice cried out. Hancock turned to see a short, square-jawed man rising from his seat.

"Be reasonable now…" Monsieur George protested, but the man refused to back down. She had survived the battle, he said. She was all that remained of their old lives. She *was* the community now. She was God's grace; their salvation. Who was this outsider, this… American, to tell them what to do? She should stand as she always had, in the cathedral. Even if most of the cathedral was gone.

"I agree with the *notaire*," the mason said.

A few others squirmed. Hancock looked around the room at their gaunt faces and visible bandages. The Madonna wasn't art to them, he realized; it represented their lives, their community, their collective soul. Why hide her in a cellar, they were thinking, when we need her now more than ever? She had triumphed. They couldn't acknowledge, after all they had been through, that the danger could return.

But Hancock knew the danger was already there, at

least for the sculpture, in the form of a splintered roof and badly damaged walls. "Let's go to the cathedral," he suggested. "Perhaps we can find a solution."

The small procession trudged across the empty town, picking its way around snowdrifts, ice clumps, shattered artillery, and debris. Someone had the key so they entered the cathedral through the door, despite the fact that only a few feet away there was no wall. Snow was falling in large flakes and settling on the Madonna. The little party crowded around her, as if warmed by her glow. Hancock looked into her face. Sadness, peace, and maybe surprise.

He started to speak on her behalf, and that's when the roof gave way. With a sudden sawing, a huge piece of wood came crashing to the floor, shattering the stillness. Snow and dust exploded upward in a cloud, and great chunks of ice rained down. As the air cleared and the debris settled, the *notaire* slowly came back into focus, his face as white as the snow. He was standing almost directly under the collapsed beam. It had been a very near miss.

"Well..." Hancock started, as another chunk of ice slid from the roof and hit a few inches from the *notaire*'s foot.

"I propose that the statue be moved to the cellar of the house of Monsieur George," the *notaire* said.[2]

The mason was right, it was impossible to separate the statue from its base. So two broken roof beams were lashed to the stone pedestal, and a few of the men began to rock the statue back and forth to loosen it from the floor. Even though the base of the Madonna was only about four feet tall, it took eight of them to carry her out of the cathedral and down the slippery slope through the center of town. All were stooped by the weight, watching their feet and picking their way carefully through the ice. Hancock wore his combat uniform and helmet; the townspeople wore fedoras and berets, a few of the older men in suits and long coats. A young woman led the procession in a cape and hood. The Madonna rose a full head above them all, solemn and peaceful. It was the strangest parade La Gleize had ever seen.

After the Madonna was safe in the cellar, a young man invited Hancock and his driver to dinner. Accepting gratefully, Hancock was surprised to find himself once again sharing the hospitality of Monsieur Geneen, the farmer-innkeeper whose daughter had entertained and fed him on his first visit to town. Hancock wanted only his K-rations and some hot water to dissolve his coffee powder, but again the family insisted on a full meal. This despite the fact that the rear half of the house was gone, leaving the living area open to the cold. Through one gap, he could see a large pile of grenades, Panzerfauste (handheld antitank rockets), and other live ammunition the family had cleared from the grounds; through the other, nothing but darkness. Everything seemed wrong, unreal. And yet here were the same people, looking older and more tired, but alive and well and spreading before him nothing less than a feast. In all that destruction, freshly cooked meat and vegetables were the most wondrous and unexpected sights of all.

They talked about the failure of the German advance; the ingenuity of the American soldiers; their possible futures. Hancock ate heartily. He looked from face to face, from the gaps in the wall to the pile of explosives to the two small rooms, and finally to the wonderful plate of food before him. A realization hit him.

"This isn't the house I visited before," he said.[3]

Monsieur Geneen put down his fork and folded his hands. "In the middle of the night," he said, "I awoke and from my bed I saw the sky through a shell hole in the wall. And when I began to realize where I was and why I was there I thought to myself, 'Isn't this a hard thing to come to me at my age after a life of unbroken labor! Not even to have four solid walls around me and my family!' Then I remembered that this was not even my house; that my friend who had owned it was dead; that of the house that I myself had built not a wall remained. And I was very sad. And then suddenly the truth came to me. We had come through the battle. During all that time we had enough to eat. We were all well and we could work." He nodded toward his family, then at the two American soldiers seated across the table. "We," he said, "were the lucky ones!"[4]

The battle had passed. Hancock was certain now the fighting would not come back to La Gleize. But out to the east, in Germany, the war was grinding on.

CHAPTER 26

The New Monuments Man

Luxembourg and Western Germany
December 5, 1944–February 24, 1945

In early December 1944, George Stout received word
that several new men would be assigned to the MFAA
for U.S. Twelfth Army Group. They were all enlisted
men intended as assistants to the Monuments officers
in the field, but they were all accomplished cultural
professionals. As usual, it would take weeks to get official assignments for them, but at least he knew more
help was on the way.

Sheldon Keck, assigned by Stout to assist the newest
U.S. Ninth Army Monuments officer, Walter "Hutch"
Huchthausen, was an esteemed art conservator. He had
served as a soldier in the army since 1943, but had only
recently been assigned for monuments duty. Married
with a young son—"Keckie" was only three weeks old
when his father reported for duty—Keck was exactly
the kind of professional man Stout had envisioned for
the conservation effort.

Lamont Moore, a curator at the National Gallery
who had helped evacuate its prized works to the Biltmore Estate in 1941, remained to help George Stout
run the Twelfth Army Group MFAA office, an essen-

tial responsibility since he was so often away on trips to
the front.

Walker Hancock was supposed to receive a ranked
assistant, Corporal Lehman, but his transfer was tied
up in army bureaucracy. For now, Hancock was going
it alone—but with the frequent advice and assistance of
George Stout.

The last new man was, without a doubt, the most
impressive. Private First Class Lincoln Kirstein, thirty-
seven years old, was a well-known and well-connected
intellectual gadfly and cultural impresario. The son of
a self-made businessman who had risen from obscurity
to become an associate of President Roosevelt, Kirstein
had shown extraordinary promise from a young age. As
a Harvard undergraduate in the 1920s, he had started
the Harvard Society for Contemporary Art, a direct
predecessor of the Museum of Modern Art in New
York City. He also cofounded a literary review, *Hound
and Horn*, which was so well respected that it published
original pieces by world-renowned writers like the novelist Alan Tate and the poet e.e. cummings. *Hound and
Horn* also published America's first warning (written
under an assumed name by Alfred Barr, the first director of the new Museum of Modern Art) about Hitler's
attitude toward art.

After graduation, Kirstein became a novelist and
artist. But it was as a patron of the arts, not a cre-
ator of them, that he was to make his name. A highly
respected critic, by his early thirties he was a leading
figure in the New York City cultural scene, counting
among his close friends the poet laureate of the United
States Archibald MacLeish and the writer Christopher

Isherwood, whose chronicle of Nazi Berlin, *I Am a Camera*, would catapult him to international fame (and eventually become the basis for the musical and movie *Cabaret*).

Kirstein's major contribution to the art world, however, had occurred quietly and had, as of the outbreak of war, proved only moderately successful. In 1934, he had convinced the great Russian ballet choreographer George Balanchine to emigrate to the United States. The two men had founded the School of American Ballet, as well as several traveling ballet "caravans" and the American Ballet Company in New York City.

But like everyone else, Kirstein put his plans on hold in 1942. Chronically short of money to support his various projects, unsure of his future, and determined not to become a simple enlisted soldier, he had applied for the Naval Reserves. He was turned down because, like most Jews—as well as blacks, Asians, and southern Europeans—he didn't meet the racially suspect requirement of being at least a third-generation American citizen.[1] He was rejected by the Coast Guard for faulty vision. So he joined the army as a private in February 1943. "At 36 I did with difficulty what wouldn't have been so tough at 26, and fun at 16," he wrote his good friend Archibald MacLeish, then Librarian of Congress, about his experiences in boot camp.[2] To another friend he confessed, "I am an old man and find the going very hard....I am so tired I can't sleep, but I believe they only care if you get 4½ hours....I learned (almost) to shoot and disassemble a rifle, roll away from a not very big tank, do very slow an awful obstacle course and fall into assorted water hazards. I don't think it's fun—although most do."[3] At least, he joked, he managed to lose forty-five pounds.

After completing basic training, Kirstein was rejected for the third, fourth, and fifth time: by the War Department division of counterespionage, Army Intelligence, and finally the Signal Corps. He ended up training to be a combat engineer at Fort Belvoir, Virginia, where he wrote instruction manuals. Bored by the slow pace of the army, Kirstein began documenting artwork created by soldiers, first his fellow combat engineers at Fort Belvoir, then in all branches of the service. With the aid of his many friends and correspondents, the tireless Kirstein built the War Art Project into a full-fledged, army-supported operation. In the fall of 1943, nine paintings and sculptures by soldiers, selected by Lincoln Kirstein, were featured in *Life* magazine. He then organized those works and others into American Battle Art exhibitions to be held at the National Gallery of Art and the Library of Congress in Washington, D.C.

By then, the Roberts Commission had offered Kirstein a position in the MFAA. He wasn't an officer, but the commission had pressed his case because of his outstanding qualifications. Kirstein was torn by his love of the War Art Project and his respect for the importance of the MFAA mission, but in the end he chose conservation and preservation. He arrived in England in June 1944, along with the three other noncommissioned Monuments Men, eager to join an efficient, well-defined military operation.

He found nothing of the sort. The original fifteen Monuments Men were all either in Normandy or awaiting passage across the channel. The base at Shrivenham was filled with civilian experts and Civil Affairs officers, but there was no military structure in place for the MFAA. In fact, with the trained officers on active duty, there was no real MFAA organization at all. Arriving in London, Kirstein and his companions discovered no one had been informed they were coming, and no one they spoke to had ever heard of Monuments, Fine Arts, and Archives. They were told to wait while their paperwork was straightened out. Preoccupied with the battle for Normandy, the army promptly forgot about them.

Kirstein managed to contact Monuments Man James Rorimer, who as a Metropolitan Museum curator mingled in the same New York social arena as Kirstein. Rorimer wrote his wife:[4]

> It's strange to think of men like Lincoln, an author of 6 books and numerous articles, 6 years at Harvard, responsible for the original "Hound and Horn," director of the Amer. Ballet School, etc. still doing fatigue as a private. "Screwy"—we calls it. But then Saroyan is a private. He will make war plays, though. One can hardly expect 10,000,000 or more men to be properly used to the last man. I hardly know what matters most—luck, direction, friends, pull, etc. Certainly ability isn't apt to have a high premium placed on it per se.

Unfortunately for Kirstein, Rorimer was just reaching the end of his own months-long battle for an assignment with the MFAA, and he could do nothing for the brilliant but ignored private. The tireless, well-connected Kirstein managed to get himself transferred to France, and eventually on to Paris, but even there he had no assignment. With nothing else to do, he set up an office on packing crates and woke up early every morning to write letters, poetry, and magazine articles.

He was restless and increasingly depressed by the uselessness of his tasks. This was a common recurrence in his life: manic activity followed by a grinding sense of despair. His manic periods had resulted in astonishing cultural successes, but they usually ended in a gathering gloom and sense of wasted opportunity. These depressive states resulted in a persistent wandering of attention, a seeming inability to stick to things. He was a large, hulking man with deep, penetrating eyes and a hawk nose, the kind who could intimidate paint off a wall with his stare but who could also be a matchlessly charming dinner guest or friend. Beneath his intimidating exterior, Lincoln Kirstein was an insecure, sometimes bullying genius, constantly on the hunt for a creative outlet.

Trapped in the army bureaucracy, Kirstein's mood blackened throughout the early fall of 1944, even as the Allied armies rushed across Europe. In October, in the depth of depression, he began a blistering series of correspondence with the Roberts Commission. Explaining that he had turned down a master sergeancy in the air force to work in the MFAA, he lamented the futility of being a thirty-seven-year-old private and that "Skilton, Moore, Keck and myself were quite simply either too much trouble for the Commission, or else were forgotten....I for one think the behavior of the Commission has been, to put it mildly, callous and insulting."[5] Unless an assignment was forthcoming, he wrote, he had "absolutely no desire to remain on [the personnel] lists."

The letters were only moderately successful. The Roberts Commission wanted Lincoln Kirstein at the front, but had been shocked to discover that military rules didn't allow privates to serve in the MFAA. This necessitated new procedures working their way up and down the chain of command, while the officers at the front ran themselves ragged and their assistants rotted away with nothing to do. Kirstein's orders finally came through in December 1944, more than six months after his arrival in England, and he reported to U.S. Third Army on temporary duty on December 5. The long delay seemed even more frustrating when he discovered how badly the Monuments Men of Twelfth Army Group needed help.

George Stout, who had taught Kirstein at Harvard during his graduate years, was aware of the brilliance of the new private. He was also, probably, aware of his shortcomings: his easy frustration, his mood swings, and his distaste for army life. Whether by accident or design—and knowing Stout it was almost surely by design—Kirstein was assigned the perfect partner: Monuments Man Robert Posey of George Patton's Third Army.

If ever there was an odd couple, it was Posey and Kirstein: a quiet, blue-collar Alabama architect and a manic-depressive, married yet homosexual, Jewish New York bon vivant. Posey was steady, while Kirstein was emotional. Posey was a planner, Kirstein impulsive. Posey was disciplined, his partner outspoken. Posey was thoughtful, but Kirstein was insightful, often brilliantly so. While Posey only requested Hershey's bars from home, Kirstein's care packages included smoked cheeses, artichokes, salmon, and copies of the *New Yorker*. But perhaps most importantly, Posey was a soldier. Kirstein chafed at the rigidity and bureaucracy of the army, and found most officers a frustrating bore. Posey understood and respected the military and its rules. He loved them, in fact. He had been wounded in the Battle of the Bulge, and he had gone immediately back to his duties out of loyalty not just to the mission, but to his fellow soldiers in Third Army. Together, the two men could go a lot further in the army than either could go alone.

There were also more practical reasons to put them together. Posey was one of the most experienced MFAA officers. He understood how the job needed to be done, and he was also an expert on buildings and building materials. But he was not highly cultured or well-read, and he didn't speak any foreign languages. Kirstein's familiarity with the cultures of France and Germany and his extensive knowledge of the fine arts were a perfect complement, and his fluency in French was invaluable. Unfortunately, there was one hole in their armor: Neither of them spoke fluent German, although Kirstein knew enough to get by.

Even though there was no doubt Kirstein was highly qualified for the Monuments job, arguably more qualified than his superior officer Captain Posey, he was still an enlisted man and his tasks included those typical of a newly arrived private: pumping water from a flooded basement; finding a muzzle for a colonel's dog; tracking down and delivering a load of plywood; serving meals; digging latrines; and, of course, writing reports and filing paperwork. The paperwork was the worst. Each sheet had to be typed in eight copies, and if anyone along the line discovered a typo, he had to start all over again. But even that didn't get Lincoln Kirstein down. After seven months of limbo, he was interested, active, and happy to be near the front.

Kirstein received his education in Monuments work at Metz, France. Posey and Kirstein spent the last weeks of January traveling the icy road between Third Army headquarters at Nancy and the citadel town of Metz, which had been captured by Third Army in the fall after a vicious struggle. During the Bulge, Posey told him, the Germans had parachuted troops behind Allied lines dressed in American uniforms. The only way to find them out was to ask questions on strictly American topics, like baseball. The Germans were always clueless.

Not long after, on an excursion down a side road to some out-of-the-way villa or town, Kirstein heard gunfire from the trees. Since they had not quite reached the front lines, he thought it was Allied target practice. He didn't find out until the next day that Germans had been shooting at them. Posey seemed unconcerned; just part of the job. Kirstein wasn't so sure. His only comfort was his realization the old saw must be true: the "Jerries," army slang for Germans, couldn't shoot straight. Still, he never cared much for the back roads after that.

For much of January, at least, they stuck to the main road. Since the end of the Bulge, Robert Posey had been trying to figure out where the treasures of Metz had been taken. This involved primarily interviewing clerks and lesser art officials in the city and the nearby overcrowded Allied prison camp, the true Nazi gangsters having fled east into the Fatherland. It was a tiring exercise given how little these minor functionaries really knew. When pressed, they could usually give only another name, another address of someone that might, just possibly, know something.

This, Lincoln Kirstein learned, was the MFAA grind: finding and interviewing reluctant officials until the right person was found. It was a little like a game of ping-pong: Posey would get a name, find that person, gain a little information and a few more names, find the new people and ask more questions until, through hard work and repetition, he began to figure the situation out. Rarely would the answer come from one source. More often, through a series of mostly unhelpful interviews, a complete picture would slowly, ever so slowly, emerge.

For the most important sources, like Dr. Edward Ewing, an archivist whose name came up repeatedly in interviews, Posey called Twelfth Army Group Monuments Man George Stout. Kirstein would soon realize that Stout, an instigator of the conservation effort as far back as the meeting at the Met in 1941, was the resident expert upon whom all the other Monuments Men relied. If something had to be done, Stout would know the way.

Stout was called on January 15. Two days later he questioned Dr. Ewing, while Kirstein took notes. At first there wasn't much to record. Dr. Ewing sat quietly and answered quickly. German propaganda had long claimed the Allies, and specifically the Americans, planned to confiscate European art and, being too boorish to appreciate it themselves, sell it to the highest bidder. One of the MFAA's most insightful early decisions had been to exclude art dealers from Monuments work, focusing instead on cultural officials in the public and academic sphere. It was a trust of their fellow civil servants that usually won over European art officials, even those who were Nazis. And no one was more trustworthy than George Stout. He exuded knowledge, professionalism, and the pure love of and respect for cultural objects.

Eventually, Ewing began to talk. In the eyes of the Nazis, he told them, Metz was a German town. Germany had lost it to the French at the end of World War I, so that must be its true lineage, yes? Its history was far more complicated than that, of course, but the Nazis liked to keep things simple. He quoted Hitler: "The crowd will succeed in remembering only the simplest concepts repeated a thousand times."[6]

In a course of twenty minutes or so, Ewing opened Kirstein's eyes to the challenges ahead. It was punishable by death, or at least assignment to the Eastern front, which was worse than death, to suggest the Allies could ever breach the Fatherland. Even to prepare for such a possibility was treason. So the art experts in Metz catalogued the treasures but made no provisions to move them. Only when the danger of the Allied advance became undeniable had they begun the evacuation. Ewing didn't call it an evacuation, of course. He called it temporary custody for the safety of the objects, all of which would be returned when Germany won the war.

"The denial is standard," Stout told Kirstein afterward. "The use of the word 'they,' not us. The insistence that someone else committed the crimes. It doesn't matter. Our job isn't to judge; our job is to save the art."

The treasures of Metz had ended up in various locations: a hotel, a cathedral crypt, a mine. Ewing pointed out the towns on a map Stout gave him. Kirstein saw Stout stiffen with interest at only one location: Siegen.

What about the Ghent Altarpiece?

Ewing knew of its appropriation and was sure the altarpiece was still in Germany, possibly in an underground bunker near Koblenz. Or at Göring's residence, Carinhall. Or Hitler's Berghof, in Berchtesgaden. "Or perhaps," he said, "the *Adoration of the Mystic Lamb* was taken to Switzerland, Sweden, or Spain. Honestly, I cannot say."

Kirstein's realization came sometime later, although he could never say exactly where or when. *There is not one type of German*, went the thought. *There are many who were never Nazis, but remained silent out of fear. Nor is there one type of Nazi. There are those who went along to survive, or for career advancement, or out of a sheepish devotion to the status quo. Then there are the hardcases, the true believers. It is possible we will find what we are looking for only when the last true believer is dead.*

CHAPTER 27

George Stout with His Maps

Verdun, France
March 6, 1945

Monuments Man George Stout looked at the battered packages, one stamped "Received in Defective Condition" by the army postmaster. He picked up the first one and turned it over. There was an ominous rattle, as if something had broken in transit. The writing on the shipping label was definitely his wife Margie's, but otherwise the package carried no hint of home. The postmark read early December 1944; it was now March 6, 1945. George Stout was pretty sure he had finally received his Christmas presents. They made him think again how much had changed in three months.

The Bulge, for one thing. And the Western Allied advance. And the bitterly cold winter. And of course his transfer to U.S. Twelfth Army Group, the command group for the bulk of the American army. The transfer had necessitated his leaving the combat zone for France, but at least it provided a warm bed. Not that warm, actually—he cursed his "stiff conscience" all winter because he had balked at picking up a quilted bedroll abandoned by the Germans last fall[1]—but it was far better than the procession of trenches and foxholes the army had used to hopscotch its way to Germany. Back in France, he had even been getting real eggs for breakfast and a little captured wine with dinner. The Twelfth Army Group assignment also offered a desk, a small office, and authority over four armies numbering 1.3 million men—of which exactly nine were frontline MFAA personnel.

It might have been a promotion, but to George Stout the posting felt like his worst nightmare: middle management. France had been all paperwork, meetings, passing messages back and forth from SHAEF to the men at the front. "MFAA administration posts," read a typical diary entry, "vetting, selection, qualifications, pay, tenure, accountability to authority; problem of centralization of museum administration; procedure in microfilming any MFA&A documents in field; information required on MFA&A and other civilian personnel; information on repositories in Germany."[2]

He felt much better since being back at the advanced headquarters at Verdun, France, near the German border and the combat zone. With his move east, the advantages of his position had become clear to him, and he was becoming more and more comfortable with his new role. As the lead MFAA officer, he was no longer limited to the area in front of him. He could travel anywhere in Twelfth Army Group territory—with the proper pass, which could take several days to receive—and as a consequence his officers had begun to call him to important finds. He had recently been in the Amblève Valley of Belgium with Walker Hancock, surveying damage done to the small villages there during the Bulge. At Metz with U.S. Third Army to

interrogate prisoners. In Aachen, Germany, to review
the state of the damage caused by U.S. First Army's
assault on the city in October 1944. He was drawing
the effort together, solidifying it. For the first time, the
men in the field could understand that, at least through
one officer, they were part of a larger organization, and
that they weren't out fighting for Europe's cultural heritage alone. With his unwanted promotion to Twelfth
Army Group, George Stout had become quite by accident the indispensable man, the rock upon which the
northern European monuments conservation effort
was built.

Or perhaps it wasn't an accident at all. Perhaps it was
inevitable. For from the initial meeting in New York
City in December 1941, through Shrivenham, England, and the hedgerows of Normandy and the race to
the German border, George Stout had always been the
indispensable man. The only difference now was that
he had an official position.

And none too soon, because on March 6, 1945, the
toughest work lay ahead. Stout put aside his packages
from home—he would open them later, when he could
truly savor them—and unrolled his map.

British Second Army was on the northern edge of
the advance in the Netherlands. His old roommate, the
British scholar Ronald Balfour, no doubt had the situation well in hand, even though he had yet to locate his
primary objective: Michelangelo's *Bruges Madonna*.

On the southern edge of the advance, U.S. Seventh
Army had not yet been assigned a Monuments Man.
The only consolation Stout could take from that was
that the Seventh was headed for the heavy industrial

region of southwestern Germany, an area with relatively few monuments. They would need a Monuments Man soon, though, and Stout hoped fervently that the officers back at SHAEF had someone exceptional in mind.

Between those two armies lay Stout's command: First, Third, Ninth, and Fifteenth Armies.

The conservation effort in Fifteenth Army was being run by Monuments Man Everett "Bill" Lesley, who had been transferred from First Army.

To the south, in the Moselle River valley, was General Patton's Third Army. On January 29, 1945, Third Army had finally broken through the Siegfried Line outside Metz and was advancing toward the heart of Germany. From what he had seen during the last few weeks, Stout felt confident Posey and Kirstein were the right pair for the job.

Ninth Army, meanwhile, was now responsible, among other things, for holding the important German city of Aachen. Their Monuments Man was Captain Walter Huchthausen, an architecture professor at the University of Minnesota. Stout had never met "Hutch" before his arrival at the front, and he wasn't sure how or when the young man had joined the MFAA. All he knew was that Hutch had been wounded in a Luftwaffe bombing run on London in 1944, which might explain why he hadn't spent time in Shrivenham before D-Day. For all Stout knew, Hutch had been intended for the first wave of Monuments Men.

He certainly had the credentials: knowledgeable, worldly, professional, driven. He had studied architecture as well as design, and he was familiar with European culture. He had recently turned forty, a typical age for a Monuments officer, but Stout couldn't help but think of him as a young man. And it wasn't just the paternal feelings of a superior officer. Hutch had the sandy blond, boyish good looks of an all-American kid, acquired no doubt during his upbringing in the small town of Perry, Oklahoma.

But more than his mild manners and boyish charm, what stood out to George Stout about the new Monuments Man was his dedication. Already, he had organized the citizens of Aachen into a *Bauamt*—building authority—to oversee emergency repairs, and had turned the Suermondt Museum, where back in the fall of 1944 Walker Hancock had discovered the catalogue of German repositories, into a collecting point for artwork found in Ninth Army territory. Now cultural objects were pouring in not just from the field, but from the hiding places ordinary Germans had used to protect them from their own Nazi government. On a recent visit, Stout had seen more altarpieces in the Suermondt Museum than he had imagined existed in the whole Rhineland. And if the Monuments Men had anything to do with it, they would all be inspected, repaired, and given back to their rightful owners.

Stout's primary concern at the moment, though, was First Army, where he had been replaced as lead Monuments Man in December by his colleague Hancock. First Army was finally fighting its way through the forests of western Germany and into the Rhineland, the well-populated area along the Rhine that comprised a major German cultural region. Stout rolled up his large campaign map and unrolled his map of the Rhineland. Every few days, he updated the overlay, so this map was filled with circles and triangles, each marking the rumored location of a German art official or art repository. All were on the German side of the front line, but so many were just across the river, so tantalizingly close. He knew there was a chance the Germans would try to move the artwork farther east as the Allies approached, as they had before Metz and Aachen fell. But packing and transporting that much material took trucks and gasoline and men, all things the Germans couldn't afford to spare. He believed, or hoped, that the objects were still there, just across the Rhine.

He ran his finger south from the major city of Cologne, First Army's next objective, along the Rhine to the big triangle at Bonn. It represented the last known location of Count Franz von Wolff-Metternich, former head of the Kunstschutz in Paris and now *Konservator* of the Rhine Province. Wolff-Metternich was probably one of the most knowledgeable fugitive art officials in Germany, and if reports from Paris could be believed, one of the most likely to cooperate with Allied officials.

But Stout's finger didn't stop at Bonn, just as his mind never stopped thinking ahead to the next step, and the next step, and the one after that. Beyond the Rhine, a few inches to the east, was Siegen.

He tapped the word twice. Siegen. The city came up again and again. At Aachen, at Metz, from other Nazi sources. Stout felt sure an art repository was there, probably a sizable one. It had to be. In every liberated territory, from the Brittany coast to Germany itself, artwork was missing. And not just any art, but works by the immortals—Michelangelo, Raphael,

Rembrandt, Vermeer. They were gone, but they had to be somewhere.

And then there were the religious relics, altars, Torah scrolls, church bells, stained-glass windows, jewelry, archives, tapestries, historic objects, books. Even the trolley cars from the city of Amsterdam were rumored to have been stolen. The variety of items stolen was exceeded only by the volume. After all, five years was an eternity to commit robbery, and there were thousands of people involved in the looting operations: art experts, guards, packers, engineers. Thousands of trains, tens of thousands of gallons of fuel. Could a million objects have been taken? It seemed impossible, but Stout was beginning to think the Nazis had done it. Their appetite for plunder was boundless, and they were, after all, a model of efficiency, economy, and brutality.

But the Nazis, for all their artistic zeal, were not careful conservators, at least not from what he had seen. In Western Europe, the government repositories were clean, well-lit places marked on maps and prepared years, or even hundreds of years, in advance. It took a full year for the British to retrofit their great underground art storage facility at Manod quarry in Wales. Nazi art officials Stout had interrogated in Metz had claimed the Germans only started preparing their repositories in 1944. Most of the stolen works already found by the Allies had been simply stashed in damp basements, where some yellowed and others became covered with mold. The canvases of some paintings were punctured or torn. Objects were improperly crated, or not crated at all. Urgency always seemed to have superseded planning.

What was it Walker Hancock always repeated during their days on the road? *The Germans were wonderfully disciplined and "correct" while they had the upper hand—and went berserk when it was obvious their visit was at an end.*

What if the Germans damaged artwork out of spite? Or destroyed the evidence of their crimes? What if rogue Nazi gangs or common criminals stole prized pieces? After all, works of art were often used as barter for a meal, safe passage, even a life during times of conflict. This was especially true during the Nazi rise to power.

And what if the Nazis did try to move them? Paintings could be destroyed by Allied pilots strafing a column of German trucks, only to discover afterward they contained a sculpture by Michelangelo, not German troops. What if the trucks hit mines? Or got caught in a bombing run? And a new consideration was beginning to loom: The Soviets had launched a two-million-troop advance on the Eastern front. Who was to say they wouldn't get to the artwork first?

Stout thought of his old partner, Squadron Leader Dixon-Spain, who had departed the MFAA contingent but left him one nugget of wisdom: "In war, there is never a reason to hurry."[3] After Cologne, the Monuments Men might very well be in a race: against Hitler, against rogue elements of the Nazi Party, against the Red Army. They would be tempted to run, but they needed to be prepared. Doing something once, and doing it right, was better than doing the same thing quickly but having to do it twice. That was one lesson George Stout had learned quite well over the years.

He put away his maps and turned to his paperwork.

The monthly reports had gone out two days ago to the army. His monthly report to the navy had been dispatched soon after. The report on his recent inspection tour, completed a few days ago, was signed and filed. He had reviewed the field reports for February from Lesley, Posey, Hancock, and Hutch, then tallied the numbers. There were 366 MFAA-protected monuments currently in the occupied zone, but only 253 had been inspected.

Almost four hundred sites, and that was west of the Rhine. Once Twelfth Army Group jumped the Rhine there could easily be a thousand square miles of front, and he still had only nine Monuments officers to cover it. At least they'd finally gotten four men for the enlisted staff. It seemed SHAEF agreed with Dixon-Spain: There was never any need to hurry.

At least he had his old reliable captured Volkswagen; most of the Monuments Men still didn't have their own vehicles. They'd have to be satisfied for now with the new cameras delivered from SHAEF. This time they'd even been given film. The cameras were French hand-me-downs, but they would have to do.

Damn the Germans. Why did they continue to fight? The war had been decided when the Western Allies broke through the Bulge. Everyone knew that. It was not *if* victory now, but *when*—and at what cost… to soldiers, civilians, guilty, innocent, old, young, not to mention historical buildings, monuments, and works of art? Victory on the battlefield was far different than a victory in the preservation of mankind's cultural legacy, and the results would be measured far differently, too. Sometimes Stout felt he was fighting another war entirely, a war within a war, a backward-circling eddy in a downward-rushing stream. *What if we win the war*, he thought, *but lose the last five hundred years of our cultural history on our watch?*

"You ask why the Germans don't give up the fight and stop the slaughter," Stout would write his wife. "You know I have never put that nation on any pedestal and my low esteem of them drops lower as we go along. I think they are immature, mean, and scheming at the top, and immature and incredibly stupid at the bottom. They have nothing to gain by surrender, in their own idiotic view, but by fighting on they can hold up to themselves the illusion of military glory."[4] And yet George Stout would do everything he could to protect German culture.

He looked at his watch. It was past dinnertime, the mess hall was closed. Again. His stomach rumbled, but he knew it wasn't hunger, it was the grippe he'd been suffering for the last few days. Carefully he rolled up his map of Germany, slid it into its tube, and placed it back on the shelf. Then he moved the brown box to the center of the table. It was an artifact from another world, a connection with his old life, and he stared at it fondly. Finally, he removed the tape and opened the flaps. Inside, surrounded by wrapped gifts, was a fruitcake. He thought of his kitchen back home, and of his wife over the mixing bowl, and of his sons—one still clutching his mother's apron strings, the other recently enlisted in the navy. He believed in duty and honor, but like everyone, he was homesick. He wanted to break off a chunk of the fruitcake and shove it into his mouth, but propriety told him a knife was better. He pulled out his dagger and carefully cut himself a slice. The cake was still good, moist and delicious. *It is amazing how the world can change*, he thought, *during the life span of a fruitcake.*

That night, as he often did at the end of a long day, he picked up his pen.[5]

Dear Margie:

It's half past eight and I've knocked off work for the day except for a telephone call I'm waiting on. And while waiting I take the great pleasure to report that your two Christmas packages reached me this afternoon. They got somewhat battered...but it all made me very happy. The fruit cake was entirely unharmed and is now largely consumed. They were very nice things. I needed the socks, I relish everything else. Bertha's handkerchief nearly made me bawl; and all the pretty ribbons and wrappings. The Christmas candle is not a frill. They are valuable things and hard to get....

There is a lot to do. Right at the moment we're pushed somewhat, but it will get itself worked out. In methodical procedure these things straighten out. And there's always the comfort of knowing that you're dealing with the necessities of a situation and not with the vagaries of some fool's whim. It was that latter which always got me down at the Fogg. I wonder what it will be like next.

Thank you darling.
Love,
George

CHAPTER 28

Art on the Move

Göring's Estate at Carinhall
March 13, 1945

The Soviet Red Army, having wrested Poland from Nazi control, crossed the Oder River into Germany on February 8, 1945. Days before, a line of buses and trucks had begun an evacuation from Carinhall, Hermann Göring's hunting lodge/art gallery/imperial palace located in the Schorfheide Forest northeast of Berlin. At a nearby train station, the evacuated items were loaded for transport on the rail system, filling both of Göring's private trains, plus eleven extra boxcars. The shipment was predominantly art.

A month later, on March 13, 1945, Walter Andreas Hofer, the man in charge of Göring's art collection, filled a second train with more of the Reichsmarschall's precious art collection. Göring, more concerned with the fate of his personal possessions than the loss of eastern Germany, had visited Carinhall personally and chosen the pieces to be sent in each shipment. His inclination had been to leave behind the artwork he had acquired through his ERR operation in Paris. Göring prided himself on his honesty, and these pieces—viewed from a certain perspective—might appear less than legitimately acquired. Hofer had argued vehemently with the Reichsmarschall and eventually had won out. Most of the works that had made their way from the Jeu de Paume to Carinhall were now en route, along with hundreds of others, to Göring residences farther south, away from the Red Army.

Several astonishing small paintings—including six by Hans Memling and one by Rogier van der Weyden—went with him and his wife. They were her financial safety net, Göring told her, in case of disaster. She also carried with her the Reichsmarschall's prized possession, Jan Vermeer's *Christ with the Woman Taken in Adultery*. Having lost out to Hitler on two previously available Vermeers (of only thirty-eight believed at the time to have been painted by the master), Göring wasn't about to let this one slip through his hands. He had traded an astonishing number of valuable paintings for it: 150.

Other pieces remained behind. After years of "acquisitions"—Hofer could not bring himself to even *think* the word "looting"—the Reichsmarschall had amassed thousands of valuable artworks. The walls of his galleries and living quarters at Carinhall had been lined with paintings, sometimes with two or three hanging right above each other because of a chronic lack of space. Paintings had even been clustered over doorways and around the furniture, with little attention to period or style. It was a frankly ostentatious display of abundance over quality, for the Reichsmarschall had no eye for true genius. Most art dealers in Europe knew he couldn't resist a famous name and pawned off on the unsuspecting Nazi inferior works by well-known artists. He had thirty paintings by Dutch master Jacob van Ruisdael, almost an equal number of works by the Frenchman François Boucher, and more than forty paintings by the Dutch artist Jan van Goyen. He possessed a staggering sixty paintings by his favorite artist, the great German master Lucas Cranach the Elder.[1] Hofer had helped him deepen and enhance the collection, moving the lesser-quality works to Göring's secondary residences at Veldenstein and Mauterndorf, and storing the best of his collection in the air raid bunker at Kurfürst, but there was still no chance that two trains, even extra-long trains, could empty the volume of art treasures of Carinhall. With the Red Army less than fifty miles away, Hofer knew the second shipment might very well be the last train out, and the thought of leaving all that art behind made him sick.

A final shipment would eventually take shape in early April, but even after those traincars were packed Carinhall wasn't empty. Much of the heavier statuary and decorative works had been buried on the grounds. A few exceptionally large paintings and numerous pieces of ERR-looted furniture were still in the vast rooms. The body of Göring's first wife, Carin, for whom the estate was named, was left buried in the nearby forest.[2] The artifacts were joined on the estate by several hundred pounds of explosives. On Göring's orders, Luftwaffe experts had rigged the estate for destruction. The Reichsmarschall had no intention of letting his prized possessions fall into Soviet hands—even if that meant blowing up his imperial hall and everything left in it.

CHAPTER 29

Two Turning Points

Cleves, Germany
March 10, 1945

∗

Paris, France
March 14, 1945

In Cleves, Germany, Ronald Balfour, the British Monuments officer attached to First Canadian Army on the northern flank of the Western Allied advance, inspected the packing and crating of the treasures of Christ the King Church, which had been heavily bombed and was in danger of collapse. Supplies were tight, as always, and the only transportation available in the city was a wooden handcart. Now four German civilians had to pull the loaded handcart to the Cleves train station for temporary evacuation.

This would be a lot easier with a truck, Balfour thought. But since his truck accident in late November 1944, which knocked him out of commission for almost two months, things had gotten complicated. The two officers he knew at First Canadian Army headquarters had been replaced, and the new men always had an excuse. First they said the army didn't have any spare vehicles. Then he was told he couldn't get a new truck because he had lost the old one. He found the old truck in the camp lot, only to be told that locating the old truck wasn't enough; he needed a "BLR certificate"—whatever that was!—to requisition a new one. The new officers, of course, refused to give him a BLR certificate. He finally received one, but he was never given a truck since the latest allocation of vehicles didn't include any for the MFAA.

Meanwhile, he had heard nothing about the *Bruges Madonna*. This wasn't surprising given the chaotic situation in Belgium. In some weird way, the absence of information merely added to the intrigue of this particular work. It seemed appropriate, as the statue had long been shrouded in secrecy. Michelangelo had insisted, as an item of the sale, that no one be allowed to view it without permission. In other words, it could not be simply placed out for public viewing. Some scholars thought this was out of shame at the quality of the finished product, but there's a more likely explanation. The sculpture had been promised to the pope, but was sold secretly to a Flemish merchant family, the Mouscrons, when the young Michelangelo, only in his early twenties, received a financial offer he couldn't refuse.[1]

The Mouscrons spirited the sculpture out of Italy to their hometown of Bruges in 1506. In the 1400s, Bruges had been a center of commerce and the home of three of Belgium's most celebrated artists—the Van Eyck brothers, creators of Hitler's coveted Ghent Altarpiece, and Hans Memling, a Göring favorite. But by 1506 the city had begun a rapid decline in importance as its harbor, vital to commerce during that era, silted up and became impractical for shipping. Stuck

in a floundering northern European city, where the
city's inhabitants had never even heard of a young artist named Michelangelo, the *Madonna* dropped into
obscurity. The famous artist biographer Giorgio Vasari,
writing in the mid-1500s, knew so little about the
statue—the master's only work located outside Italy
during his lifetime—that he thought it was made of
bronze, not white marble.

And yet to look at the *Madonna*—the beautiful
face of the Virgin, the carved robes so reminiscent of
Michelangelo's contemporary masterpiece the *Pietà*,
the Christ Child not cradled in his mother's arms, but
standing within the folds of her gown, still protected
by her—was to know immediately you were in the presence of greatness. By the 1600s, with Michelangelo
elevated to exalted status, the Belgians had come to
regard the statue as a national treasure, and a century
later the French had begun to covet its glory. In 1794,
after conquering Belgium in the Napoleonic Wars, they
demanded that the *Bruges Madonna* be shipped to
Paris. It was returned only after the defeat of Napoleon
two decades later. Would the *Madonna*, and the world,
be as lucky this time?

The answer, Ronald Balfour had believed, lay in
Flushing, Holland, a port city near the outlet of the
Rhine. If evacuated by sea—and how else would it have
gone with the Allies blocking the roads and rails and
the piece too heavy for many airplanes?—the *Bruges
Madonna* would have had to travel through Flushing. Balfour had been making enquiries all along the
Rhine, with little success. Flushing, he felt, was his last
good chance to generate a solid lead. But it took him

until the last few days of February to reach the city, and by then the trail was cold. The Dutch knew nothing. Any German official high enough placed to know of the shipment had fled. The *Madonna*, moving east, had eluded his grasp again.

But the disappointment he felt in Flushing was relieved, to some extent, in Cleves. It was still cold, but the snows of early March made the historic town, the home of Henry VIII's fourth wife, Anne of Cleves, more beautiful. He had a scholar's appreciation for historic papers, and it was a personal honor to rescue the archives and treasures of Cleves. He looked across the street at the four Germans pulling the cartload of gold chalices, silk robes, and silver relics. The world might marvel at such grandeur, but Balfour would trade it all for the soft warmth of old paper.

Balfour looked up and noticed the train station was now only half a block ahead. "Hold on," he called to Hachmann, the sexton of Christ the King Church, who was following the cartload on the other side of the street. "I'll be right over." Out of habit he looked both ways, although there was no traffic in the deserted town. And then, just as he stepped off the curb, the world exploded.

Across the street, the sexton staggered from the effect of the blast. A cloud of smoke engulfed him, and his ears rang like fire alarms. As the smoke cleared, the world came rushing back. The buildings stood as they always had, but he was alone in the street. The four Germans had lunged for shelter. A dozen yards away, Monuments officer Ronald Balfour was leaning against a railing, covered in blood.

———————

On March 14, 1944, four days after the explosion in
Cleves and the day after the second evacuation of Carinhall, recently promoted First Lieutenant James Rorimer
rode his bicycle to Rose Valland's apartment in the fifth
arrondissement, an ancient section of Paris known as
the Latin Quarter. The quarter had been popular with
tourists before the war, but few tourists, Rorimer suspected, had ever visited Valland's middle-class residential area, a lonely and secluded stretch just beyond the
site of a massive fire started by German bombardment
in August 1944. As he used his flashlight to navigate
the dark stairwell—even seven months after liberation
there was still no electricity in parts of Paris—Rorimer
was reminded of how easy it would have been for the
Nazis to make Rose Valland disappear.

He was heading to the front. Finally. He had discussed a transfer with his superior officers on December
28, 1944, just after his conversation with Valland over
champagne. He had not been surprised to discover the
French had already approached the Americans suggesting just such a transfer, especially as he recalled hearing that when Jaujard held a reunion of his staff at the
Louvre on August 26, 1944, and described Rorimer's
early entry into Paris, tears were said to have flowed.[2]
He was sure this long-hoped-for development was the
behind-the-scenes work of Jacques Jaujard and Rose
Valland. She had been telling him he was needed at the
front, and he knew her well enough to know that, in
her low-key, unobtrusive way, she had been advocating

his transfer within her own bureaucracy as well. Still, it had taken more than two months, until March 1, 1945, for Rorimer to receive official word that he would soon become the Monuments officer for U.S. Seventh Army.

Valland called him soon after, and invited him to her apartment. For the last few months, she had been ladling information to him in dribs and drabs. Rorimer had wanted to know everything, and Valland knew that. But as their relationship evolved, he accepted that she would provide him the information he wanted and needed, when needed, not sooner. The more he learned, the more excited he became. He had visited Lohse's apartment in Paris with Valland, but it had been taken over by a French colonel who knew nothing of the previous tenant. Undaunted, he returned the next day and spent an hour outside the building trying to "fix" the flat tire of his bicycle, from which he had removed the air. But this wasn't a movie, and no one suspicious entered or left the building.

This time, when he arrived at Rose Valland's apartment he could sense a change in her demeanor. She knew about his assignment to U.S. Seventh Army; she was almost as excited as he was. She had all the information he needed.

"Here is Rosenberg," she said, showing him the first photograph in a large stack, "the man Hitler selected to oversee the spiritual and philosophic training of the Nazis. In other words, the chief racist."

He was sitting in her living room, which was lit only by the small fire and one dim bulb. There were flowers in a vase on the coffee table; a bottle of cognac on the bureau. As Valland showed him each photograph— Göring, Lohse, von Behr, and the other key Nazi and ERR figures—Rorimer tried to appear interested in the small cakes she had baked for his visit. But the ordinary nature of the scene could not diminish the extraordinary nature of the discoveries.

She showed him more photographs of Göring, inspecting artwork with Walter Andreas Hofer, Bruno Lohse, and Colonel von Behr at his side. In another he was manhandling a small landscape, a silk scarf around his neck and a cigar in his hand. There was Lohse handing his patron a painting; von Behr in uniform behind his enormous desk, his lackeys sitting on the nearby chairs. Usually, Rorimer recognized them before she even told him their names. He knew them, he realized, because Valland had spoken about them so descriptively many times before.

She's grooming me, he thought. *She's been grooming me all along.*[3]

She disappeared and came back with more material. Receipts, copies of train manifestos, everything the Western Allies would need to prove which items had been stolen and shipped to Germany through the Jeu de Paume. She got up and returned with another stack: photographs of some of the works themselves, many stripped of their frames for ease of transport and hung carefully on the walls. Behind a curtain out of sight, another photograph showed artwork squeezed onto every inch of wall space and stuffed viewing stands.

"Vermeer's *Astronomer*," Valland said, stopping on one particularly important work. "Stolen by the ERR right off the wall of Edouard de Rothschild's sitting room. Göring had a mania for paintings by Vermeer."

Even after everything he had seen, Rorimer was stunned. *The Astronomer* was one of those rare works that had become an acknowledged masterpiece.

"This went into Göring's private collection?"

"No. This one went to Hitler. They say he coveted it more than any work in France. So Göring sent it to him in November 1940, soon after he decided to assume control of the ERR operations from Rosenberg. Göring wanted to prove to Hitler the operation would redound to the glory of Germany, and that the very best works, those reserved for the Führer, were being located and transported home. Many others, though, went into Göring's private collection."

"And the rest?"

"They burned some of them," she said. "In the summer of 1943. Mostly works by modern masters, considered by the Nazis degenerate for their depictions of the world. They kept several they thought could be sold. The 'worthless' pieces were slashed with knives and trucked to the Jeu de Paume, then burned in the adjacent gardens. I would estimate one military truck full, about five or six hundred works. Klee, Miró, Max Ernst, Picasso. The frames and stretchers crackled first. Then the paintings would explode into flame, burn hotly, and dwindle swiftly into ash. It was impossible to save anything."[4]

"Just like Berlin in 1938," Rorimer said, remembering a bonfire of modern art that had, in those more innocent times, shocked the world. By now the world understood there was nothing the Nazis wouldn't do.

"What about the rest?" he said.

Valland got up and went to her bedroom. When she returned, she had yet another stack of evidence. "The rest is in Germany," she said, handing him documents on the Nazi art repositories at Heilbronn, Buxheim, Hohenschwangau, all names he had heard from her before. As she explained their locations and importance, Rorimer had a realization: the repositories were in southern Germany, which meant they were all going to fall into Seventh Army territory. His army. His territory. Suddenly, he could feel the weight. For more than four years, the preservation of these treasures had been Rose Valland's responsibility; today, she was sharing that burden—that privilege, that obligation—with him.

She picked up a photograph and handed it to him. It didn't require an extensive knowledge of art history for Rorimer to immediately recognize the soaring fairytale towers of the enormous castle at Neuschwanstein.

"At this castle," Valland said, "the Nazis have gathered thousands of works of art stolen from France. Get there, and you will find all the records and documentation of the ERR along with the works of art." She paused. "I only hope the Nazis will not make our treasures suffer for their defeat."

Rorimer stared at the photograph. The world knew Neuschwanstein as the great romantic folly of Mad Ludwig, a nineteenth-century king of Bavaria. Valland was telling him it was perhaps the greatest treasure house in the world. But Neuschwanstein was high on a rocky outcrop in the Bavarian Alps, isolated and barely accessible to modern vehicles. It would take a tremendous effort to transport hundreds of heavy crates containing works of art to such a location, so much of which would have to be carried, much less the twenty thousand pieces Valland had documented moving through the Jeu de Paume.

"How can you be sure?" he said finally.

"Trust me," Rose Valland replied. "This is more than a woman's intuition."[5]

CHAPTER 30

Hitler's Nero Decree

Berlin, Germany
March 18–19, 1945

Albert Speer, Hitler's personal architect and the Nazi minister of armaments and war production, was at a loss. Speer was not an early joiner of the Nazi Party—he was official party member number 474,481—but he had been close with Hitler since the mid-1930s. The Führer fancied himself an amateur architect, after all, and always had a special fondness for fellow "artists." In their decade of working together, Speer had never disobeyed a direct order. But recently, Hitler had developed a plan to destroy Germany's infrastructure—bridges, railroads, factories, warehouses, anything to impede the progress of the enemy. For weeks, Speer had successfully argued for prudence and restraint.

Then on March 18, 1945, Speer received word that four officers had been executed on Hitler's orders because they had not blown up the bridge at Remagen, allowing the Western Allies their first advance across the Rhine. Fearing the failure at Remagen was the excuse the Führer needed to implement his "scorched earth" policy, Speer hurriedly composed a twenty-two-page memo on the apocalyptic effects of the planned destruction. "If the numerous railroad bridges over the smaller canals and valleys, or the viaducts, are blown up," he wrote the Führer, "the Ruhr area will be unable to handle even the production needed for repairing the bridges."[1] He was even more pessimistic about the effect on German cities. "The planned demolition of the bridges in Berlin would cut off the city's food supply, and industrial production and human life in this city would be rendered impossible for years to come. Such demolitions would mean the death of Berlin."

On March 19, only one day later, he received the Führer's response. It came in the form of a command to all military officers:[2]

The Führer
Führer's Headquarters
March 19, 1945

The struggle for the very existence of our people forces us to seize any means which can weaken the combat readiness of our enemy and prevent him from advancing. Every opportunity, direct or indirect, to inflict the most lasting possible damage on the enemy's striking power must be used to the utmost. It is a mistake to believe that when we win back the lost territories we will be able to retrieve and use these transportation, communications, production, and supply facilities that have not been destroyed or have been temporarily crippled; when the enemy withdraws he will leave us only scorched earth and will show no consideration for the welfare of the population.

Therefore, I order:

1. All military, transportation, communications, industrial, and food-supply facilities, as well as all resources within the Reich which the enemy might use either immediately or in the foreseeable future for continuing the war, are to be destroyed.

2. Those responsible for these measures are: the military commands for all military objects, including the transportation and communications installations; the Gauleiters and defense commissioners for all industrial and supply facilities, as well as other resources. When necessary, the troops are to assist the Gauleiters and the defense commissioners in carrying out their task.

3. These orders are to be communicated at once to all troop commanders; contrary instructions are invalid.

Adolf Hitler

CHAPTER 31

First Army Across the Rhine

Cologne, Germany, and Bonn, Germany
March 10–20, 1945

Walker Hancock, the Monuments Man for U.S.
First Army, pushed down on the accelerator, urging the
jeep through the outskirts of Bonn, Germany. For the
last several days, he had been traveling with his new boss
(and former colleague) George Stout, and it was exhila-
rating to share both his company and his expertise. In
Aachen, Hancock walked the city. On one block was an
open restaurant, a few people on the sidewalk, one with
a bag of groceries on her hip. Around the next corner,
Aachen was a dead city, a graveyard of snapped wires,
rusted metal, and rubble filthy with dog droppings.
He imagined, looking down some streets, that no one
would ever come back. Perhaps, he thought, they were
all dead. At that moment, he had thought Aachen was
as bad as it could get. Then he saw Cologne.

As a matter of policy, Germany was being pounded
into submission. Hancock knew that fact, had heard it
many times, but didn't understand what "massive aerial
bombardment" meant until he entered Cologne. The
city had been hit by repeated Allied bombing runs—
262 to be precise, although Walker Hancock had no

way of knowing that—and the downtown area had been decimated. Not broken, but gone, knocked to the ground and then hit again and again until it was pulverized. It was "more devastation," he wrote Saima, "than is possible for the human imagination to grasp."[1] George Stout estimated 75 percent of the monuments in the area were destroyed, but that didn't tell the whole story. Those spared were on the outskirts of town. In the center of the city, there wasn't even anything to examine. The only thing standing was the cathedral, the Dom, untouched in the middle of a wasteland. It should have been an inspiring sight, an example of Western Allied compassion, but Hancock couldn't see it that way. The scale of the destruction—the brutality of the Allied campaign to break the German will—was painful to contemplate. It was almost as if there was a message in this madness. *We could have spared any building*, the untouched cathedral seemed to imply. *This is the only one we chose.*

"All this has made me spend more time," Hancock confessed to Saima, "escaping in my thoughts to *our* world, *our* plans and our hopes. Somehow they seem more actual to me than what my eyes have been seeing."[2]

The Allies were angry. There was no other conclusion. The Allies were angry at Germany and everything in it. The anger had been building for months, maybe since Normandy, but it had accelerated during the terrible winter. Before the war, Cologne had a population of nearly 800,000; Hancock figured there were fewer than 40,000 citizens still left in the city. Those left seemed scarred and bitter, or worse. "I felt [their] bitterness, hatred, the way you feel a raw, north gale," Stout would write of the citizens of Cologne. "Out of curiosity, I kept looking for some kind of feeling in their faces. It seemed always the same. A kind of hate and something like despair—or else a blank."[3]

Looking at those blank and broken faces, Walker Hancock thought of Saima, and of their plans to build a house (he was saving his army paychecks), to settle down, to have a family. He couldn't help but wonder: If he had dinner with a family in Cologne, would he feel the same about them as he had about Monsieur Geneen and his family in La Gleize? Or were his feelings tied to the fact that Geneen was Belgian, a victim, and not an aggressor?

The thought came back to him, as it often did: To save the culture of your allies is a small thing. To cherish the culture of your enemy, to risk your life and the life of other men to save it, to give it all back to them as soon as the battle was won...it was unheard of, but that is exactly what Walker Hancock and the other Monuments Men intended to do.

The treasures of Aachen lay out there somewhere. It was his duty to find them. But he wouldn't drive himself like this, he knew, just for duty. Success took conviction, a belief that the Monuments mission was not only right, but *necessary*. It couldn't be just a duty; it had to be a passion. And the more Hancock saw of destruction, the more passionate he became.

Cologne had produced no clues. The movable works of art were gone, evacuated before the worst of the destruction. He and Stout had arrived with the names of a few local officials, culled from past interviews in other broken cities, but none could be found. The monuments were dust. After only a day, Stout left to inspect some smaller towns in the area; Hancock headed to Bonn and the last known office of the former Paris Kunstschutz leader Count Wolff-Metternich. Word had filtered up from Paris that Wolff-Metternich was a good man, that he had been not just sympathetic but active in the French cause. In fact, he had lost his position for siding one too many times with the French against his Nazi bosses. If anyone had information, it would be him. And if he was gone, there was always the paperwork. The Nazis were fastidious about paperwork. The long months of not knowing, Hancock felt, were coming to an end.

On the outskirts of Bonn, the sun was shining. The buildings were untouched. But like so many other cities, the farther toward the center he drove, the more damage he saw. The town center was mostly destroyed, the result of Western Allied bombing runs, but even here he saw cherry trees in bloom, twisting up among the ruins. He stopped outside an eighteenth-century house. The arched stone doorway was just a few feet from the street, spiral metal grillwork hanging from the keystone but the door open for access. Entering the dark hallway, he ascended a small wooden staircase and moments later stood awestruck in the tiny upper room where Ludwig van Beethoven had been born. In the countryside outside town, he had seen peasants with their whole lives loaded on rickety carts, coal mines on fire, the world black from their smoke. But this sanctuary, this artistic reliquary, stood. He thought of the cherry trees among the ruins. Even in Germany, slivers of hope and beauty—and happiness, and art—survived.

The office of the *Konservator* was in a neighborhood that had been ignored by Allied pilots. Hancock felt confident, jubilant even, filled with the peace of Beethoven's room. Then he turned the corner and saw the gap in the row of houses. He didn't need to check the address; he knew immediately what had happened. Only one building on the block had been leveled, and it was 9 Bachstrasse, the office of the *Konservator*. What had he been thinking? Of course the Nazis would blow it up rather than letting it fall into enemy hands. Hancock sat in his jeep in dismay and frustration. Then he fastened on his helmet and began to knock on doors.

"*Nein. Nein.*" Nobody wanted to talk. "*Wir wissen nichts.*" They had nothing to say.

He finally found a man willing to speak to him, but he didn't know much about the building, only that it had been an office and that it was destroyed by a bomb.

What about paperwork, he asked? Files? Inventories? The man shrugged. He didn't know. He assumed it had been moved. "They left weeks ago for Westphalia," he said. "They took everything."

Hancock frowned. Westphalia was still behind enemy lines. And when the Allies got there, he had no doubt Wolff-Metternich and his files would again be gone.

"I know of one man who stayed," the man continued. "An architect, the assistant to the *Konservator*. He's in Bad Godesberg. His name is Weyres."

"Thank you," Hancock said with relief. No dead

ends, at least not yet. He started to turn away, but the man stopped him.

"Do you want his address?"

Walker Hancock called his boss, George Stout, from Bonn. Stout had just received devastating news. His old roommate, British Monuments Man Ronald Balfour, had been killed by shrapnel to the spine while working in the German town of Cleves.

Walker Hancock didn't know Balfour well, but he no doubt felt the sudden shock at the loss of a brother in the Monuments mission. He remembered his wry smile from their days in Shrivenham, the glint off his scholar's glasses, the surprising force that moved his small frame. The "gentleman scholar" had been a true gentleman, a good bloke for a pint. But Hancock hadn't known him, not really. He wondered if the dead man left a wife, a child, a grieving parent, a string of unfulfilled promises or lost desires.

Walker Hancock thought of his beloved Saima, his bride now for more than a year, although they had spent only a few short weeks together as man and wife. Balfour's death was a reminder of the danger of the mission; his time apart from her, he knew, could very well be more than a temporary respite than the long life of love and happiness he hoped for.

And Balfour's death no doubt reinforced the loneliness of the job, the isolation from friends and companions even in the middle of a million-man army. It had been ten days since Ronald Balfour died, and this was the first time any of his fellow Monuments Men on the front had heard of it. Hancock had no assistant to travel with him. After all their time in separate fields of combat, he wondered if he would recognize Robert Posey or Walter "Hutch" Huchthausen were they to walk in the door. After the compressed events of war, where nine months seemed like nine years, they were simply names on reports to him. But always, when he needed him, in the flesh and blood, there was George Stout.

At least Hancock had excellent news for his boss, even as they shared their sorrow. He had found Weyres, Count Wolff-Metternich's assistant, in Bad Godesberg, Germany. The man was a treasure trove of information, and Hancock wanted to know how to handle him. Stout, perhaps preoccupied himself with thoughts of Ronald Balfour, told him simply, "I don't need to tell you what to do, Walker."

By the next morning, Hancock was passing detailed information on art repositories to the advanced units of First Army. Within a few days, he had transmitted to frontline troops the location of 109 repositories east of the Rhine, doubling the number of known repositories in all of Germany.

A week later, on March 29, 1945, an American commander pushed straight through the fighting and pounded on the door of the *Bürgermeister* of Siegen. When the astonished mayor opened the door, the commander said simply, "Where are the paintings?"

CHAPTER 32

Treasure Map

Trier, Germany
March 20–29, 1945

By late March 1945, Captain Robert Posey and Private Lincoln Kirstein, the brilliantly mismatched Monuments Men for Patton's U.S. Third Army, were rolling through the Saar Valley along the border between France and Germany. Around them, they could see the effects of the Nazi occupation in the fallow fields and rusted, broken factories. Meat, it was said, was so hard to find that rutabagas were now the dietary staple. The citizens, most of whom were sympathetic to the Western Allied cause, would offer assistance for a mere cigarette, which were so scarce that many people had calmed their cravings for years with the butts thrown down by prisoners of war being marched to prison camps deeper in German territory. It was a land impoverished by war, used by Third Army as a warehouse and supply area, but Kirstein saw the beauty: the rolling hills beginning to green as the snow melted, the lazy river valleys, the dark forests so reminiscent of Grimm's fairy tales. The small farms seemed as old as the dirt, and the ancient town gates and towers reminded him of the fantastic realms lurking in the background of Albrecht Dürer's engravings.

"One gets a chance now to observe the attitude of the German people toward us," Robert Posey wrote his wife, Alice, after crossing the Moselle River into Germany itself:[1]

The advance is so fast that many towns are not badly damaged. In these, and even in the damaged ones, the people line the sidewalks to watch our convoys go by just as they did in Normandy. They of course are not cheering but one almost thinks it is simply because they are less emotional than the French. They all have a look of lively curiosity. The older men light up with admiration of our superb equipment manned by spirited, healthy soldiers. Children shout to us and the tiny girls smile brightly and wave. Though we are supposed to ignore them I am too soft hearted not to return those waves. Large crowds mill about and watch our engineers build a new wooden bridge alongside of one their own soldiers blew out a few days before so as to retard the inevitable destruction of their arms. Instead of the newly unfurled tricolor as in France, each house flies the white flag of unconditional surrender....One old woman wiped a tear from her eye with the corner of her apron but the frail, bent, white haired creature was probably thinking of her own boy who may have been sacrificed for Hitler....When our bull dozers push the long pole road blocks out of the ground the people watch until it is finished and then saw the logs up and split them into firewood. Bobby sox girls try to flirt a bit when they are sure no one is watching. It is not an altogether dismal picture but why do they fight.

On March 20, 1945, the Monuments Men arrived at the Third Army base in Trier, one of the most historic cities in northern Europe. "Trier stood one thousand three hundred years before Rome; may it continue to stand and enjoy eternal peace," read a famous inscription on a house on the main market square. The founding date was a fabrication, but Trier indeed had been a garrison town even before the arrival of Roman legionnaires in the time of Augustus Caesar. Unfortunately, it had not fared as well in this war as the "smooth and conquered" Saar valley.[2]

Posey, in a summary of Third Army's progress, referred to Trier as "smashed."[3] Kirstein suspected the city was in worse shape than at any time since the Middle Ages. "The desolation is frozen," he wrote, "as if the moment of combustion was suddenly arrested, and the air had lost its power to hold atoms together and various centers of gravity had a dogfight for matter, and matter lost. For some unknown reason one intact bridge remained.... There was only enough room for one way routing as everything had fallen into the street. The town was practically empty. Out of 90,000, about 2,000 were there, living in a system of wine-cellars. They looked very chipper, women in slacks, men in regular working suits. The convention is to look right through them. Some of the houses have white sheets or pillow cases hanging out. Hardly a whole thing left. 15th century fragments of water spouts, baroque pediments and gothic turrets in superb disarray mixed up with new meat cutters, champagne bottles, travel posters, fresh purple and yellow crocusses and a lovely day, gas and decomposition, enamel signs and silver-gilt candelabra, and appalling, appalling shivered, subsided blank waste. Certainly Saint Lô was worse, but it didn't have anything of importance. Here everything was early Christian, or roman or romanesque or marvelous baroque."[4]

The Nazis had poured money into restoring Trier, especially the Market Place, now mostly ruined, and the Simeonstrasse, known as the "Street of German History." The façade of the Dom and connecting cloister and the surrounding district was heavily damaged. The baroque palace of the counts of Kessel was demolished. The home of Karl Marx, who was born in Trier in 1818, had been turned into a newspaper office by the Nazis. The Allies flattened it in an aerial bombardment.

And yet what remained was, in itself, a world-class collection of buildings. "The interior of the Dom was intact," Kirstein wrote, "except that the bell fell through the tower, the Liebfrau[en]kirche was badly burnt, but standing, St. Paulinus, an absolute orgy of pink and blue rococo marvels, was only hit, because the idiot Nazis put tanks in a corner of the façade, the Porta Nigra [ancient Roman gate] untouched except where the idiots had put machine guns, the Matthias Abtei, intact except for the rifled sacristy."[5] The treasures of the Dom, including the "Seamless Cloak" said to have been stolen from the dying Christ by Roman soldiers, were found hidden in secret bunkers built into the city's ancient stone foundations.

Posey and Kirstein immediately set out to educate the soldiers on the wonders of the city. Posey's previous historical notes on Nancy and Metz had proven popular, so by the time Third Army reached Trier, he and Kirstein had compiled a treatise on the history and importance of the city and its buildings. They feared the troops, having crossed into enemy territory, would be less careful with historic monuments and more inclined to casual looting. By educating them about a grander, pre-Nazi German culture, the Monuments Men hoped to create interest and appreciation, which would translate into good behavior.

Not that they were above picking up a few souvenirs. Posey often sent small things home to Woogie—mostly cards and German coins. In Trier, he added an aluminum flagstaff ornament, telling Woogie the Nazi flag had been burned and that the staff "must have gone all through the war. The Germans have not had enough of this metal even for airplanes in the last three or four years."[6]

Posey and Kirstein knew the names of most of the town officials from their interviews in Metz and other cities, and they used this information to create a five-person board of experts to "salvage fragments, barricade damaged walls, make temporary repairs wherever possible, gather scattered documents, open secret passages…and advise upon necessary emergency care" under the direction of the Allied Military Government.[7] Two days after Trier fell to Third Army, the board was at work. These officials, one of whom proved to be a Nazi Party member and was thus dismissed, in turn passed on information about German officials farther east. The model established in Trier—education coupled with local participation—would be used by the Monuments Men of Third Army for the rest of the campaign.

But by March 29, 1945, the last thing on Robert Posey's mind was the next city farther east. By then, his one consuming thought was his toothache. Like many soldiers, he had been in pain for much of his tour of duty. He had injured his back at Normandy when a sergeant stepped on his hand as the troops went over the rigging into their landing craft, causing him to fall several feet onto a machine-gun turret. He had broken the arch of his foot in the Bulge. A Third Army officer had suggested a Purple Heart for that one, but Posey refused it. Purple Hearts were for troops wounded *by the enemy* in combat, not for soldiers who fell into snow-covered holes.

But neither injury was as painful as the toothache. Unfortunately, the nearest army dentist was a hundred miles away in France. He tried to work through it, but the constant pain was too much to ignore. Neither he nor Kirstein spoke German very well, so finally Kirstein stopped a little blond boy in the street—children were usually the best sources of information—and pantomimed a sore tooth. For three sticks of Pep-O-Mint gum, the boy grabbed Kirstein's hand and directed him to a Gothic door a few blocks away, above which hung a sign in the shape of a tooth.

The dentist, an older man, spoke fine, heavily accented English and "gabbled more than a barber."[8] He seemed to know everyone in Trier, and he seemed as interested in the Monuments Men's mission to save German culture as he was in fixing poor Posey's impacted wisdom tooth.

"You might talk to my son-in-law," he said, putting away his tools at the end of the procedure and wiping the blood from his hands. "He's an art scholar, and he knows France. He was there during the occupation." He paused. "But he lives miles from here, I'm afraid. I can only take you there if you have a car."

The three men drove east out of the city. The roads were littered with ammo and artillery and some of the farmhouses still smoldered. The trees were green and half full of spring leaves, but the fields were bare and brown, the grapevines untended. They passed a child, grim-faced and still, staring at them as they passed. The dentist was in high spirits. "Wonderful," he'd say when they entered each small town. "Wonderful. It feels like a lifetime since I left Trier." He kept excusing himself to stop at a farmhouse to visit friends or a small store to buy supplies. "Wonderful," he'd say, coming back with food in hand. "We haven't had fresh milk in months."

"Is this a good idea?" Kirstein asked Posey as the Monuments Men waited for the dentist outside an inn in another shattered village. They were twelve miles from Trier, and with each mile the surrounding hills seemed increasingly hostile. Every village looked abandoned, and the white pillowcases of surrender no longer flew from the houses. *Sudden vacancies*, Kirstein thought. *Nobody wants to be seen.*

"Probably not," Posey said. But instead of saying anything else, he just stared out at the ridge that formed the end of the valley. His mouth felt like someone had taken a sledgehammer to it, but discomfort was part of the job. He was thinking instead of the thin line between doing that job and the essential interest in making it home for supper. What would Woogie do without a father?

The dentist approached, smiling, fresh vegetables in hand. "Wonderful," he said. "Simply wonderful."

"No more stops," Posey said gruffly, running his tongue along his swollen gums. He suspected the dentist was a harmless fraud, but the more stops he made, and the more the end of the valley loomed, the more the whole excursion seemed like a trap.

Finally, at the base of the valley, the dentist told them to pull over. A large white-plastered house stood at the foot of a hill, a forest rising beyond it. "This way," the dentist beckoned, walking behind the house. Halfway up the hill was a small building, an isolated weekend cottage perfect for an ambush of careless art experts. Posey and Kirstein looked at each other. How stupid was this? Even if the son-in-law was an art scholar, and even if he was alone in the house, what could he possibly know? Almost reluctantly, Posey started climbing the hill.

Inside, the cottage was bright and clean, an homage to France and to a life of beauty and intellect. The walls were lined with photographs of the Eiffel Tower, Notre Dame, Versailles, and other famous Parisian landmarks. A few vases were stuffed with flowers, probably picked from the surrounding hills. The bookshelves were filled with books on art and history, both common and obscure. It evoked, especially in Kirstein, the "agreeable atmosphere of a scholar's cultivated life, domestic, concentrated, a long way from war."[9] This was the first owner-occupied private residence he had entered in Germany, and it made him feel at home.

The scholar was handsome and surprisingly young, probably in his mid-thirties. He should have been fresh and enthusiastic, at the start of his career, but something about him was stooped and worn. The war had poisoned everyone, Kirstein thought, even this country scholar. Nonetheless, the young man smiled at the sight of the Allied art officials. "*Entrez*," he said enthusiastically in French. "I have been eagerly awaiting you. I have spoken with no one since I left Paris twenty-four hours before your army arrived. I have missed that great city every day."

He beckoned to two seats, then turned to introduce the other occupants of the cottage. "This is my mother. And my wife, Hildegard." He glanced nervously at her father the dentist. "My daughter, Eva. And my son, Dietrich," the scholar said proudly, indicating the baby in his wife's arms.

Posey reached out a finger for the child to grasp, but the baby shrank back. He didn't look anything like Woogie, but every child reminded him of the boy he had left behind.

"My father-in-law tells me you are art scholars in the service of the American army," the man said, taking a seat. "You must find Trier a marvel. I understand the Paulinerkirche was unharmed, thank God. The ceiling is one of a kind, a true work of art, though only two hundred years old. My own area of study is the Middle Ages: the end of the old world, the birth of our own. Or perhaps that is too dramatic. I am only an art scholar, after all, a figure of some authority on medieval French sculpture. I am completing a book on the twelfth-century sculpture of the Île-de-France. I began writing it with Arthur Kingsley Porter, an Englishman, you may have heard of him?"

"Of course," Kirstein replied, picturing the old professor who had taught him art history as an undergraduate. "I remember him from Harvard."

"As do I," the German scholar said. "Graduate work. I have fond memories still of his wife. The cleverest mad woman I've ever met."[10]

He turned suddenly to his wife. "*Kognak*," he said. When she, the children, and the dentist had left the room, the scholar's tone changed. He bent forward and, talking swiftly, began to tell them a bit of his history.

"I won't lie to you," he said. "I knew Göring in Paris. And Rosenberg. I worked with them. As a scholar, you understand, no one important, but I observed them and their operation. I was there when Göring hauled away his first trainload of art. I told him his treatment of the confiscated Jewish art treasures was in contradiction to the Hague Rules of Land Warfare and the army's interpretation of Hitler's orders. He asked for an explanation. When I concluded he said simply, 'First, it is my orders that you have to follow. You will act directly according to my orders.'[11]

"When I told him the military command in France and the Juristen—meaning the legal representatives of the Reich—would probably be of a different opinion, he told me, 'Dear Bunjes, let me worry about that; I am the highest Jurist in the State.'

"He told me that directly, gentlemen. Word for word, on February 5, 1941. What was a simple art scholar to do? And besides, the art was safer in the hands of Göring than spread through the hands of the thousand lesser Nazi officials clamoring to obtain it.

You see, I acted to protect the art. It was conservation by acquisition."

His wife entered with the cognac. "*Ich danke Dir Darling*," he said, pouring a glass for himself and Kirstein. Posey demurred, lighting a cigarette instead. Both men needed the distraction. It was all they could do to keep their mouths from hanging open. This man, this country scholar, had been in Paris. He knew the angles. He might provide answers to questions they had been sweating over for months.

"I have knowledge," the scholar said after a few swirls of the snifter, "but I also have a price: safe passage out of Germany for myself and my family. I want nothing more than to complete my book, to live in peace. In return, I will tell you not only what was taken, but where it is."

"Why do you need safe passage?" Kirstein asked.

"I was an SS captain. For five years. Yes, it's true. Only for professional purposes, you understand, always in the service of art. But if the citizens of this valley knew...they wouldn't understand. They'd probably have me shot. They blame us for...all of this."

Posey and Kirstein looked at each other. They had interviewed many art officials, but never an SS officer. What kind of scholar was this?

"I don't have the authority to offer deals," Posey said, as Kirstein translated. The German sighed. He drank cognac, seemed to consider his options, then abruptly rose and left the room. He came back minutes later with a bound booklet. It was a catalogue of artwork stolen from France: title, size, exchange rate, price, original owner. He explained it to them, translating from the German text. Then he told them to spread their maps on the table, and he began to show where the objects could be found. He seemed to know it all from memory, right down to the smallest detail. "Göring's collection is no longer at Carinhall," the scholar said confidently. "It is in Veldenstein. Here. But I cannot be sure if it is going to stay there for long."

He told them the inside works of the German art world. How the treasures of Poland and Russia had been distributed to various German museums. Which art dealers in Berlin were actively trading in looted works. Which stolen French masterpieces were hidden in Switzerland, and which had made it farther into Germany itself.

"What about the Ghent Altarpiece?" Posey asked.

"Van Eyck's *Adoration of the Mystic Lamb?*" the scholar said, picking up the name of the work despite Posey's English. "The panels are in Hitler's extensive collection of artistic masterpieces." He moved his finger southwest into the deepest part of the Austrian Alps, not far from Hitler's boyhood home of Linz. "Here, in the salt mine at Altaussee."

Hitler's collection? Posey and Kirstein didn't say anything. They didn't even look at each other. All those miles driving, all those fruitless interviews, all those months of painstakingly fitting information together piece by piece, and suddenly they were being given everything they had always hoped for and more. They hadn't just been given information; they had been given a map to the treasure room of the Führer. And until that moment, nobody on the Allied side had even known the Führer had a treasure room.

"The Nazis are boors," the scholar said. "Complete frauds. They don't understand the beauty of art, only that it is somehow valuable. They robbed the silver service from the Rothschilds, then used it like ordinary flatware in their Aeroclub in Berlin. To see them dribbling food off those priceless forks made me sick."

The scholar rose and poured himself another cognac. When he returned, he began to talk about his own work, about Paris and cathedrals and the twelfth century and its remarkable funereal statuary, about how much had been lost since then to the ravages of time and the senselessness of war. "Here," Kirstein would write, "in the cold Moselle spring, far from the murder of the cities, worked a German scholar in love with France, passionately in love, with that hopeless, frustrated fatalism" so characteristic of the Germans.[12] Kirstein couldn't help but like the man.

"I offer you my services, gentlemen," the scholar said finally. "Anything you ask. All I want is for my family to return to Paris." As if waiting for their moment, his wife and baby suddenly appeared in the doorway.

"I'll see what I can do," Posey said, as he and Kirstein stood up to leave. They appeared calm, but inside they were buzzing. They had learned more in the last twenty minutes than they had in the last twenty weeks. And they had a mission now; a big one: to find and recover Hitler's secret hoard of masterpieces.

The German scholar smiled, extended his hand. If he was disappointed at the lack of safe passage, he didn't show it. "It has been a pleasure, my friends," he said genially. "Thank you for coming."

"Thank you, Dr. Bunjes. You have been a great help." They had no idea that they had spent the afternoon speaking with Göring's corrupt Kunstschutz official, and one of the top men in the notorious looting operation at the Jeu de Paume.

CHAPTER 33

Frustration

Northern European Theater
March 30–31, 1945

Private First Class Richard Courtney was frustrated. Like most of his fellow soldiers in U.S. First Army, he had been slugging it out on the ground since Normandy. He had been through the German ring of fire around the beaches, and he had survived the Siegfried Line. He had fought to take Aachen in September, then fought to take it again after the Battle of the Bulge. Now he was searching a country estate—what the army called "clearing"—on the other side of the Rhine, near the small town of Breidenbach, and even after nine months of fighting he couldn't believe his eyes. The house, the soldiers had been told, belonged to a Nazi Party leader, and as they moved from room to room they stared in awe at the extraordinary collection of paintings, crystal, silverware, and statuary. Art collecting was in vogue among the Nazi elite, no doubt fueled by their desire to curry favor with the Führer and the Reichsmarschall. This particular Nazi had clearly been "collecting" from all over Europe.

But Private Courtney wasn't truly mad until he entered the cellar and saw, stacked floor to ceiling, Red

Cross care packages intended for American prisoners of war. Why were they here? What did a high Nazi official need with hardtack biscuits and Band-Aids? The longer he looked at those packages, the more he became enraged. Finally, he picked up a crowbar and started smashing things: boxes, mirrors, china, artwork, chandeliers. He was so mad, he even knocked the light switches off the wall. Nobody tried to stop him.

"What was that about?" a fellow soldier asked once the swinging had stopped.

Private Courtney threw down the crowbar and looked at the destruction around him. "That was for our boys in the camps," he said.

———

Meanwhile, in a "repple depple" in Liège, Belgium, Private Harry Ettlinger played craps. He had resisted for a month, but there was nothing else to do. During the first week, he won $1,500 with funds from his $60 monthly army salary. A day later, he lost it all. He went outside and looked at the night sky. Everything seemed a million miles away. It had been two months of nothing. He wasn't eager to be at the front, but the long-termers in the "repple depple" were depressing. One soldier had bought perfume while stationed in Paris, and was now selling it at marked-up prices. The perfume stunk up the whole camp, but all the man could think about was getting back to Paris to replenish his supply. Harry Ettlinger didn't want to be that kind of soldier. Somewhere out east, the war was grinding on without him. He felt sure he had a part to play—he must—but he still had no idea why they'd pulled him off that truck on his nineteenth birthday. No one had told him a thing.

In Paris, James Rorimer received his notice to report to the front as Monuments Man for the U.S. Seventh Army, which had thus far been without the services of a Monuments officer. Seventh Army territory in Germany alone stretched 280 miles with an average width of eighty miles. He would be the only Monuments Man in those 22,400 square miles. But he had something no other Monuments Man had ever possessed: the information Rose Valland had given him two weeks earlier, and the knowledge she had imparted to him during the last few months. Thanks to Valland, he knew exactly where to go: the fairytale castle at Neuschwanstein. For months, the name would echo in his dreams. Exactly what he should find, and how exactly to get there quickly... that was something as yet unknown.

"General Rogers came out of his way at my dinner last night in Paris to tell me what a fine job I had done," Rorimer wrote his wife. "My boss Lt. Col. Hamilton gave cocktails to our group and all but wept when I was taken from his staff for Germany. Yes, I made my place and now must build a new under very different conditions."[1]

He had no doubts. This was the important mission; this was the one he wanted more than anything to be given. As he prepared his gear for departure, he no doubt looked back fondly on his days in the City of Light, but looked ahead even more eagerly to the adventures ahead: the great ERR repositories, the Nazi villains, the chance to save the patrimony of France. And despite his excitement—or perhaps because of it— he wondered about Rose Valland. Jacques Jaujard was right. She was a hero. Perhaps *the* hero of French culture. But what would she do now? She had turned over to her protégé the work for which she had risked her life. What does the teacher do once the student is gone?

Rorimer thought more deeply about it and realized he knew the answer. Rose Valland, often underestimated but never deterred, was angling for a commission in the French army. She was convinced she had found the right man in James Rorimer, but the importance of rescuing France's patrimony was too great to rely on any one person to do the work. Rose Valland was no timid art official or wilting flower; she was a fighter hiding behind a façade. And she had every desire and intention of making it to the front and finding France's precious art.

———

In Berlin, Albert Speer stood once more before his Führer. Soviet artillery and Western Allied bombers were pounding the city, and Adolf Hitler, the indispensable man, had descended into his vast, impenetrable bunker beneath the Reichschancellery. He had cut himself off from the world, from even the catalogues of artwork destined for Linz that in better times had brightened his dark days. He could no longer, for instance, gaze at the photograph of Vermeer's *The Astronomer*, his most cherished painting, with its image of a great man of intellect, turned slightly away from the viewer with the light streaming in through his window, reaching a hand to his globe as if grasping the world. But Hitler still had his building plans for Linz, which had descended with him into the bunker. (The scale model of Linz was nearby in a cellar of the New Chancellery.) He still had his vision. He may have been pale and drained, but he was still iron-willed, a man aware of his predicament but not yet capable of grasping that his empire was doomed.

He was not one to delay. He had been informed by his personal secretary, Martin Bormann, that Speer had been to the Ruhr to convince the gauleiters to disobey Hitler's Nero Decree and leave intact the infrastructure of Germany.

Speer did not deny it. Hitler, a man of lethal anger but not yet debilitating paranoia, suggested his friend and minister of armaments take a sick leave. "Speer," he said, "if you can convince yourself the war is not lost, you can continue to run your office."

"I cannot," Speer replied, "with the best will in the world. And after all I do not want to be one of the swine in your entourage who tell you they believe in victory without believing in it."

"You have twenty-four hours to think over your answer," Hitler said, turning on his heel. "Tomorrow let me know whether you hope that the war can still be won."[2]

As soon as Speer left, Hitler ordered his chief of transportation to issue a teletype reaffirming the "Nero Decree." "Included in the list of facilities slated for destruction," Speer wrote, "were, once again, all types of bridges, tracks, roundhouses, all technical installations in the freight depots, workshop equipment, and sluices and locks in our canals. Along with this all locomotives, passenger cars, freight cars, cargo vessels, and barges were to be completely destroyed and the canals and rivers blocked by sinking ships into them."[3] Hitler was asking for nothing less than the complete destruction of the Reich.

That night, Speer wrote Hitler a letter. "I can no longer believe in the success of our good cause," it said in part, "if during these decisive months we simultaneously and systematically destroy the foundations of our national existence. That is so great an injustice to our people that should it be done, Fate can no longer wish us well. . . . I therefore beg you not to carry out this measure so harmful to the people. If you could revise your policy on this question, I would once more recover the faith and the courage to continue working with the greatest energy. It no longer lies in our hands to decide how Fate will turn. Only a higher Providence can still change our future. We can only make our contribution by a strong posture and unshakable faith in the eternal future of our nation. . . . May God Protect Germany."[4]

Hitler refused to accept the letter and demanded a verbal answer. On March 30, 1945, standing before the Führer he had loved and served so well, Albert Speer lost his resolve. "*Mein Führer*," he said. "I stand unreservedly behind you."[5]

———

Three days later, 350 miles west of Berlin, Monuments Men Walker Hancock and George Stout approached the town that for months had tantalized them with its mystery and its promise of artistic treasures: Siegen, Germany.

Letter from Walker Hancock
To his wife, Saima
April 4, 1945

Dearest Saima:

The last few days have been the most incredible of my whole life. For *instance*, the other day I made a long trip with George Stout and the vicar from Aachen to see a place where the greatest art treasures of western Germany are hidden. We entered the town the same day that it was taken. Only one road into it could be used as there were still "pockets of resistance" in the surrounding hills. Shelling and machine gun fire were heard intermittently. (No real danger, but it all added to the excitement.) The town had been solidly bombed for three months, and for two weeks battles had raged in the streets, so you can (or can't) imagine how the place looked. An occasional civilian ventured out of hiding, but mostly it was empty desolation—a pool of blood with an American helmet beside it told a story—the ruin that we know so well was everywhere.

Our priest-guide found us the entrance to the tunnels where the works of art were hidden. In contrast to the deserted town, here all was teeming with wretched humanity. We entered the narrow passage into the dark, suffocating mine. People were packed in so tightly that survival under such conditions for a day seemed a miracle. None of them had left the place for a fortnight.

We went deeper and deeper into the hillside and when our eyes became accustomed to the darkness, and our ears to the hushed words we became somewhat aware of the drama of the situation. (Our noses did *not* become accustomed to the sickening smells.) We were the first Americans these people had seen. There were gasps— "Amerikaner! Amerikaner! Sie kommen!" Mothers called their children to them in fear.

But some others were not afraid. One little tot took George by the hand and held him for a long part of the way. Some tried to talk in English. There were the old, and young, and the sick of the city, piled on bunks or huddled together. We walked on and on—more than a quarter of a mile into the hill.

Walker

Dear Margie:

I've not written for four days—a field trip
and every hour used up . . . [but] there was an
occurrence day before yesterday which was of such
a character that it deserves better than the poor
sketchy account that I am now able to give of it.
I cannot tell you the name of the city—it is well
east of the Rhine—because as yet the fact of what
it holds is not allowed out. We had known about a
storage depot there from information we got last
November [in Aachen] and since then more had come
in. We knew it was somewhere in an iron mine at
the edge of the city. We found a German priest, a
really dauntless fellow, who had been there and
offered to go as our guide.

An armored force had been in, and elements
of an infantry regiment had followed. There was
fighting during the day, but most of the German
troops had pulled out. We came in at 4:30 (1630),
Walker Hancock, two enlisted men, the priest and
I. The streets were not very safe for a vehicle
because of debris and fallen trolley lines. There
was very little artillery shelling, sporadic
and weak. The German soldiers were being round
up with no evident resistance. We saw three
civilians, two German nurses, and a man who
walked with a limp, a young man. He said he was

trying to find his sister on the other side of town and wanted to know if it was dangerous to go there. All this was commonplace and had happened many times before.

One of the enlisted men had been left with the vehicle. The rest of us walked about a half mile across the broken town and came to the mine. Our intrepid priest was then not too sure of the entrance. What followed was not commonplace.

Around a hole in the steep hill stood some twenty people. They fell back and we went in. The tunnel—an old mine shaft—was about six feet wide and eight high, arched and rough. Once away from the light of the entrance, the passage was thick with vapor and our flashlights made only faint spots in the gloom. There were people inside. I thought we must soon pass them and that they were a few stragglers sheltered there for safety. But we did not pass them.

It was a hard place to judge distance. We walked more than a quarter mile, probably less than half a mile through that passage. Other shafts branched from it. In places it had been cut out to a width of about twenty feet.

Throughout we walked in a path not more than a foot and a half. The rest was compressed humanity. They stood, they sat on branches and on stones. They lay on cots or stretchers. This was the population of the city, all that could not get away. At one time the priest had to stop and speak to a woman who was ill. Many must have been ill. There was a stench in the humid air. Babies cried fretfully.

We were the first Americans they had seen. They had no doubt been told that we were savages. The pale grimy faces caught in our flashlights were full of fear and hate. Children were snatched out of our path. And ahead of us went the fearful word, halfway between sound and whisper—"Amerikaner." That was the strange part of the occurrence, the impact of hate and fear in hundreds of hearts close about us and we the targets of it all.

Yet, there was some indifference. There was a boy of about ten blowing at a cup. Somewhere out of the damp and the stink he had got something hot to drink and he was trying to bring it down to a tolerable temperature. He paid us no attention at all. And there was some little sign of a thing, not fear and not unconcern. We must have been more than halfway through. I felt a touch on my free hand, and turned my light there. It was a boy of about seven. He smiled and took hold of my hand and walked along with me. I should not have let him do it, but I did and was glad. I wonder why he felt that way. What could have made him know that I was not a monster. He and another followed us out into the good air.

We found our storage depot through another
entrance and I'm not really sorry that we made a
blunder on the first.

This has been quite long and quite
inadequate, but I thought you would like to hear
about it.

Much love, darling,

George

CHAPTER 34

Inside the Mountain

George Stout raised his fist and knocked on a locked door buried half a mile inside a hill. It had been a long walk, through a broken town, then down the wrong tunnel for half a mile, and finally down this lesser passage, but after months of anticipation it was well worth the trouble. As the door swung open, Stout almost expected to see artistic and cultural riches come flowing out into the tunnel. What he saw instead was a stern little man.

After what they had just been through, there was almost nothing that could have surprised the Monuments Men, but that was clearly not true of the guard. He looked in wonder at the American soldier, then the vicar of Aachen beside him, and then finally at the two other American soldiers accompanying them.

"Hello, Etzkorn," the vicar said. The Monuments Men had wasted precious hours that morning doubling back at the request of headquarters to pick up a "guide," but Vicar Stephany had turned out to be worth the trouble. He was none other than the man who had met Hancock at Aachen Cathedral and requested his help in freeing the cathedral's fire brigade. He had been surprised to see his old visitor, and he was embarrassed to acknowledge that, yes, he had known about Siegen all along, even as he told Hancock he had no idea where the treasures of Aachen Cathedral had been sent.

"Welcome back, Vicar," the little man known as Etzkorn replied gruffly, reluctantly stepping aside to allow the soldiers through. As he swung the door closed, a group of uniformed Germans, apparently guards, roused themselves to attention, but they too let the Monuments Men pass. Beyond them was a vault door. Herr Etzkorn arrived with the key before being asked.

As the door swung open, Hancock caught a glimpse, just visible in his flashlight beam, of a massive brick-vaulted gallery. Then he felt the air: warm and humid. The ventilation system had been damaged beyond repair by Allied bombs, and water was dripping from the ceiling. George Stout entered the room first, his flashlight beam falling on a series of enormous wooden racks. The racks, Hancock noticed, went all the way to the ceiling. And every nook was filled with art: sculpture, paintings, decorations, altarpieces, all packed as tightly as the townspeople had been in that terrible passageway outside. In the beam of his flashlight, Hancock recognized works by Rembrandt, Van Dyck, Van Gogh, Gauguin, Cranach, Renoir, and especially Peter Paul Rubens, the great seventeenth century Flemish painter who had been born in Siegen. On some of the canvases he noticed mold, while the paint on several wood panels was noticeably bubbled and flaked.

"It's still here!" the vicar cried from a dark corner.

Stout and Hancock hurried to the last of the fourteen

giant wall bays. Inside were six enormous crates marked "Aachen Cathedral."

"The seals haven't been broken," Stout observed.

"Two weeks ago the *Oberbürgermeister* of Aachen..." the stern little guard known as Etzkorn began.

"Ex-mayor," Vicar Stephany corrected.

Etzkorn seemed not to notice the vicar's hostility toward a party functionary. "The *Ex-Oberbürgermeister* of Aachen," he started again, "tried to remove the treasures when the Americans approached. The crates were too heavy."

Hancock ran his hands over the wood. Inside were the silver-gilt bust of Charlemagne containing part of his skull, the Virgin Mary's robe, Lothar's processional cross set with the cameo of Augustus Caesar, numerous gilt and wrought metal shrines. Carefully, he slid the lid off an unmarked crate. Inside was the twelfth-century shrine of Saint Heribert of Deutz.

"Is that gold?" whispered an awed voice.

Hancock had forgotten about the enlisted soldier who had escorted them into the mine. The Monuments Men had known for months the repository was here. They had some idea of what to expect, but even for them the presence of all these vital connections to mankind's past was hard to fathom, especially in such strange and lousy surroundings.

"Gold and enamel," Hancock said, signaling for the soldier to help him with the large heavy lid.

"How much is it worth?"

"More than either of us could imagine."

Etzkorn gave them a quick tour. Most of the bays held the works of western German museums, especially those in Bonn, Cologne, Essen, and Münster. Others contained the treasures of Rhineland churches. Much to their disappointment, the only foreign works at Siegen were from the French city of Metz, which they had already been told to expect. The stolen cultural heritage of the rest of Western Europe was hidden somewhere else, perhaps in some other mine, waiting to be found.

Etzkorn pointed to forty boxes. "From Beethoven's house in Bonn. The original manuscript of the Sixth Symphony is in there somewhere."

"I visited that house," Hancock whispered, remembering the cherry blooms among the ruins.

Two enormous oak doors stood near the entrance. Hancock recognized the rough shallow relief of the numerous panels depicting the life of Christ. He wanted to put his sculptor's hands on them, to feel the ancient chisel marks. The carvings were primitive, but they were also history, magic beyond words for the medieval people who originally beheld them.

"The doors of Sankt Maria im Kapitol in Cologne," Etzkorn said, genuinely moved. "I know that parish well."

Hancock nodded, but said nothing. Sankt Maria had been destroyed. These doors, he suspected, were all that remained.

"I know what you're thinking," Stout said to Hancock when their cursory examination was complete. "It seems foolish to leave it all here. The moisture, the stale air, the…unreliable guards. But we have no trucks, no packers, no movers. We don't even have a better place to take it. We'll post an armed guard from the infantry division, come back tomorrow and study what we've found. But we can't take it out. Not until proper arrangements are made. But don't worry, Walker, this much at least is safe. Nothing will harm it now."

They left through an even shorter tunnel than the other two, which was apparently the main entrance to the repository. Like the first, it was filled with displaced persons who had taken shelter there from the Allied assault. Most of these displaced people, however, wore uniforms. There were all different styles and colors, most of which Walker Hancock didn't recognize. As the Americans passed, many of them sprang to attention and saluted.

"*Quand pourrons-nous rentrer en France?*" someone cried.[1]

Hancock turned to find a group of French prisoners looking at him expectantly. Were the Allies coming to rescue them? Hancock didn't know, so he told them only that for the past few weeks he had seen truckloads of former prisoners heading west. At the entrance, an old man grabbed Hancock's sleeve, babbling about the cruelty of the Nazis. He became so agitated over the fate of his family that foam flew from the corners of his mouth. He tried to follow them, but he was too weak. Hancock left him at the foot of the hill with the others. When he looked back, the man was still standing there, watching them leave. Hancock felt terrible, but he was dead tired, and there was nothing he could do. He had been underground for an afternoon, and it seemed like a lifetime.

He looked back one last time. In the slanting evening light, the hill looked like any other in Germany, beaten and desolate and strewn with debris. There was nothing to indicate the marvels and the horrors inside.

CHAPTER 35

Lost

East of Aachen, Germany
April 4, 1945

North of Essen and east of Aachen, in the area known as the Ruhr Pocket, Captain Walter "Hutch" Huchthausen and his assistant Sergeant Sheldon Keck, the Monuments Men for U.S. Ninth Army, drove toward the battle front to investigate reports of an altarpiece. Hutch was a gregarious bachelor, now fully recovered from the wounds he suffered during the bombing of London and at forty years old just starting to come into his own. Keck, a married conservator, had started his military service in 1942 when his son "Keckie" was only three weeks old. He hadn't seen his child since, but his wife, Caroline, also an art conservator, never complained. She had been a student in Berlin during the 1930s, when food was scarce, employment nonexistent, and corruption endemic. At her university, fifteen students a month committed suicide until, finally, they closed the school. Twice she heard Hitler speak in person, and his words still shivered her bones. She wanted Sheldon back, but knew the importance of his mission. Besides, she reasoned at least for a few years little Keckie wouldn't even realize his father was gone.

"Not much traffic out here," Keck observed after twenty or thirty minutes on the road. The maps had proved useless, as usual, since so many of the roads were impassable because of damage or enemy combatants. The Monuments Men were used to being lost, but they were also used to passing jeeps, tanks, and trucks, the usual support vehicles for the front. Out here there was nothing.

"Let's ask for directions," Keck said.

There were no Allied military posts alongside the road, but a mile or two farther on Hutch spotted American soldiers peeking over the top of a highway embankment.

"Thank God," he said, slowing down.

But as soon as he hit the brakes, the gunfire erupted. Sheldon Keck, in the passenger seat, heard the sudden explosion at almost the same instant he felt a hard force push him backward to the floor. He glimpsed American soldiers rising over the embankment, and then adrenaline took over, the world went black, and everything disappeared. The next thing he knew friendly hands were pulling him into a foxhole. The jeep was shot to hell in the road. The soldiers could only tell him that Hutch had been taken away in an ambulance, "bleeding from the ear, and that his face was snow white."[1]

For two days, Sheldon Keck rushed frantically from field hospital to field hospital, searching for his senior officer. There was no news anywhere; no wounded soldiers who matched the dog tags of his friend. He found him eventually not in a field hospital, but on the rolls of the dead. Walter "Hutch" Huchthausen had been hit by gunfire and died instantly on the road east of Aachen.

His body had been the force that knocked Keck to the floor of the jeep, shielding him from the bullets and saving his life. It was a moment Shelden Keck—and his son Keckie, who thanks to Hutch was raised by his loving father—would always remember.

Word of Hutch's death, like that of Ronald Balfour's, spread slowly through the MFAA ranks. Out of a force of nine officers on the front lines, they had lost their second good man. The reaction was one of quiet, of resignation, of a slow-moving contemplation that matched nothing so much as the slow walk of the officer who approached a small house in Dorchester, Massachusetts, to tell Walter Huchthausen's elderly mother that her son was dead.

"He was a wonderful chap," Walker Hancock wrote his new wife, Saima, many months later, when he feared Hutch's work would be forgotten, "and really believed in the fundamental goodness of everybody. Bill [Lesley] knew him better than I—was an old friend—but Hutch's attitude toward his mission in the war was one of my best memories. . . . The buildings that he hoped, as a young architect, to build will never exist . . . but the few people who saw him at his job—friend and enemy—must think more of the human race because of him."[2]

CHAPTER 36

A Week to Remember

Merkers, Germany
April 8–15, 1945

On April 6, 1945, two days after Walter Huchthausen's death, an American jeep crept up behind two huddled figures walking slowly along the dusty road. "Good morning, ladies," one of the MPs said, his finger on the trigger of his gun. "You know there's a strict curfew, right? General Patton's orders." Then he noticed one of the women was pregnant.

They were French displaced persons, walking to the nearby town of Kieselbach to visit the midwife. After questioning at U.S. XII Corps Provost Marshal's Office confirmed their story, the MPs offered to drive the women back to town. Just outside Merkers, the driver noticed the scars on the hillside and asked what kind of mine they were passing. One of the women pointed to a small door and said, "*Or.*" The French word for gold.

The MPs stopped. "*Or?* Are you sure?"

The woman nodded. "*Lingots d'or.*" Gold bars.

Robert Posey and Lincoln Kirstein, the Monuments Men for U.S. Third Army, arrived at the mine two days later, on the afternoon of April 8, 1945. They couldn't have missed the entrance if they tried. Every few steps, they passed another group of soldiers standing guard, and anti-aircraft guns were positioned along the narrow road. Posey guessed a whole company was on duty (more than a hundred men), but as he passed more inspection posts and sentry points he decided it was half a battalion (at least two hundred men). In fact, Merkers was being guarded by two entire infantry battalions, supported by elements of two more tank battalions.

The elevator, stuffed with officers sent from headquarters in Frankfurt to assess the gold and currency, smelled like sulfur and creaked like the wooden planks of an old stairwell. Soon, Kirstein's ears were aching from the pressure. "How deep is this mine?" he asked the operator.

"Twenty-one hundred feet, almost half a mile," an officer said. "Operator's a Kraut, by the way. Can't understand a word."

"I hope he's not one of those stay-behind SS officers."[1]

"Don't worry, Private. There are three-stars all over this place. He doesn't give a damn about you."

The elevator opened into a scene out of Dante's Inferno: darkness, shadows, men running in every direction, steam, water, wires, sprawling insectlike metal equipment, officers barking orders, and every sound echoing over and over again off the stone. The lights, at least the ones operational, threw deformed images on the walls and revealed layers of white rime on the necks and arms of most of the men. Hoses were being used to spray down men and equipment, and the water was collecting in slushy puddles on the floor. Within seconds, it seemed, Kirstein was wet from the humidity. He reached up to wipe his brow, then massaged his aching throat.

"It's the mineral salts in the walls," someone said, handing him a rag. "Take this to cover your nose. Use it to wipe down your boots when you're back up top. That salt water will eat through the leather in a day."

They passed more soldiers on guard, and a group hauling away a big pile of paper currency that had been dumped near the elevator. Nazi bank officials had tried to evacuate the currency the week before, but it was Easter Sunday and no one was on duty at the train station. Beyond the currency was a sandbagged artillery emplacement manned by a couple of silent GIs in flak helmets. Beyond them was a great steel bank vault door. Apparently nobody had a key, because a hole had been blasted in the three-foot-thick brick wall that surrounded it. Posey and Kirstein crawled through the opening. The first thing they saw was an American officer getting his picture taken. In his hands was a helmet overflowing with gold coins; behind him was Room #8, the great Nazi treasure room.

Lincoln Kirstein looked up. Above him, the massive stone ceiling gleamed with the reflection of a hundred lights. He estimated 150 feet long at least without a single support column, and another seventy-five feet across. How high? Maybe twenty feet, with a row of hanging lights down the center of the room. Beneath the lights ran a railroad track. A few carts were down at the far end of the room, being loaded with boxes. Posey thought the rows of boxes looked short and unimpressive; then he realized it was all perspective. They were taller than the soldiers loading the carts. In front of the

boxes, covering most of the floor, were thousands of
bags. They were all identical: plain brown, about the
size of a loaf of bread, and tied off at the top. They
were piled four high and five across, twenty rows per
section, with a footpath between each section. Kirstein
tried to count the sections, but it was impossible. The
last sections were so far away he couldn't see the paths
or the individual bags. They just looked like dots in the
distance. And every one of those bags, all thousand or
ten thousand or one hundred thousand of them, was
filled with gold.

The artwork, stored in a nearby room, was mostly
paintings. Some were boxed; some were in marked con-
tainers with hinged covers and padlocks; others were
wrapped only in brown paper. A large number were
stacked upright in wooden holding pens like posters at a five-and-dime. Kirstein flipped through them.
A lovely Caspar David Friedrich painting of a distant
schooner had a nasty rip in the sky, but the others
appeared unharmed.

"Not much, considering," Posey said.

"Oh, that's not all of it," a passing officer said with a
laugh. "There are miles of tunnels down here."

The outside passages were less spectacular than
Room #8. There was also less activity, and one could
experience for the first time the claustrophobia of being
in a small stone tube half a mile underground. Kirstein imagined hidden detonators, the Jerries waiting for
the art experts to arrive so they could blow the tunnels
and trap them in an underground tomb. Luring their
victims underground, like the villain with his cask of
amontillado in that old story by Edgar Allan Poe.

"I wonder how many tons of dirt are above us right now?" Kirstein said as he squeezed through a narrow passage. He was thinking of Caspar David Friedrich's little schooner under the massive sky.

"The only thing worse than being a soldier in these tunnels," Posey said, "is being the miner who dug them." He had no way of knowing there was something worse: All those tons of gold and artwork had been brought underground by conscripted labor, mostly Eastern European Jews and prisoners of war.

Slowly, the Monuments Men began to realize just how much was hidden in the Merkers mines. Crated sculpture, hastily packed, with photographs clipped from museum catalogues to show what was inside. Ancient Egyptian papyri in metal cases, which the salt in the mine had reduced to the consistency of wet cardboard. There was no time to examine the priceless antiquities inside, for in other rooms there were ancient Greek and Roman decorative works, Byzantine mosaics, Islamic rugs, leather and buckram portfolio boxes. Hidden in an inconspicuous side room, they found the original woodcuts of Albrecht Dürer's famous *Apocalypse* series of 1498. And then more crates of paintings—a Rubens, a Goya, a Cranach packed together with minor works.

"There's no order," Kirstein said. "Time periods and styles mixed together, masterpieces alongside novelties, boxes from different museums. What happened here?"

"They were packed by size," Posey said, pointing out the uniformity of the paintings in one of the crates.

They left the mine in the evening and drove back to Frankfurt to report their findings. With them was

Major Perera, an officer sent by Third Army to examine the gold and currency. Perera reported an initial count of 8,198 gold bars, 711 bags of American twenty-dollar gold pieces, over 1,300 bags of other gold coins, hundreds of bags of foreign currency, and $2.76 billion in Reichsmarks, along with various foreign currencies, silver and platinum, and the stamping plates the German government used to print money.[2] A bank official found in the mine, Herr Veick, had confirmed that it represented most of the reserves of Germany's national treasury.

Posey reported that, from preliminary evaluation, the artwork had also come from Berlin. The packing was sloppy, hurried, probably a case of simply grabbing what was portable. Nonetheless, the mine held thousands of works of art. None of it appeared to have been looted from other countries.

The next morning, Robert Posey called George Stout. MFAA commanding officer Geoffrey Webb, the British scholar, happened to be in Verdun meeting with Stout, and Posey suggested they both come down immediately. Then he and Kirstein left for the nearby town of Hungen, which had been recently overrun by Third Army. A few hours later, in Schloss Braunfels, a castle erected in 1246 as a fortress, they discovered enough incunabula, ancient manuscripts, and sacred Jewish texts to fill a museum. The looted material had been destined for ERR mastermind Alfred Rosenberg's Racial Institutes, whose purpose was to prove the inferiority of the Jewish race.

"I presume it is better to write a short dull letter than to not write," Posey wrote his wife, Alice, that night. "The situation is that I am so busy that my work drives me each day until I am exhausted and too tired to exercise a few thoughts in a letter. About sixteen hours a day seven days a week doesn't leave one much spare time."[3]

The closer the Monuments Men got to the end of the war, and the more important their work became, the less time or freedom they had to tell their loved ones back home of their experiences.

———

George Stout arrived at Merkers on April 11, 1945. Fresh from his tour of the repository at Siegen, where he had prevailed upon the Eighth Infantry Division to post a sufficient guard, he expected to find a half-forgotten mine. Instead, Merkers was crawling with Western Allied officers, German guides, and experts from all branches of Civil Affairs. The guards now totaled almost four battalions (more than 2,000 men), including an infantry battalion called back from the front, and still it seemed the soldiers were outnumbered by the war correspondents. As Kirstein wrote, "Due to the fact that the works of art…were discovered as an adjunct to the uncovering of the Reich's gold-reserve, the story was given unusual press treatment."[4] In other words, the reporters didn't care much about Germany's great works of art—in fact, they kept getting the information wrong, such as referring to a famous sculpture of the head of Queen Nefertiti as a mummy—but a mine full of Nazi gold was an irresistible headline. Patton was so furious that word of the find had leaked to the press, he fired the responsible censor, even though he had no authority to do so. But the damage was done. *Stars and Stripes* ran a story on Merkers every day for a week, and newspapers around the world followed suit. Three days later, an even larger, more spectacular discovery made international headlines, at least until someone realized the new "Mercedes" mine was actually a misspelling of Merkers.

Stout had been told to arrive at 1500 hours, without the higher-ranking (but British) Geoffrey Webb. Webb had been denied permission to enter by the financial branch of Civil Affairs. Stout arrived at 1445 in a jeep provided by Third Army and was immediately ushered into the presence of a lieutenant colonel, who assigned him to a billet and told him he couldn't leave until further notice. The billet was filled with financial staff. At 2115, Colonel Bernstein, Ike's financial advisor for civil affairs and military government, arrived to inform Stout he had been designated the MFAA officer for this operation. When Stout complained about the exclusion of his boss Geoffrey Webb, Bernstein showed him a letter from Patton stating that Bernstein was in charge of the mine area. No arguments, and no mistaking the message: This was an American operation—with apologies to Webb, no British officers allowed. And it was an American *financial* operation as well. The artwork was secondary. A glum Stout, having dispatched Lincoln Kirstein to give Webb the bad news that Patton wanted "no damn limeys" in the mine,[5] spent the rest of the evening interviewing Dr. Schawe, a German librarian he found "clumsy and unnecessarily vindictive."[6]

The next morning, Stout met Dr. Paul Ortwin Rave, a German art expert who had been living on the premises since April 3 with his family, his personal library, and his prized collection of rugs. The press had reported that Rave was the assistant director of the Prussian state museums; in fact, he was the assistant to the director. But he was no mere underling. A dedicated and professional museum man, his career had been stymied by his refusal to join the Nazi Party.

At the beginning of the war, Rave explained, the treasures of the German state museums had been removed from their galleries and placed in bank vaults and anti-aircraft towers in and around Berlin. In 1943, Rave suggested evacuating the collections from the Berlin area, which was beginning to come under Allied aerial bombardment. He was told this was dangerously defeatist thinking...perhaps fatally so. Nonetheless, he tried again the next year; he was again dismissed, and his life once again threatened. It wasn't until Soviet long-range ground artillery started battering the city that authorization was obtained to remove the artwork to Merkers. Four hundred of the largest paintings— including works by Caravaggio and Rubens—were to be left in the Berlin towers, along with numerous sculptures and various antiquities. Rave had estimated it would take eight weeks to move everything else; he was given two. The final shipment arrived on March 31, 1945. Five days later, Third Army overran the area.

"Two weeks to move this massive amount of art," Stout commented at the end of Rave's tale. "What a luxury. We've been given six days."

———

The generals—Dwight Eisenhower, the Supreme Commander in the European theater; Omar Bradley, commander of U.S. Twelfth Army Group; Manton Eddy, commander of XII Corps; and George Patton, the irrepressible titan of Third Army—flew to Merkers late in the morning of April 12. Brigadier General Otto Weyland, commander of XIX Tactical Air Command for Ninth Army, met the other generals there. Together with a few staff members and a German elevator operator, the generals rode the ancient elevator down twenty-one hundred feet into the main Merkers mine. The slow trip, undertaken in complete darkness, lasted several minutes. Halfway down, with only the groaning of the solitary elevator cable for company, Patton joked, "If that clothesline should part, promotions in the United States Army would be greatly stimulated."[7]

"OK, George, that's enough," came Eisenhower's voice out of the darkness. "No more cracks until we are above ground again."

Going into a potassium mine—or a copper mine, or a salt mine, or any other type of German mine—was an uncomfortable experience. These were working mines, not tourist sites, and the passageways were rough, narrow, and cramped. Much of the equipment was old and, because the war had drawn away men and materials, poorly maintained. The Germans had chosen the safety of deep mines for their repositories, so the soldiers often traveled a quarter mile into the ground, and another quarter mile laterally at the bottom. To exist in perpetual darkness, far below the earth, without a map of the mine or assurance the next passageway wasn't booby-trapped or the next holding bay not full of dynamite, was a nerve-jangling experience. Even worse, most of the mines were in areas that had been bombed or shelled, knocking out their power supplies. They were dark, cold, and damp.

Understandably, the generals moved quickly. In Room #8, now evacuated of all but essential personnel, they looked over rows and rows of gold bars and banknotes worth hundreds of millions of dollars. In the next room, they flipped through the paintings. Patton thought they were "worth about $2.50 and best suited for saloons";[8] in actuality, he was looking at pieces from the collection of the world-famous Kaiser-Friedrich Museum in Berlin. Other rooms, reserved for the SS, were crammed with gold and silver platters and vases, all flattened with hammer blows to make them easier to store. Entire trunks were filled with jewelry, watches, silverware, clothing, eyeglasses, and gold cigarette cases, the last vestiges of an enormous hoard the SS had not yet been able to smelt. There were eight bags of gold rings, many of them wedding bands. A soldier opened another bag and lifted out a handful of gold fillings. They had been pulled from the teeth of Holocaust victims.

"What would you do with all that loot?" Eisenhower asked over lunch, referring to Germany's bullion and paper currency.

Patton replied, in his usual gruff fashion, that he'd spend it on weapons or a gold medallion "for every son of a bitch in Third Army."[9] The generals laughed, but the question was far from academic. Much to the dismay of Stout and the Monuments Men, Bernstein was proceeding under the assumption that everything in the mine, including the artwork, was captured enemy loot. It would be months before he was disavowed of that notion.

The lightheartedness stopped for good that afternoon when the generals visited Ohrdruf, the first Nazi work camp liberated by American troops. Ohrdruf was not a death camp, like Auschwitz, where "undesirables" were sent for extermination, but a place where human beings were systematically worked to death. In silence, the generals and their staff officers walked the camp. "The smell of death overwhelmed us," General Bradley wrote, "even before we passed through the stockade. More than 3,200 naked, emaciated bodies had been flung in shallow graves. Others lay in the streets where they had fallen. Lice crawled over the yellow skin of their sharp, bony frames. A[n Allied] guard showed us how the blood had congealed in coarse black scabs where the starving prisoners had torn out the entrails of the dead for food.... I was too revolted to speak. For here death had been so fouled by degradation that it both stunned and numbed us."[10]

Several survivors, shrunken to mere skeletons, pulled themselves up on shriveled legs and saluted the generals as they passed. The generals walked on in stony silence, their lips drawn tight. Several members of their staff, all of them hardened by war, openly wept. The hard-nosed Patton, "Old Blood and Guts," ducked behind a building and threw up.

Every American soldier, Eisenhower insisted, every

man and woman not on the front lines, must see this. "We are told the American soldier does not know what he is fighting for. Now, at least, he will know what he is fighting against."[11]

Patton put it more bluntly: "You'll never believe how bastardly these Krauts can be, until you've seen this pesthole yourself."[12]

It wasn't until midnight that Patton, exhausted from two of the most remarkable and terrible tours in history, lay down to sleep. Before turning off the light, he noticed that his watch had stopped. Tuning in to BBC radio for the correct time, he heard one last bit of news: President Franklin Delano Roosevelt had died.

————

While the generals toured the main chambers of Merkers, Stout toured the nearby mines. The Merkers complex included more than thirty-five miles of tunnels and a dozen entrances.[13] There was no inventory of the works in the mines, but Dr. Rave had a list of the museums and collections from which they had come. The Berlin museum collections were the first to arrive and had been stored in the Ransbach mine. Rave had found the mine unsatisfactory and subsequent shipments had gone to Merkers. This worried Stout since the damp, salty Merkers was a less than ideal place for art, but the elevator was out of service at Ransbach so he couldn't inspect its contents.

No matter, there was plenty to do. Descending into the Philippstal mine, he found reference books and maps. Lincoln Kirstein descended into the Menzengraben mine, only to have the power fail, leaving him trapped in complete darkness and silence thousands of feet under the earth. "Rather than walk up to the height of two Empire State buildings," he wrote home, "I explored a vast Luftwaffe uniform depot and chose a parachute knife as a souvenir."[14]

On the morning of April 13, George Stout worked out the materials needed to pack all the artwork for shipment: boxes, crates, files, tape, thousands of feet of packing materials. His conclusion: "No chance of getting them."[15]

With the elevator back in service, he descended into the Ransbach mine with the disagreeable Dr. Schawe. The mine was almost twice as deep as the main shaft at Merkers, and significantly more cramped. The books alone took up most of the space. Stout estimated a million volumes, maybe two. The forty-five cases of artwork from the Berlin museum sat where Rave had left them. Seven had been rifled, but major pieces by Dürer and Holbein had not been touched. The collection of costumes from the State Opera had been ransacked. "Russian and Polish laborers," one of his German guides grunted. Stout knew he meant *forced* laborers, and found it hard to blame them for their thievery.

Back at Merkers, Stout learned from Bernstein the plans had changed. Instead of evacuating on April 17, they would be leaving on April 15. "A rash procedure," Stout noted in his diary, "and ascribed to military necessity."[16]

Military necessity was too strong. Military convenience, the thing Eisenhower warned against in his initial orders on cultural preservation, was probably more apt. General Patton was charging ahead, and he didn't want to leave four battalions behind to guard a gold mine. Bernstein, meanwhile, had his own reasons for haste. At the Yalta Conference in late February, Roosevelt, Churchill, and Stalin had partitioned the German state into zones of control. Merkers, and all its treasures, were in the Soviet zone. If Soviet troops arrived before the mine was evacuated—and there were persistent rumors of contact between American and Red Army advanced patrols in the "no-man's land" of central Germany—its contents would disappear into the hands of the Red Army. The Soviets were in no mood for equanimity, and understandably so. They had suffered millions of casualties in the Nazis' brutal and devastating invasion of their country, including more than 1.5 million dead in the siege of Stalingrad alone. Their forces, currently hacking and slashing their way into German territory, included Trophy Brigades: art and finance officials whose job it was to find and seize enemy assets, looted or otherwise. Stalin expected to be restituted in kind in gold, silver, carved marble, and works of art for what his people had lost.

Thirty minutes after midnight on April 15, George Stout finished his plans for the evacuation of Merkers. Unable to secure packing materials, he had requisitioned from the Luftwaffe uniform depot Kirstein found in the Menzengraben mine a thousand sheepskin coats, the kind German officers used on the Russian front. Most of the forty tons of artwork would be wrapped in the coats, recrated with similar works, then organized into appropriate collections. He met with

Colonel Bernstein. The gold was too heavy to be loaded to the tops of the trucks, so crates of paintings would be mixed in to maximize the load. Loading would start in an hour, at 0200, thirty-six hours ahead of the original schedule. By 0430 the artwork already in crates or boxes was brought to the surface and loaded. "No time to sleep," Stout wrote.[17] He had to prepare invoices and detailed instructions for the unloading and storage of the artwork in Frankfurt.

At 0800, an hour before the first convoy left, Stout started on the uncrated paintings. He planned to move them to a building above ground for temporary storage, but even with twenty-five men, the work proved impossible. By noon, the crew had reached fifty, and Stout had decided to crate the paintings underground. Unfortunately, the large crates were awkward to handle, especially in the confusion of the mineshafts. Jeeps had been brought down to help transport the gold, blocking some passages. Their exhaust fouled the air, and the occasional backfire of an engine echoed ominously in the rocky corridors. The gold was being sprayed with water to remove the corrosive salt of the mine, and the main shaft to the elevator was ankle-deep with the runoff. Soldiers were scurrying in all directions, carrying stacks of money, bags of gold, and ancient art, and it was all Stout could do to keep his men from wandering off in the confusion and not returning to work.

At 0005, five minutes past midnight on April 16, Stout reported "all paintings on ground level, in 3 places. All print boxes on ground level in 2 places. Cased works below ground somewhat rearranged and piled in part ready to load at elevator shaft."[18] The loading at Ransbach started at 0830; the loading at Merkers a half hour later with seventy-five men and five officers. At 1300, prisoners of war were brought in to assist the operation. By 2100 all the paintings were loaded. Stout went to the Dietlas mine, reached by an underground passage from the main shaft at Merkers, and found photographic equipment, modern paintings, and racks of archives. One set from Weimar was marked 933–1931, a thousand years of municipal history. "Inspection finished 2300," he wrote. "Returned Merkers, ate supper, reported."[19]

The art convoy—thirty-two ten-ton trucks with a motorized infantry escort and air cover—left for Frankfurt at 0830. It arrived at 1400. Stout noted only "complicated unloading. L. Kirstein a great help. All handled by 105 PWs [prisoners of war] in poor health. Storage in temporary arrangement 8 rooms basement level, one large room underground." Stout's inventory listed 393 paintings (uncrated), 2,091 print boxes, 1,214 cases, and 140 textiles, representing most of the Prussian state art collection. "Job finished and area secured 2330."[20]

"The last time I saw them," Lincoln Kirstein wrote in his account of the operation, "Lieutenant Stout was gravely whirling a swing aerometer in all corners of their new home, determining the humidity."[21] He had been up for almost four straight days, but as always with George Stout the job got done—and done right.

"I felt badly that I could not get to write to you during those five days," Stout wrote Margie on April 19 with his usual understatement. "It was really busy… a queer job and outlandish—in and around some salt mines from 1200 to 2500 feet below ground. You've read about some of it in the papers. A mistake that it ever got there, and could have been a very serious mistake. The publicity was naturally clamped down on and I can't tell you more now.

"It was really warm here today, and I walked for an hour and a half. The sun is fine and, after the rat race, I begin to remember that I am myself and not merely a set of functions. At times it is good to be only a piece of machinery, for then you do not dream of home or wish for delights that you cannot have. But I'm not morbid. The job is interesting. And it has got to be done. And I am very well."[22] He ended by telling her of his prize acquisition from Merkers: two fur-lined coats from the Soviet front he could use as bedrolls. Those coats and a paratrooper's knife were his only souvenirs.

Robert Posey, who had worked with Stout on and off at Merkers, was even more matter-of-fact about the operation. "At the gold mine they filled my helmet with twenty dollar American gold pieces and said I could have it," he wrote Alice on April 20, a few days after emerging from the mine. "I couldn't lift it off the ground—it contained $35,000—so we poured it back in the sacks and left it. I seem to have absolutely no greed for money for I felt no thrill at seeing so much of the stuff. Your poem means more to me."[23]

It had been a remarkable few weeks, but no Monuments Men were celebrating. If the Western Allied forces could stumble on Merkers, they could easily stumble on something just as extraordinary and unexpected, as Monuments Man Walker Hancock would discover. And still out there, somewhere in Nazi hands, were known to be two great treasure troves of looted European art: the cream of the French artistic patrimony, according to Rose Valland stored in the castle at Neuschwanstein; and Hitler's treasure chamber deep at Altaussee, in the Austrian Alps, which contained many of the greatest works of art in the world.

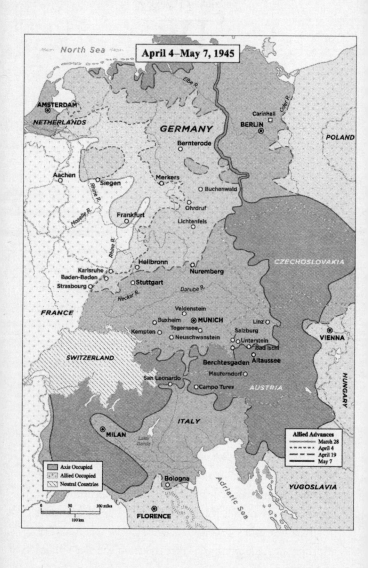

April 4–May 7, 1945

North Sea

AMSTERDAM

NETHERLANDS

GERMANY

Elbe R.

Carinhall

BERLIN

POLAND

Bernterode

Aachen

Siegen

Merkers

Buchenwald

Rhine R.

Moselle R.

Frankfurt

Ohrdruf

Lichtenfels

Rhine R.

CZECHOSLOVAKIA

Heilbronn

Nuremberg

Karlsruhe

Baden-Baden

Strasbourg

Stuttgart

Neckar R.

Danube R.

FRANCE

Veldenstein

Buxheim

MUNICH

Linz

Tegernsee

Salzburg

VIENNA

Kempten

Neuschwanstein

Unterstein

Bad Ischl

SWITZERLAND

Berchtesgaden

Altaussee

HUNGARY

Mauterndorf

San Leonardo

AUSTRIA

Campo Tures

ITALY

Lake Garda

MILAN

Adriatic Sea

YUGOSLAVIA

Bologna

Allied Advances
March 28
April 4
April 19
May 7

FLORENCE

Axis Occupied
Allied Occupied
Neutral Countries

0   50   100 miles

100 km

CHAPTER 37

Salt

Altaussee, Austria
1100–1945

The Alps, the tallest and most rugged mountain range in Europe, rise about a mile above sea level along the German-Austrian border. They form a land of steep rocky peaks, full of snowcapped mountains and picturesque chalets. The road from Salzburg, the most important entry point from the north, winds like hairpins up the mountains and down into deep green forested valleys, each one seemingly more remote than the next. For miles, the forests are so thick there is nothing to see but trees. Then, suddenly, an alpine lake will appear, and across it a gingerbread town of steep roofs and carved decorations wedged against a mountain slope. About forty-four miles from Salzburg lies the Pötschen Pass. The road over it is so steep, twisting, and precarious that it is almost unfit for driving, but the pass eventually levels out into a high alpine valley, at the end of which is the tiny village of Bad Aussee and finally, a few miles beyond, tucked against the banks of another spectacular alpine lake, the even smaller village of Altaussee.

From there, the road begins a climb so steep that

the Pötschen Pass seems a mild slope by comparison. Along the road runs a clear, crashing alpine stream, and beyond are the immense and breathtaking mountains. They are limestone deposits, formed in the depths of an ancient sea, and even on the sunniest day they are pale gray beneath their caps of snow. A bleak stone building, perched precariously above a thousand-foot precipice, marks the beginning of the end. Beyond is only a low irregular building and a wall of rock, the steep side of the Sandling Mountain. Bored into the mountain is a small tunnel, the main entrance to an ancient salt mine. Local legend holds that salt had been mined here for three thousand years—before the founding of Rome, at the height of the ancient Egyptian empire. Local written records, however, only date back to the 1100s.

In those days, at the turn of the first millennium, salt was one of the foundations of civilization. Without it, food couldn't be preserved or transported, so whole societies survived because of salt. Roman legionnaires were sometimes paid in salt (the basis of the English word "salary"), and merchants trod the salt roads in large caravans, linking the Western world of Europe with the Eastern world of Asia and Arabia. In Tibet, Marco Polo noticed that salt was pressed into wafers, imprinted with the image of the Grand Khan, and used as money. Timbuktu, the great lost civilization of Africa, valued salt as highly as gold. The early Germans, whose Visigoth ancestors sacked Rome and threw civilization into darkness, were economically dependent on their salt mines, and especially the taxes from their salt trading routes. The city of Munich, an early base of power for the Nazi Party, was founded in 1158 so the ruler of Bavaria could more easily collect a tax on the salt being transported from the city of Salzburg (German for "Salt Castle").

And throughout the centuries, as cities and empires rose and fell, the Steinberg mine in the Sandling Mountain of Austria, just above the village and lake known as Altaussee, continued to produce salt. The salt was not mined with picks and shovels, but dissolved by the flow of water through special pipes and sluices. The water came from the mountain above, especially during the spring snowmelt, and descended by gravitational force through the mine. There it was inundated with rock salt, then sent down the mountain to Bad Ischl, more than seventeen miles away, where the brine was evaporated to form pure crystal salt. It was left to 125 miners to maintain the pipes and sluices, shore up the catacombs against the pressure of the mountain, and make sure the vast labyrinth of rooms and tunnels didn't merge together and destabilize the entire structure.

Since the 1300s, this job had been performed by members of a small group of families, all living in the hills near the mine. Over the centuries humans grew larger, but the miners stayed the same size, until they eventually seemed dwarfed by the demands of the mine and their time underground (diet and inbreeding were more likely causes). Even in the early twentieth century, this small isolated community spoke a dialect last popular in the Middle Ages. They explored their tunnels with acetylene torches, and wore the white linen suits and peaked caps of medieval miners.

But in the winter of 1943–1944, the salt mine at Altaussee was assaulted by the modern world. First came the tracked vehicles necessary for maneuvering over the roads in the winter, when the five meters of snow were almost level with the treetops. They were followed by supply jeeps, and eventually a seemingly endless line of trucks going back and forth through the steep mountain passes. Nazi officers descended on the mine as guards. Workers arrived, expanding catacombs and building wooden floors, walls, and ceilings in dozens of salt chambers. Giant wooden racks were assembled in workrooms deep within the mountain and hammered into position, in some places three stories high. Experts and clerks moved in; a shop was built deep inside the mine where technicians could work and even live for days at a time. And it was all done for art.

Viennese museums had been the first to store their art treasures at Altaussee, but the mine was soon requisitioned by Hitler for his personal use. Worried by increasing Allied air raids, the Führer ordered all the treasures destined for his great museum at Linz, scattered until that time in several locations, sent deep into seclusion. It wasn't just the remoteness, or the relative convenience to Linz, which was only about a hundred miles away, that made Altaussee ideal. Dug straight into the side of a massive mountain, the horizontal mine was impregnable to aerial bombardment—even if the bombers could locate it in the vast Sandling mountain range. The salt in the walls absorbed excess moisture, leaving the humidity constant at 65 percent. The temperature varied only between 40 (in the summer, when the mine was coolest) and 47 degrees Fahrenheit (in the winter). The environment helped to preserve the paintings and prints, and metal objects such as armor could easily be protected against its corrosive effect by a thin layer of grease or gelatin. No one, not even Hitler, could have devised a more ideal natural hideaway for tons of stolen loot.

And still, the miners mined as they had for a thousand years, diverting water into empty corridors, washing their rock salt down the mountain to Bad Ischl. Even as artwork continued to arrive through 1944 and into 1945, the miners worked. Often they were called upon to help unload shipments, many stamped "A.H., Linz." From May 1944 to April 1945, more than 1,687 paintings arrived from the Führerbau, Hitler's office in Munich. In the fall of 1944, the Ghent Altarpiece was transferred from Neuschwanstein. Michelangelo's *Bruges Madonna* arrived soon after, having been transported out of Belgium by boat, in October 1944.

On April 10, 1945, and again three days later on April 13, eight more crates were moved into the mine. They were the property not of the Nazi leaders in Berlin but of August Eigruber, the local Nazi gauleiter (governor). The crates were marked "*Vorsicht—Marmor— nicht stürtzen.*" Attention—Marble—Do Not Drop.[1] But they didn't contain statues, as the miners who moved them deep into the mine assumed. Gauleiter Eigruber, a fanatical Austrian Nazi, was enthusiastic in his support of Adolf Hitler's Nero Decree. The crates contained not artwork, but 500-kilogram bombs (approximately 1,100 pounds), each one large enough to comfortably seat six men. Eigruber was determined to destroy the mine...and its priceless contents.

———

Supreme Allied Commander General Dwight Eisenhower looked at the map of Germany with trepidation. The crossing of the Rhine by Western Allied forces, combined with the Red Army advance to the Oder River, had sealed Germany's fate. Churchill, among others, was urging the Western Allies to consider postwar objectives, which in the short term meant above all else beating the Soviets to Berlin. Eisenhower had at first agreed, but circumstances on the ground were leading him to reevaluate the wisdom of a march on Berlin. At a March 27 news conference, Eisenhower was asked if he thought such a march could even be accomplished. The Western Allies were still two hundred miles from the German capital; the Soviets were just over thirty miles away. "Well," Eisenhower admitted, "I think mileage alone ought to make [the Soviets] do it."[2]

But it wasn't the Red Army he was worried about. The Germans, while perhaps doomed, were far from defeated. The Wehrmacht was still fighting on all fronts, with a strong fortress at their back: the Alps.

For months, many Western Allied war planners had assumed the German-Austrian borderland—the area from Salzburg in the north, Linz in the east, and the Brenner Pass near the Italian border in the west—would be the last stronghold of Nazism. The region, Hitler's home territory, was known to contain stockpiles of weapons and food, and it was believed to be rife with fortified, entrenched defensive positions. As one SHAEF report had summarized the situation, "The area is, by virtue of its terrain, almost impregnable."[3]

Eisenhower's fear, and that of his top advisors like General Bradley, was that Hitler would slip out of Berlin and take refuge in the mountains. Intelligence agents confirmed that for weeks crack SS divisions had been moving south from Berlin, west from the Soviet front, and north from the Italian theater. They seemed to be converging on Berchtesgaden, the small mountain town where Hitler and his top aides had summer homes and often conducted government business. With Hitler at the helm—or even without him—Eisenhower feared even a modest number of well-trained, die-hard troops holed up in the nearby mountains could hold off Allied forces for years.

Eisenhower despised the Germans. He blamed them for the war, and for its often inhuman destructiveness. And he was still smoldering about the Ohrdruf work camp, which he visited with some of his generals the same day as Merkers. "The things I saw beggar description," he wrote to his boss, General Marshall. "While I was touring the camp I encountered three men who had been inmates and by one ruse or another had made their escape. I interviewed them through an interpreter. The visual evidence and the verbal testimony of starvation, cruelty, and bestiality were so overpowering as to leave me a bit sick. In one room where they [had] piled up twenty or thirty naked men, killed by starvation, Patton would not even enter. He said he would get sick if he did so. I made the visit deliberately, in order to be in position to give *first-hand* evidence of these things if ever, in the future, there develops a tendency to charge these allegations merely to 'propaganda.'"[4] He wrote more simply to his wife, Mamie, "I never dreamed that such cruelty, bestiality, and savagery could exist in this world! It was horrible."[5] Eisenhower had no intention of allowing the Nazis any refuge or scrap of hope.

On April 12, 1945, the same day he toured Merkers and Ohrdruf, the Supreme Allied Commander told General Patton that U.S. Third Army would be turning south toward Nuremberg and Munich. Their primary job now was to secure southern Germany and rout the remaining Nazis from the Alps.

Patton vehemently disagreed. "We had better take Berlin and quick," he argued, "and move on to the Oder"—Germany's eastern border.[6] Eager for the Americans to win the war's great prize, Patton claimed U.S. Third Army could reach Berlin in forty-eight hours.

Eisenhower countered that it was true the Western Allies could take Berlin, but he doubted they could get there first. And if they did, who would want it? General Bradley estimated the effort to capture the city would result in 100,000 casualties—too steep a price for a "prestige objective."[7]

So in April 1945, U.S. Third and Seventh armies found themselves heading not east toward Berlin, but south toward Austria and the Nazis' last refuge, an area known in military parlance as the "Alpine Redoubt." Only the Monuments Men—and in particular Robert Posey, Lincoln Kirstein, and James Rorimer, the men assigned to those armies—understood that Eisenhower's decision had brought into their paths the two most important art repositories in the Fatherland: Neuschwanstein and Altaussee. But even they didn't know the intentions of Gauleiter August Eigruber, or of Hitler's retreating SS troops.

CHAPTER 38

Horror

Central and Southern Germany
Second Week of April 1945

Walker Hancock felt, once again, as if he had entered another world. U.S. First Army was working its way east across central Germany through a sparsely populated area of deeply wooded forests. The German Wehrmacht had melted away, except for the occasional mortar attack or small firefight, and many of the villages seemed untouched. Actually, some were littered with military debris and even broken buildings and houses, but compared to what Hancock had seen near the German border, this world seemed whole. "We have outrun the region of total destruction," he wrote Saima, "so that I missed my guess about *never* seeing an unruined city in Germany."[1]

He lamented, however, that he had become emotionally and physically detached. "The army is moving so rapidly that our stands now are like the stands of an itinerate show company," he wrote in another letter to his wife. "It *is* odd being present in a place like this and not being allowed to enter into the life of it in the least degree. Like being in a vaccum jar, looking at the outside world."[2]

He seemed unaware that his numbness was perhaps not just the inevitable hardening of the fighting man, but a deliberate attempt to distance himself from the German world. The concentration camp at Buchenwald had been liberated by U.S. Third Army on April 12, 1945. Walker Hancock had been in the town of Weimar when word reached him of the horrors that had taken place only a few miles away. He heard for the first time descriptions of death camps and gas chambers, and was sickened by stories of emaciated survivors huddled under the bodies of their friends and loved ones. It was inhuman. Beyond comprehension. Hancock felt the sight of such horror would change him forever—this man who saw blossoms growing out of destruction—and made a deliberate decision not to visit the camp.

"A number of our officers went up to see the camp," he wrote. "I did not go, because much of my work depended on friendly relations with German civilians, and I feared that after seeing the horrors of the camp my own feelings toward even these innocent people would be affected. (Numbers of our officers who did go could not eat for some time afterwards; some survived on whisky alone for days.)"[3]

A few days later, he had a chance meeting with his friend, a Jewish chaplain. The chaplain had recently been to Buchenwald to conduct a service for the survivors, their first since being interned. The story the chaplain told was "heartrending—emotional beyond description," especially when he mentioned the anguish over the lack of a Torah.

"I have no idea where to get one," he lamented. "They have all been destroyed."

"Not all of them," Hancock said. He had one in his office; it had been brought in that very day from the local SS headquarters.

"A miracle," the chaplain said, before dashing off to Buchenwald with the scroll.

"He was soon in my office again," Hancock wrote, "to tell me how it had been received—the people weeping, reaching for it, kissing it, overcome with joy at the sight of the symbol of their faith."[4] Walker Hancock had again found his rose in the ruins, but at what cost?

Fortunately, Monuments work kept him so busy he never had to contemplate that question. The army was moving quickly toward a rendezvous with the Red Army in Dresden and, still without an assistant, it was all Hancock could do to complete the basics of his assignment. His sixteen-hour days, he told Saima, were spent half in the "pain at seeing beauty needlessly destroyed by those we might have hoped would show more signs of being civilized" and half in the joy of spring days returning to rural German towns.[5] At night he lay awake thinking of his new wife, and of the home they would one day buy together, and of the monuments he simply couldn't find time to visit, and of the ridiculous quantity of coffee he had consumed, but coffee was all that kept him going sometimes.

"How can I describe the strange, strange combination of experiences each day here in this beautiful place brings!" he wrote Saima. "The eyes have one continual feast. It is late in the spring. Flowering trees are everywhere and the charm of the romantic little towns and the fairy tale castled countryside is enhanced by all this freshness. And in the midst of it all—thousands of homeless foreigners wandering about in pathetic droves. Germans in uniform, mostly with arms and legs—or more—missing. Children who are friendly, older ones who hate you, crimes continually in the foreground of life. Plenty, misery, recriminations, sympathy. All such an *exaggerated* picture of the man-made way of life in a God-made world. If it all doesn't prove the necessity of Heaven, I don't know what it means. I believe that all this loveliness showing through the rubble and wreck are just foreshadowings of the joys we were made for."[6]

––––––––

Farther south, Lincoln Kirstein had fallen into one of his black moods. The energy and optimism he had felt before Merkers was gone. Like Hancock, he had avoided Buchenwald when Posey had visited it the day after its liberation. But there was no escaping the horror. It was in the air he breathed, the German soil over which he walked. In his mind, he could see the marks in the dirt where the survivors had been dragged away. Posey had seen men dying before his eyes from the effects of their treatment. They were so starved they couldn't digest the meat the American soldiers gave them to eat. They simply collapsed, holding their stomachs in pain. Just to hear about it secondhand was to make a grown man want to clutch his own stomach and fall to the ground.

It didn't help that he had entered "the void," a world defined by anarchy, seemingly without reason or rules. The Nazi government was collapsing; the German army was splintered; there was no semblance of authority or societal structure. He knew it was a temporary situation, a time interval between the end of one reality and the beginning of another. *Götterdämmerung*, they called it in German, the period when the clash of the gods brings an end to the world. The villages were on fire, the civilians standing in the street hoping to be told what to do next. Often, they were joined there by German soldiers in uniform waiting to be captured or led, whatever the case might be. And yet the war ground on. Without a front line, without a way to tell friend from foe. Days passed without incident, then out of nowhere the Wehrmacht was entrenched at a bridge or the road was strafed by machine-gun fire. And everywhere, there was destruction.

"It's always more of the same complete and total annihilation of the centre portions of any town that had any faint interest," Kirstein wrote. "Most of the interior memorials have been given kunstschutz protection and will come out ok, but the baroque palaces and churches which were the real glories of southern sections [of Germany] are gutted and don't even make romantic ruins. I wonder what they'll figure out for the rebuilding of the towns, where the rubble is twenty feet deep packed, where they have no machinery or man power, and where they can't move into the suburbs which are just as bad or worse."[7]

He felt little pity. He had practically stopped trying to learn German, he admitted, because he didn't want to have anything to do with the German people. He had no sympathy for them, and he resented every minute spent in their country. He knew the void was a time interval, the last phase of a long and painful tour of duty, but that didn't mean he could see an end.

"The worst of it," he wrote his sister, "is that there will be no even half-peace for five years, and even as far as Germany goes I think they'll be fighting for some time. In spite of the collapse of the wehrmacht and the triumphant newspapers, there has been so far no place where a great many people were not killed winning it.... Hoping to see you before my retirement pay starts."[8]

And yet, despite his disgust with the German people, Lincoln Kirstein was horrified by the destruction of German culture. The sight of the burned-out monuments, and especially the bits of edifice that somehow had survived, made him sick. "The horrid desolation of the German cities, should, I suppose, fill us with fierce pride," he wrote:[9]

If ever the mosaic revenge was exacted, lo, here it is. The eyes and the teeth, winking and grinning in hypnotic catastrophe. But the builders of the Kurfürstliches Palais, of the Zwinger, of Schinkel's great houses, and of the Market Places of the great German cities were not the executioners of Buchenwald or Dachau. No epoch in history has produced such precious ruins. To be sure, they are rather filigraine, and delicate in comparison to antiquity, but what they lack in romance and scale is made up by the extension of the area they cover....

There is little use in trying to figure out now what can eventually be done,—should the cities be built again around the focus of surviving cathedrals, can the Church summon enough strength to restore. Where will the transport, the gasoline, the manpower, the materials come from to clear away the solid ruins, even before any work can be considered to rebuild?...

To make a loose summation: Probably the State and private collections of portable objects, have not suffered irreparably. But the fact that the Nazis always intended to win the war, counting neither on retaliation or defeat, is responsible for the destruction of the monumental face of urban Germany. Less grand than Italy, less noble than France, I would personally compare it to the loss of Wren's London City churches, and that's too much elegance to remove from the surface of the earth.

CHAPTER 39

The Gauleiter

Altaussee, Austria
April 14–17, 1945

August Eigruber's office in Linz was packed with petitioners. As Dr. Emmerich Pöchmüller, the general director of the Altaussee mining operations, pushed his way through the crowd, he saw not only businessmen but army commanders and SS officers, all gesturing and clamoring for an audience with the gauleiter. One of them was an old friend, the director of the power plant at Oberdonau (Upper Danube district). The poor man, Pöchmüller noticed, looked sweaty and pale.

"He's going to blow up the power plant," the man said.

Pöchmüller's heart sank. "You're here to convince him otherwise, aren't you?"

"I am. What about you?"

"I'm here to convince him not to blow up the salt mine."[1]

On April 14, 1945, Pöchmüller had discovered that Eigruber's crates contained bombs, not marble. He had called the gauleiter to complain, but no one would take his call. Two days later, Eigruber's adjutant had called to say the gauleiter's decision was final. The mines were to be destroyed.

On April 17, Pöchmüller decided to drive to Linz. After all, new orders from Albert Speer had stated that destruction wasn't necessary if the facilities could be "disabled" and made unusable by the enemy. Then Martin Bormann, Hitler's personal assistant, confirmed by radiogram—after Pöchmüller appealed to his assistant Dr. Helmut von Hummel—the Führer's wish that "the artwork was by no means to fall into the hands of the enemy, but in no event should it be destroyed."[2] Surely, this was reason enough for Eigruber to relent. But now that Pöchmüller was in the gauleiter's office, he realized everyone in the Oberdonau district had a reason their particular facility should be saved. Which probably meant none of them would.

In the end, he got five minutes. Eigruber did not offer him a seat. The gauleiter was an ironworker by training and a fierce party loyalist, having been a founding member of the Upper Austrian Hitler Youth. By age twenty-nine, he was the district leader. His loyalty lay with the Führer, or at least with the man he knew the Führer to be: a force for annihilation, without pity or remorse. Eigruber was suspicious of "unpure" orders from Speer or others who would soften the Führer's Nero Decree. And it was inconceivable to him, a man who had pounded iron in the factories of rural Austria, that the Führer would have made exceptions, especially for the preservation of art. If orders from Berlin were confusing or contradictory, then it was August Eigruber's right—no, his duty—to interpret them. And he knew the Führer's mind. Hadn't the great man preached his whole life about destruction: of the Jews, the Slavs, the gypsies, the sick, and the infirm? Hadn't he courageously ordered their extermination, an order obeyed with enthusiasm by Eigruber at the Mauthausen-Gusen concentration camp and by thousands of others at camps scattered across Eastern Europe? Hadn't he condemned the corrupting, degenerate nature of modern art? Hadn't he burned artwork in a great pyre in the center of Berlin? Hadn't he destroyed Warsaw and Rotterdam instead of letting them fall to the enemy? Hadn't he scarred the face of art-rich Florence? But for that weak fool General von Choltitz, Paris would be a disease-ravaged ruin. Eigruber was determined that, in his domain at least, weakness would not prevail. Absolutely nothing of value, he swore, would fall into the hands of the enemy. He never doubted that his Führer would approve.

"Do what you think is absolutely necessary," Eigruber said, as Pöchmüller prattled on about the blast area of bombs. "The main point is total destruction. We will stay bullheaded on this."[3]

CHAPTER 40

The Battered Mine

Heilbronn, Germany
April 16, 1945

James Rorimer finally arrived at the southern German town of Heilbronn, his first objective as Monuments officer for U.S. Seventh Army, on April 16, 1945. The journey had been, to put it mildly, a complete disaster. Seventh Army had hopped the Rhine River and was moving so rapidly that no one was sure where their headquarters was currently located. The Railroad Transportation Office routed him first to Lunéville, then an officer recommended he go to Sarrebourg, which was the end of the line. A sympathetic GI overheard his story and gave him a ride to Worms on his two-and-a-half-ton truck. From there he hitched a ride to Military Government headquarters, which informed him that Seventh Army was now south of Darmstadt, across the Rhine. "I've been expecting you for months," Lieutenant Colonel Canby snapped when Rorimer reported for duty at Seventh Army headquarters. "I concurred with the order to assign you to this headquarters in January."

"There's no need for monuments work over here," Canby told Rorimer bluntly, once he had settled in.

"The Army Air Forces have completely destroyed every major city in southern Germany, and our ground troops are taking care of the rest. Your job, as far as I'm concerned, is to locate art looted from Western Allied countries. Third Army has come in for more than its share of publicity"—referring to Merkers, which was still making worldwide headlines—"and it's time that Seventh Army had a salt mine or two of its own."[1]

Rorimer realized what Canby meant by complete destruction when he reached the outskirts of Heilbronn. Elements of VI Corps, Seventh Army, had arrived at the city on April 2, the day George Stout and Walker Hancock entered the mine at Siegen. They had been barreling through the industrial centers of south-central Germany on their way to Stuttgart, and they expected little resistance from this typical midsized town. Heilbronn was just another broken city, they figured, shattered by British air raids; a devastating raid in December 1944, in particular, had destroyed 62 percent of the infrastructure and killed seven thousand civilians, including a thousand children under the age of ten.

But looks could be deceiving, especially in the void of southern Germany. When Seventh Army tried to cross the Neckar River on the morning of April 3, the broken city exploded with life. The Neckar was a hundred meters wide and the Wehrmacht, hidden in the hills east of town, had perfect sightlines down on the plodding assault boats. Time and again the boats were sunk or driven back. When army engineers tried to launch a pontoon bridge, the Jerries took it out with mortar fire, sinking two tanks. Those who made it to the far bank were pinned down by enemy fire. The German mortars fired every three minutes, more frequently when targets showed themselves on the river or bank. When the soldiers crept into the streets, they discovered the angry citizens had formed the rubble of their homes and businesses into barricades, and crack German troops had taken up defensive positions along every line. For nine days the city was the site of one of the most brutal battles of the war, as Seventh Army fought block to block, then house to house, then room to room through the collapsing town.

James Rorimer, stuck in Paris for most of his time in Europe, hadn't seen anything like what remained since his inspection of Saint-Lô in Normandy. "What you read in the newspapers is not exaggerated," he would write his wife. "The ghost towns are fantastic. They are particularly bad just after they have surrendered."[2]

One route had been cleared; every other street looked impassable. Other than the Allied bulldozers working to clear the rubble, the city was deserted. Of the Germans, it seemed only the dead remained. The stench was overpowering.

According to captured German intelligence, the artwork could be found in the town's salt mine, whose superstructure—a grid of metal that supported the lift mechanisms—was visible from a mile away. Rorimer scrambled down Salt Street, then Salt Works Square and finally Salt Ground Street, where he was able for the first time to glimpse the brick and concrete building that housed the mineshaft. The fighting had been savage; several buildings were still smoldering. But there were people on the street, huddled and beaten but still alive. Rorimer pulled up beside two men and asked about the mine.

They shook their heads. "*Russo*," they said. They were Soviet slave laborers.

"*Deutsch*?" he asked. Did they know anyone who spoke German?

They shrugged. Who knew anything these days?

Rorimer finally located two terrified German women in an employee housing complex. The Nazis had wanted the mine destroyed, the women told him, but the miners refused. "We can live without the Nazis," they said, "but we cannot live without salt." There were twenty square miles of minable salt under Heilbronn, enough to provide work for generations. This was not something the miners were willing to destroy; the Nazis, fortunately, were too busy with other concerns. In the end, the fierceness of the battle saved the mine.

But there was still the water.

The mine, excavated to an average depth of six hundred feet, consisted of dozens of large chambers in two levels, one on top of the other. Much of the extensive tunnel system was beneath the Neckar River. Water seeped continuously down through cracks in the rocks. This seepage had to be pumped out eight hours a day to keep the mine from flooding, but because the power had been out, the pumps were not working. The lack of power had also knocked out the only elevator. No one had entered the mine, but the women assumed the lower level was full of water by now.

Rorimer had anticipated a quick stop. There were numerous repositories on the road to Neuschwanstein, and he couldn't afford to spend time at each one. But

Heilbronn, he realized, was a disaster in the making, and it was worth the investment of time. So he went immediately to Military Government headquarters with the mayor of Heilbronn to secure an engineering team. All the army would do was post a guard, so the next day he returned to headquarters in Darmstadt, where the colonel told him bluntly, "Nobody can be spared. The mine is your responsibility. Fix it yourself." Seventh Army wanted the glory of a major repository, but they didn't want to spare more than a single man— James Rorimer—to secure it.

Rorimer returned to Heilbronn, where he appealed directly to the mayor. The mayor sent runners to find the mine's chief engineer and its vice director, Dr. Hans Bauer, who had fled the city. Bauer confirmed the mine had been used as an art storage depot, but no inventory had been left with the mine directors. Bauer remembered a famous Rembrandt, *St. Paul in Prison*, and the stained-glass windows from the cathedral in Strasbourg, France, among other things. And although water leakage was a serious problem—the Neckar leaked 100,000 gallons of water into the mine every day—he assured Rorimer those objects might still be saved. They were on the upper level, which would probably not be flooded for days, maybe even weeks.

"Are you sure?"

"No, but there is a way to find out."

Bauer led Rorimer to a hole in the floor of the mine building. "Our emergency exit," he said. On the side of the hole was a thin, rickety ladder. Not more than ten feet into the hole, the ladder disappeared into darkness.

"How far down does it go?"

"Six hundred feet."

Rorimer stared into the darkness, wondering if a tour of the mine was absolutely necessary. "Did you hear something?" he said.

The men peered down into the hole, then stepped back as two wet, dirty men emerged from the darkness. "PFC Robert Steare, Company B, 2826 Engineers, sir," one of them said, snapping to attention.

He was just a kid. "What were you doing down there, son?"

"Exploring the mine, sir. With one of the miners."

"On whose orders?"

"No one's, sir."

Rorimer stared at his exhausted and dirty face, wondering why a kid would take it upon himself to descend six hundred feet into a flooded mine. The foolishness and bravery of youth, he supposed.

"What did you see?"

"There's nothing working down there, sir. Pitch-black. Everything's covered with three feet of water, including the pumps. There are locked storage rooms at the far end of the corridor. We didn't try to open them."

"Any indication of what was inside?"

"One of them said 'Strasbourg' in chalked letters. Others said 'Mannheim,' 'Stuttgart,' and 'Heilbronn.' But that's all I saw."

"And had the water reached them?"

"Oh, yes sir, the water was everywhere."

It took Bauer two weeks, until April 30, to implement a workable plan. The backup steam engines had not been badly damaged, and there was sufficient coal to run them for a few months. After repairs and adjustments, they could operate the elevators and skips, which were the trays that carried the salt from the bottom of the mine to the surface. By modifying the skips and welding an enormous bucket to the bottom of the elevator platform, water could be lifted out of the mine. It wouldn't stop the seepage, but it would keep the water level down while the pumps and electrical plant were repaired. Given the circumstances, it was an elegant solution. In the dead city of Heilbronn, there would be one beast alive and lumbering: the iron hands of the salt mine, hauling away water to protect the art.

By the time the plan was implemented, James Rorimer was gone. Seventh Army was nearing Munich, and he had no time to lose.

CHAPTER 41

Last Birthday

Berlin, Germany
April 20, 1945

On April 20, 1945, the Führer's fifty-sixth and last birthday, the Nazi elite gathered briefly in the Reichschancellery for a hastily arranged birthday celebration and series of "goodbyes." Most of the party hierarchy wished they were anywhere but Berlin. It may have been the Führer's birthday, but it was far from a festive occasion. That day, Western Allied troops had taken Nuremberg, the earliest base of operation for the Nazi Party, and raised the American flag over the stadium where the Nazis had once hosted the spectacles of annual rallies. The home of legendary fifteenth-century German artist Albrecht Dürer had been severely damaged; the top floors of the building that had sheltered one of Hitler's most cherished objects, the Veit Stoss altarpiece, which he had stolen from Poland at the start of the war, were demolished. Fortunately, the altarpiece was stored safely underground.

This salvation might have been a consolation to the world, but the men gathered in the Führerbunker couldn't have cared less. Their world was getting smaller by the day, and their time was short. There was no greater reminder of their impending doom than this impromptu party. In years past they had feasted, and the highest-placed among them had feted their leader with gifts, often looted artwork, his favorite thing to receive. Now the Red Army was pounding Berlin, and the explosions of their artillery could be heard even deep underground. Those not stationed in Berlin were eager to leave the city; those staying with Hitler were desperate for reprieve. For days, the mood in the bunker had been erratic. Wild hope would collapse into despair. Rumors of success would degenerate into squalid stories of defection and surrender. Hitler was rarely seen. The main topic of conversation was suicide—should it be cyanide or a bullet? The main activity was drinking.

The sight of Adolf Hitler, late for his own celebration, did nothing to cheer his followers. Suddenly, he seemed an old man, ashen and gray. He dragged his left foot, and his left arm hung weakly at his side. His posture was so slumped that his head seemed to have sunk into his shoulders. He could still be aggressive with his subordinates, especially his generals, but instead of his former fire he now exhibited an icy rage.[1] He believed he had been betrayed. He saw weakness everywhere. But at this party he could not even summon contempt. He was so depressed his doctors had to medicate him before he would appear before his most loyal associates, the men and women who had followed him onstage for the final act. His eyes, once so charismatic that they drove a nation to madness, were empty.

After shaking Hitler's hand and explaining that he needed to join his staff, Hermann Göring left the building, knowing he would never return. Albert Speer observed that "[I] felt I was experiencing a historic moment. The leadership of the Reich was parting company."[2] The next day, April 21, Göring arrived in Berchtesgaden, the Nazi retreat in the center of the Alpine Redoubt. Waiting for him there was Walter Andreas Hofer, his personal curator. His art collection had left his estate at Veldenstein in early April and, after numerous delays in the faltering German rail system, arrived in Berchtesgaden on April 16. After a few days, the eight railcars containing the artwork were sent northwest to Unterstein. When Göring arrived, the only railcars remaining at Berchtesgaden were the two or three that contained his furniture, his records, and his library. Hofer was living in one of the cars.

The situation, Göring knew, was grim. The Führer was clearly ill; anyone with a shred of common sense knew the Führerbunker was soon to become his tomb. The war was lost; the personal bounty of all those years dispersed; the Nazi movement splintered. The Reichsmarschall, momentarily safe in the German Alps, believed himself the only man capable of pulling together the last of the Reich and successfully suing for peace. And, after all, he was Hitler's designated successor.

On April 23, Göring sent a radiogram to Hitler. Aware that Berlin was surrounded and the situation hopeless, the Reichsmarschall was prepared to step in and lead the Nazi Party. If he did not hear back by 10:00 p.m. that evening, he would assume the Führer was incapacitated and take command. Hitler did not respond until April 25, 1945, but his reaction was furious and determined: He ordered the SS to arrest his second in command. The Third Reich was disintegrating.

———

Meanwhile, at Altaussee, the art restorer Karl Sieber ran his hands along the grain of his greatest work. *Here's where the panel split*, he thought, running his fingers along the wood. *And here the paint bubbled.* Before the war, Sieber had been a modest but highly respected art restorer in Berlin, a man so quiet, patient, and in love with his work that opinions of him ranged from the last honest craftsman in Germany to a complete simpleton. He had joined the Nazi Party for business reasons on the advice of a Jewish friend, and as a consequence his practice had flourished. Artwork had been pouring into Berlin from the conquered territories, and even if it was stolen or acquired through shady means, it still needed to be cared for and restored. Maybe even more so, in fact, since the Nazi officials were less art lovers than greedy hoarders, and they often treated their possessions roughly. Sieber had worked on more world-class pieces in the last four years than most restorers see in a lifetime. But never had he imagined working on a piece of this magnitude, one of the wonders of Western civilization: the Ghent Altarpiece. And he never imagined working like this: a mile within a mountain, in a remote Austrian salt mine.

He circled the panel so that he could look into the face of Saint John. What humanity in those old eyes! What skill at invoking the most exacting details! Every hair was painted with a single brushstroke from a single bristle. He could almost feel the folds of the cloak, the vellum of the Bible, the sadness and awe in the old saint's eyes. The only thing he couldn't see anymore was the split in the wood panel that had occurred while the piece was in transit, the repair he had worked so many months to make utterly and completely invisible to even the most trained eye.

It was a shame Sieber had to leave it in this unsafe chamber. But the wooden panel was taller than he was, and far too heavy for him to carry. He needed help to move it to the chambers deeper in the mountain where he and a few others had been transporting the best pieces since yesterday. So he turned to *The Astronomer*, painted by Jan Vermeer in 1668, almost two hundred and fifty years after the Ghent Altarpiece, but still showing the same delicacy of brushwork and attention to the most precise detail.

But that's where the similarities ended. The Ghent Altarpiece was an acknowledged, adored masterpiece from the moment of its creation, the centerpiece of the Dutch Renaissance. Vermeer was a provincial painter from Delft who died deeply in debt and completely unknown to the larger world. He had been rediscovered in the late 1800s, two hundred years after his death. Now he was considered a leader of the golden age of Dutch painting, the great master of light, the unsurpassed chronicler of domestic life. His *Girl with a Pearl Earring* was known as the "Dutch Mona Lisa,"[3] but this painting, *The Astronomer*, was every bit as powerful and unknowable. It showed a scholar in his chamber, an observation book open before him, studying intently the object of his obsession: a globe of the universe. What tinkerer, what scientist or art restorer, hadn't experienced such a moment, when the rest of the world disappeared and only the facts at your fingertips stood before you? Who hadn't fallen in love with discovery or felt that thirst for knowledge?

But then who could ever say what a man in such a moment was thinking? The astronomer's touch was delicate, almost shy. A natural light from the open window brushed the globe and the astronomer's outstetched hand. Was he simply measuring another in an endless series of distances, or had he found what he had been looking for? Here was a man wrapped completely in his work, a moment universal and idiosyncratic, momentous and inconsequential.

And it was untrue. There was no untouched astronomer, no detached craftsman. The lead art restorer at Altaussee knew that better than anyone. Bury a man a mile within a mountain, hundreds of miles from civilization, give him the work of a lifetime and all the resources needed to do it, and he was still subject to the whims of the world.

With one last look at the scholar—looking now, he thought, almost fearful of his discoveries—Karl Sieber picked up Hitler's favorite painting. Then, looking once over his shoulder, he disappeared into the dark passageway. He was headed back, farther into the mountain, to the Schoerckmayerwerk, one of the few mine chambers he believed—he hoped—would survive even the most cataclysmic bomb blast.

CHAPTER 42

Plans

Central Germany,
Southern Germany, and
Altaussee, Austria
April 27–28, 1945

On April 27, 1945, a young ordnance captain walked into the office of the chief of staff in the forward section of U.S. First Army. With a smile, he placed a small metal rod and ball on the desk. The commanding officer stared at them for a moment, then picked up the rod and looked at it from one end to the other. The intricately wrought, jewel-encrusted piece looked like a scepter made for a king. In fact, that's exactly what it was. The soldier had brought him the coronation scepter and coronation orb of the eighteenth-century Prussian king known as Frederick the Great.

"Where did you find it?"

"In a munitions dump, sir."

"Where?"

"In a hole in the forests in the middle of nowhere, sir."

"Is there anything else?"

"Sir, you are not going to believe what is down there."

A little more than a day later, on the morning of April 29, 1945, George Stout received a call from

First Army Monuments Man Walker Hancock. Stout had just finished sending an urgent request to SHAEF headquarters in France, begging for supplies: trucks, jeeps, packing materials, at least 250 men to guard repositories. He had received no guarantees.

"I'm outside Bernterode, a small town in the northern Thuringian forest," Hancock told him, almost tripping over his words. "There's a mine here, George, with 400,000 tons of explosives in it.[1] I can't tell you what else is down there, not over the phone, but it's important, George. Maybe even more important than Siegen."

While Hancock was exploring the mine at Bernterode, Emmerich Pöchmüller, the director general of Altaussee, was sitting in his office at the salt mine. In his hand was an order he had just typed; at the bottom was his signature. Seeing his own name there, in his own hand, made him feel sick.

He didn't want to send the order, but he could see no other option. After weeks of effort, he had been granted authority over the fate of the salt mine, but that authorization had not come from Eigruber. It had come from a minor museum official acting on third-hand information purportedly from Martin Bormann's assistant Helmut von Hummel in Berchtesgaden. It was hearsay at best, and probably an outright fabrication. If Pöchmüller's order fell into Eigruber's hands, the gauleiter would see it as insubordination, and it would mean his arrest—if not his immediate execution. But with the madman Eigruber in power, and no word from an ever more isolated Berlin, Altaussee was doomed. Something had to be done. As Pöchmüller walked toward the office of Otto Högler, the mine's chief engineer, he couldn't help but feel he was carrying his own death warrant.

"New orders," Pöchmüller said, handing Högler a sheet of paper. "I'm off to Bad Ischl. Don't wait for my return."[2]

---

28 April 1945

Mr.
Mining Engineer Högler

Saltmine Altaussee

Regarding: Depository

You are hereby being instructed to remove all 8 crates of marble recently stored within the mines in agreement with Bergungsbeauftragter Dr. Seiberl and to deposit these in a shed which to you appears suitable as a temporary storage depot.

You are further being instructed to prepare the agreed palsy as soon as possible. The point in time when the palsy is supposed to take place will only be presented to you by myself personally.

The General Director,
Emmerich Pöchmüller

The same day—April 28, 1945—*Stars and Stripes* reported that U.S. Seventh Army had reached Kempten, a town close to the castle at Neuschwanstein. It was the news James Rorimer had been waiting for since leaving Paris. He immediately phoned ahead for confirmation, only to be told by the major in charge that *Stars and Stripes* was incorrect. "But if there's any truth to it at all," Rorimer insisted, "our troops ought to be at Neuschwanstein pretty soon. That castle contains invaluable caches of looted works of art from France. I've been on the trail for months. I must get there at the earliest possible time. You must get there as soon as you can."[3]

"We're doing what we can."

If there was a hint of desperation in his appeal, it was because in the week since leaving the mine at Heilbronn, Rorimer had received a crash course in the realities of Monuments work. On one hand, he had discovered the great Riemenschneider Altarpiece undamaged in a damp basement in Rothenburg, the most famous medieval walled city in Germany. He had even convinced the Military Government officer to move the altarpiece from the damp cellar where it had been stored. With great satisfaction, he had assured the press the damage to the town had been greatly exaggerated.

A few days later, he received misinformation of a more dangerous kind when, on a mission to an ERR repository, he discovered the bridge over the Kocher River had been blown up. The area was partially in

German control, but that didn't stop Rorimer from trying to find another way across. Unfortunately, his driver soon became hopelessly lost in the thick German forests. As night approached, the men realized they couldn't even find their way back to the main road. Twice they drove through the same smoldering village, the embers the only light in a pitch-black night. Around dawn, they spotted two Allied soldiers walking alongside the road.

"Jesus," the soldiers said, after directing the two men to their encampment. "Have you been driving all night? There are Germans all through these woods."

In the late morning, after a brief nap, Rorimer and his driver forded a shallow point in the Kocher River in the company of an Allied truck. Later in the day, they finally reached their destination: a local castle. It was, as promised by Rose Valland, another Jeu de Paume way station full of priceless art.

But it wasn't the near misses that frightened Rorimer, or even the successes that inspired him. It was the big prize that had gotten away. While still headquartered at Darmstadt, Rorimer had received word that Baron Kurt von Behr, the scourge of the Jeu de Paume, was in residence at his castle in Lichtenfels, an area that had just fallen under American control. Too busy to make the long trip to Lichtenfels himself, Rorimer dispatched a telegram to Supreme Headquarters requesting that someone be sent immediately to apprehend the Nazi who knew more than anyone else about ERR looting operations in France. Days later, he discovered the telegram was being held in Heidelberg, pending his instruction on whether it should be marked "Priority" or "Routine." By the time American troops reached the castle at Lichtenfels, Colonel von Behr was gone. Aristocrats to the end, he and his wife had killed themselves in their library by drinking glasses of poisoned champagne.

CHAPTER 43

The Noose

Berlin, Germany, and
Southern Germany
April 30, 1945

On April 30, 1945, Adolf Hitler committed suicide in his bunker underneath the Reichschancellery in the city of Berlin. He had suffered a nervous breakdown during a military situation conference on April 22, admitting in a hysterical attack on his commanders that Germany was doomed. His Nazi Party was broken. His new Berlin was being blasted apart by bombs and artillery. His friends and generals had betrayed him, or so he in his paranoia believed. He was capable of terrific fits of temper, when he would become livid at those who had abandoned him, insist victory was achievable, and vow to fight on, but he had also become increasingly brooding and consumed with hatred and a will to destroy: to kill as many Jews as possible; to throw his armies, including old men and young boys, into the enemy lines as cannon fodder; to smash every brick and gut every element of infrastructure in Germany until the country that had betrayed him, that in its cowardice had proven the weaker race, not the master race, was sent back to the Stone Age. Their failure stripped everything from him until, in those final days, in his bunker deep beneath the Reichschancellery in Berlin, with the sound of Soviet artillery shells exploding overhead, one of the few things that remained in his twisted heart—perhaps the one thing that made him human and therefore truly terrifying—was his love of art.

During the preceding months he spent hours alone or with his loyal aides—Gauleiter August Eigruber had been a regular visitor—contemplating his scale model of Linz in the cellar of the New Chancellery: its great arcades and byways, its towering cathedral of art. Sometimes he would gesture energetically, pointing out a brilliant design element or an essential truth. Sometimes he would lean slowly forward in his chair, involuntarily clutching the glove in his left hand tighter and tighter, his eyes popping under the brim of his military cap as he silently stared, perhaps for the last time, at the symbol of everything that ever was or might have been.

Now it was over. During evening supper on April 28, only hours before he would marry his longtime mistress, Eva Braun, Hitler looked at his secretary, Traudl Junge, and said, "Fräulein, you are needed at once; bring your stenographer pad and pencil. I wish to dictate to you my last will and testament."[1]

[Seal]
[ADOLF HITLER]
My Private Will and Testament

As I did not consider that I could take responsibility, during the years of struggle, of contracting a marriage, I have now decided, before the closing of my earthly career, to take as my wife that girl who, after many years of faithful friendship, entered, of her own free will, the practically besieged town in order to share her destiny with me. At her own desire she goes as my wife with me into death. It will compensate us for what we both lost through my work in the service of my people.

What I possess belongs—in so far as it has any value—to the Party. Should this no longer exist, to the State, should the State also be destroyed, no further decision of mine is necessary.

My pictures, in the collections which I have bought in the course of years, have never been collected for private purposes, but only for the extension of a gallery in my home town of Linz a.d. Donau.

It is my most sincere wish that this bequest may be duly executed.

I nominate as my Executor my most faithful Party comrade, Martin Bormann.

He is given full legal authority to make all decisions. He is permitted to take out everything that has a sentimental value or is necessary for the maintenance of a modest simple life, for my brothers and sisters, also above all for the mother of my wife and my faithful coworkers who are well known to him, principally my old Secretaries Frau Winter etc. who have for many years aided me by their work.

I myself and my wife—in order to escape the disgrace
of deposition or capitulation—choose death. It is our
wish to be burnt immediately on the spot where I have
carried out the greatest part of my daily work in the
course of a twelve years' service to my people.

Given in Berlin, 29th April 1945, 4:00 o'clock.

(Sd.) A. Hitler

His family and loyal associates were practical considerations. The party, he understood, was doomed.
His newly married wife, Eva Braun, was merely "that
girl," even though she was only hours away from kill-
ing herself with poison by his side. Everything he had
worked for was gone, destroyed, but even at the end
one of the worst madmen of the twentieth century saw
one last chance at a legacy: the completion of a museum
in Linz, *his* museum in Linz, full of the plundered treasures of Europe.

The following day, within hours of Hitler's death,
three motorcycle couriers left the Führerbunker, each
carrying an original of Adolf Hitler's last will and testament.[2] They were all headed in different directions, but
each with one goal: to ensure that the dying wish of
the leader of the Nazi Party would survive the complete
destruction he himself had visited upon his people, his
country, and the world.

And yet even at that moment, Hitler's own
followers—some out of confusion and misguided loyalty, some out of self-interest, some out of fear, and

some out of a fundamental belief that the man who had asked them to annihilate millions of people and destroy entire cities would never ask them to save anything, especially something as decadent and meaningless as art—were working to thwart his wishes and destroy the stolen art collection he had held so dear.

And nowhere was this more true than in the Austrian Alps, where Gauleiter August Eigruber was as always "bullheaded" in his insistence on complete destruction of the salt mine at Altaussee. Even worse, he had discovered Pöchmüller's attempt to thwart his plans. His adjutant, District Inspector Glinz, had overheard Högler, the mine foreman who had received Pöchmüller's order, arranging for trucks to remove the gauleiter's bombs. "The crates are staying were they are," Glinz told Högler, drawing his gun. "I am completely in the picture and can see what's happening here. If you dare touch those crates, I will kill you."[3]

Högler begged Glinz to talk to Pöchmüller, who was down the mountain at another salt mine in Bad Ischl. In a tense telephone conversation with Glinz, Pöchmüller insisted the Führer's April 22 order—that at all costs they must keep the artwork from the enemy but by no means destroy it—was perfectly clear. The artwork was not to be harmed.

"The gauleiter considers the April 22 order outdated," Glinz responded, "and therefore obsolete. He considers all orders since not clean since they did not come from the Führer himself."[4]

With Hitler dead, there seemed no way to dislodge the gauleiter from his course of action, but Helmut von Hummel was prevailed upon by the mine managers one last time. On May 1, von Hummel sent a letter to Karl Sieber, the art restorer at Altaussee, stating that "last week" the Führer reconfirmed that "the artwork in the Oberdonau area are not to be permitted to fall into the enemy's hands, but shall by no means be finally destroyed."[5]

The telegram didn't work. When Pöchmüller arrived back at the mine, he found that the gauleiter had posted six more heavily armed guards at the entrance. The bombs were still inside; all that was needed now were the detonators—and they were already in transit to the mine.

———

To Robert Posey, South Germany was the worst possible place: a world without rules. Society had collapsed, and with it the battlefield. The shattered towns and villages lay one after another, destroyed either by Western Allied forces, dead-end Nazi hardcases, or local gauleiters still bent on executing Hitler's Nero Decree. Boats were sunk in the rivers; factories were on fire; bridges were severed. Civilians were wandering everywhere, searching for food and shelter. It was common to see a hundred or more ragged refugees in a group, walking nowhere in particular. They were coming from the local towns but also from the east, fleeing the vengeance of the Soviet advance.

Was he crossing the front lines? It was impossible to say. In many places, German soldiers were driving around in convoys, desperately hoping to surrender to Americans. Along the roads, Posey could see their faces behind barbed wire, most of them smiling now that their war was over. But oftentimes in the next town, German forces would be dug in, fighting to the last man. An abandoned village would erupt with sniper fire from dark windows. Unseen machine-gun emplacements would strafe the road. Some American units experienced little or no fighting; others lost more men during the void than they had in the previous six months. Both violence and peace were random and chaotic. The maps were useless. Sometimes Posey wondered if his compass still pointed north. There was no magnetism here, he figured, no force holding things together. It seemed the laws of nature, all laws in fact, were suspended. The best advice the army could give its soldiers was to stick close to their units and never wander alone. But what if you had no unit? What if your job by its very nature was defined by wandering nearly alone through this burned-out land?

Posey thought often of Buchenwald, even as the world around him deteriorated. In an abandoned office there, he had found a picture of a German officer. The man was standing at attention with an enormous smile on his face, holding up for the camera his prized possession: the noose he used to garrote prisoners to death. Posey kept the picture in his kit, and often looked at it before turning in for the night. The sight of that officer's smile would alternately make him angrier than hell, then sad beyond tears. In so many German faces Posey now saw that terrible officer, even sometimes in the children that for so long had reminded him of his son. He felt numb to the destruction, but terribly troubled. One day, caught far from camp without rations, he and Kirstein met a company of infantrymen who had just decided to kill and cook a rabbit they had spotted in a hutch behind a country home. As they entered the yard, a woman opened the door and called out to them.

"Please," she said in broken English, "that is my son's rabbit."

The soldiers were unmoved.

"Please," she said again. "My husband was an SS officer. I know, terrible, but no doubt he is dead. He gave my son that rabbit before he left for war. My son is eight, that rabbit is the only thing he has left to remember his father."

Robert Posey looked at the woman for a long time. Then he reached into his kit. He pulled out a piece of paper, but it wasn't the photograph from Buchenwald. It was one of the "Off Limits" signs he had so often posted on protected monuments. He wrote at the bottom, "By Order of Captain Robert Posey, U.S. Third Army," then hung the sign on the cage.

"No one will bother your boy's rabbit," he said, before marching off with the infantrymen.[6]

"The story [in your last letter] of the two year old colored boy," he wrote Alice a few days later, "somehow reminded me of the greatest horror I have seen. It was at the Nazi concentration camp near Weimar where I visited the day after its surrender. I still don't believe what I saw. It was simply too fantastic. Nothing that I have read about the sadistic cruelty of the Nazis now seems far fetched. It is a fine tribute to Roosevelt that he almost alone stood against them when the rest of the world was defeated. The people of Weimar, only four miles away, claim they didn't know what was going on, but he knew though four thousand miles away. But I wonder if our society is not a bit off-color when a tiny black boy is abandoned and left alone by his family. Perhaps I am just a softie. When I am billeted in a German home even for one night I go out and search for the chickens and rabbits or pets and give them water and food if possible. Generally the family has pulled out too rapidly to care for such things. I suppose the stern and the cruel ones rule the world. If so, I shall be content to try to live each day within the limits of my conscience and let great plaudits go to those who are willing to pay the price for it."[7]

CHAPTER 44

Discoveries

Thuringia, Germany, and
Buxheim, Germany
May 1, 1945

George Stout arrived at Bernterode on May 1, 1945. Just as Walker Hancock had hinted in his phone call, the mine was in a rural area, with nothing to see but forests. Even the tiny village nearby had been evacuated by Nazi officials so that no one would know about the frantic activity at the mine. The only sight of civilization, if that's what it could be called, was an internment camp for displaced persons, mostly French, Italian, and Soviet slave laborers who had worked in the mine. The mineshaft was deep, eighteen hundred feet, and the tunnels spread almost fifteen miles underground. The slave laborers had primarily been used to load and unload ammunition, since Bernterode was one of the largest munitions production sites in central Germany. The American ordnance crew that had explored it estimated the mine contained 400,000 tons of explosives. "It was a flogging or worse if you even carried a match into the mine," one of the French laborers had told Walker Hancock.

"The civilians were sent out six weeks ago," Hancock

commented to Stout as the two men took the long, slow, dark elevator ride to the bottom of the mine, "and the next day German soldiers started pouring in. They worked in complete secrecy. Two weeks later, the mine was sealed. It was April 2, George, the day we entered Siegen."

The elevator stopped at the bottom of the shaft, and the men flipped on their flashlights. There were electric lamps in the ceiling, but the light was feeble and the power intermittent. "This way," Hancock said, indicating the main corridor. They were more than a third of a mile underground, and there was no sound except their footsteps. Branching tunnels disappeared into the darkness, studded with chiseled rock chambers. Whenever Stout shone his flashlight beam into one of the rooms, it illuminated stacks of mortar shells and explosives. A quarter mile down was a newly mortared wall. There was no door—the Nazis hadn't expected anyone to enter this repository—so an even newer hole had been smashed out of the middle. Across the corridor was an enormous cache of dynamite.

"After you," Hancock said.

George Stout crawled through the wall opening and into a room even he, who had been at Siegen and Merkers, never imagined. There was a wide central passage, ablaze with light and lined with wooden racks and storage compartments. From the compartments hung 225 flags and banners, all unfurled and with decorative effects on their finials. They were German regimental banners dating from the early Prussian wars to World War I. Near the entrance to the chamber were boxes and paintings, and in the bays Stout could see carefully arranged tapestries and other decorative works. In a few of the bays, Stout noticed, were large caskets.[1] Three were unadorned; one bore a wreath, red ribbons, and a name: Adolf Hitler.

"It's not him," Hancock said over Stout's shoulder. "The ordnance men thought it was, but it's not."

Stout walked into the bay that held the decorated casket. Above him the flags hung limply, some of the older ones in nets to hold them together. He saw steel ammunition boxes on the floor nearby and swastikas on the ribbons. Hancock was right; it wasn't Hitler. A crude label, written in red crayon and held on with tape, read, "*Friedrich Wilhelm Ier, der Soldaten König.*" Frederick William I, the Soldier King, dead since 1740. The decorations, Stout realized, were Hitler's tribute to the founder of the modern German state.

He examined the other coffins, each with its crude red crayon label held on with tape. There was Feldmarschall von Hindenburg, the greatest German hero of World War I, and beside him Frau von Hindenburg, his wife. The fourth coffin contained the remains of "*Friedrich der Grosse*"—Frederick the Great, the son of the Soldier King.

Where did Hitler get these coffins? Stout wondered. Did he rob their tombs?

"It's a coronation chamber," Hancock said. "They were going to crown Hitler the emperor of Europe."

"Or the world," Stout said, examining the photographs in a small metal box. They contained photographs and portraits of all the military leaders of the Prussian state from the Soldier King to Hitler. In the next three boxes were prizes of the Prussian monarchy:

the Reich Sword of Prince Albrecht, forged in 1540; the scepter, orb, and crown used at the coronation of the Soldier King in 1713. The jewels had been removed from the crown, according to a label, "for honorable sale."[2]

Stout examined the rest of the room. The steel ammunition boxes held books and photographs from the library of Frederick the Great. The 271 paintings in the farthest holding bay were from his palaces in Berlin, and Sanssouci in Potsdam.

"This isn't a coronation room," Stout said. "It's a reliquary. They were hiding the most precious artifacts of the German military state. This room wasn't intended for Hitler; it was intended for the next Reich, so they could build upon his glory."

Hancock laughed. "And it didn't even stay hidden until the end of this one."

———

Three hundred and fifty miles to the south, James Rorimer finally received the news he had been waiting for: U.S. Seventh Army was closing in on Neuschwanstein. He immediately raced to the transportation depot only to find that, since the command unit would be leaving soon for Augsburg or Munich, there were no vehicles available.

Wily and determined as ever, especially with his objective so close after all these months, he secured a jeep from a friend in the Red Cross and was soon on his way. Since Neuschwanstein was not yet liberated, he took a detour to Buxheim, where Rose Valland had reported the Nazis had been storing the overflow items

from Neuschwanstein since as early as 1943. Without
hesitation, a German policeman offered directions
to the monastery a few miles outside of town, where
everyone in the city knew the Nazi artwork was stored.
The American soldiers there, however, seemed unaware
of the cache. The outer rooms of the monastery had
been broken into by thieves, and the Allied troops were
busy protecting looted French dry goods from hungry
displaced persons. In the back of one of the rooms,
completely ignored by the American troops, Rorimer
noticed cases containing statuary marked "D-W,"
the personal symbol of Pierre David-Weill, one of the
world's great collectors. In the main section of the
monastery even the corridors were stacked with looted
Renaissance furniture. The rooms, which housed a
priest, thirteen nuns, and twenty-two refugee children, were filled with pottery, paintings, and decorative
works. The floor of the chapel was almost a foot thick
with rugs and tapestries, many stolen directly from the
walls and floors of the various Rothschild estates.

The German overseers of the monastery were will-
fully unhelpful, but Rorimer had better luck with
Martha Klein, a restorer from Cologne and the superintendent of the repository. The monastery was, Rorimer
discovered from Klein, the primary restoration studio
for the items stolen from France by the ERR. Around
her were the tools of her trade: cameras, brushes,
paints, scrapers, lights, measuring tools, and milk,
which was used to reline canvases. Rorimer noticed a
small painting tossed casually onto one of the tables.
Klein told him it was a Rembrandt, discovered by the
Nazis in a bank vault in Munich. When Rorimer asked,

she offered the list of paintings that she and others had restored in those small rooms over the last two years.

"There are few museums in the world that could boast a collection such as the one we found here [at Buxheim]," Rorimer later wrote. "Works of art could no longer be thought of in ordinary terms—a roomful, a carload, a castle full, were the quantities we had to reckon with."[3]

And this was just the overflow. Neuschwanstein was still miles away.

CHAPTER 45

The Noose Tightens

Germany and Austria
May 2–3, 1945

The war, of course, was not just being fought by the Western Allies. In Italy, German forces officially surrendered on May 2. On the Eastern front, the more than two-million-man Soviet Red Army had ripped through Poland and was moving deep inside the Fatherland, leaving German troops and civilians fleeing west to avoid annihilation. On May 4, U.S. forces caught up with Hans Frank, the notorious Nazi governor-general of occupied Poland, at his home in Neuhaus on Lake Schliersee, just ten miles from the Austrian border.

Frank's reign in Poland had been brutal and bloody. "We must not be squeamish when we learn that a total of 17,000 have been shot [in Poland]," he said in a speech to the party faithful in 1943. "We are now duty bound to hold together; we who are gathered together here figure on Mr. Roosevelt's list of war criminals. I have the honor of being Number One."[1] Once, while visiting another territory, he noticed a sign proclaiming seven partisans had been executed; he would have to fell a whole forest, he boasted to his retinue, if he posted a sign every time he killed seven Poles.

So quick to condemn others, Frank proved too weak to face his own crimes. Powerless, and with no alternatives, the weak-willed Frank turned over forty-three volumes of his personal diaries to his captors. On his first night in captivity, he tried to commit suicide by cutting his wrists and throat. He failed even at that. Scouring his house, the soldiers found nine world-famous paintings, including two of the three masterpieces stolen from the Czartoryski Collection in Cracow: Rembrandt's *Landscape with the Good Samaritan* and Leonardo da Vinci's *Lady with an Ermine*. The third, *Portrait of a Young Man* by Raphael, was officially listed as missing.

———

In a prison cell near Trier, Hermann Bunjes fell into despondence as he contemplated his life. Monuments Men Robert Posey and Lincoln Kirstein had not returned to accept his offer of assistance; instead, Posey had sent an army interrogator to his small scholar's hideaway outside Trier. Shortly thereafter, Bunjes was arrested by Allied forces.[2] He had helped Göring pillage France; he had bullied Rose Valland at the Jeu de Paume; he had sold out every cultural, scholarly, and personal virtue in pursuit of Nazi power, and yet he had convinced himself he might somehow go free. Perhaps he imagined he could slip away in the confusion of the Allied advance, or that he could buy his freedom by telling Posey and Kirstein the location of Hitler's treasure room at Altaussee. But he had sold his soul, and that is something you can never repurchase at any price. Hermann Bunjes had craved Nazi power, wealth, and prestige, but they had been nothing but a cruel illusion for a foolish man.

————

In Bavaria, Hermann Göring rode, with all the tassels and regalia of his exalted rank (officially stripped from him by Hitler a few days before), in an open car and in the custody of SS guards. The guards had been ordered to kill the Reichsmarschall and his family, but even the SS knew Germany had entered a leaderless void, and they ignored the order. The convoy was headed to Mauterndorf, one of Göring's many estates; the Reichsmarschall was planning to wait there until he received an audience with Eisenhower. He was sure the two would meet and talk together, one military man to another.

His artwork, meanwhile, was in transit to the town of Unterstein, six miles from Berchtesgaden. In the last two weeks, it had traveled a hazardous journey over the bombed-out rail lines of Germany. First it had gone to Berchtesgaden, where three cars had been decoupled despite the fact that the bomb shelters were damp and proved too small to hold the entire collection. The remaining cars had gone to Unterstein, but once they arrived the Reichsmarschall rethought his decision and decided to deposit the collection back in the bomb shelters outside Berchtesgaden. The paintings were covered with tapestries for protection, then the doors to the bomb shelters were sealed with a foot-thick wall of concrete and disguised with timbers that looked like ceiling beams. The bulk of the artwork still wouldn't fit, of course, so while bombs fell on Germany, Allied troops rushed across the rubble of what had once been its great cities, and Nazi fanatics worked to blow up every railroad, factory, and bridgehead in the Fatherland, the Reichsmarschall sent the overflow of his massive collection of stolen paintings, sculpture, tapestries and other cultural treasures back to Unterstein. He kept in the possession of himself and his wife only the ten small masterpieces they had been holding since evacuating Carinhall, which were valuable enough for the two of them to live like royalty for the rest of their lives.

———

Across the Austrian border in the Alpine Redoubt, the defenders of Altaussee were in disarray. Eigruber had sent a demolition team to arm and detonate the bombs. A reliable source—the husband of a friend of a sympathetic miner—had seen the demo experts in a valley only a few miles away, awaiting a Gestapo escort. Pöchmüller and Högler had discussed a few days before sending someone down the mountain to Salzburg to inform Western Allied forces of the situation. They had decided it was too risky. The idea of rebellion against the armed guards seemed foolish, especially if the Gestapo was arriving with the demolition experts. And there was no time or means to move the heavy bombs out of the mine.

At this pivotal moment, one of the miners, Alois Raudaschl, came forward with an idea. Dr. Ernst Kaltenbrunner, chief of Hitler's security police and the second-highest-ranking member of the SS, had fled Hitler's bunker in Berlin and was on his way to the area to visit his mistress. Raudaschl, a Nazi Party member, knew how to contact him. Might Kaltenbrunner help?

The scenario was appealing. As the Nazi security chief, Kaltenbrunner outranked Eigruber. He had been in the bunker and knew Hitler's mind. And he had many personal traits the gauleiter would doubtlessly admire. A native Austrian, he was well known for his violent adherence to Hitler's most vile practices: the establishment of concentration camps, the execution of prisoners of war, and the disappearance of thousands of "undesirables" from German-occupied territories. In short, he was a ruthless, heartless bastard: exactly the type of man who would command the respect of August Eigruber.

But would such a man really go out of his way to save art?

CHAPTER 46

The Race

Berchtesgaden, Germany, and
Neuschwanstein, Germany
May 4, 1945

The Third Infantry Division of U.S. Seventh Army, "the Rock of the Marne," had fought its way from North Africa, through Sicily, Anzio, France, southern Germany, and finally into the Bavarian Alps. It had taken part in the capture of Munich in late April, and toured the nearby Dachau death camp. On May 2, 1945, its Seventh Infantry Regiment, known as the "Cottonbalers," advanced on Salzburg, Austria's gateway to the Alpine Redoubt. They expected a fight, but in the last few days resistance had suddenly disappeared, and they took the city without firing a shot. This left them in perfect position to push on to the last jewel in the war: the Nazi stronghold at Berchtesgaden, the heart of the Alpine Redoubt.

On the morning of May 4, the commander of Third Infantry Division, Major General John "Iron Mike" O'Daniel, visited Colonel John A. Heintges, the commander of Seventh Infantry Regiment. "Do you think we can make it to Berchtesgaden?" he asked.

"Yes sir," Heintges replied. "I've got a plan already

prepared." Heintges had ordered his engineers to work all night to strengthen a local bridge in case the division received the order to advance.

Within an hour, the First and Third battalions were moving in a pincer formation toward Berchtesgaden. While First Battalion crawled apprehensively through the mountain passes, Third Battalion swung wide and rolled down the autobahn untouched. First Battalion entered Berchtesgaden at 3:58 p.m. on May 3, 1945, followed two minutes later by the Third Battalion. The two forces found the streets lined with German officers standing at attention in their gray longcoats. One of them stepped forward, took off his pistol and dagger, and presented them to Colonel Heintges. He was Fritz Göring, the Reichsmarschall's nephew. Heintges accepted the surrender, then invited the young man to a local *Gasthaus* for a bottle of wine. The Reichsmarschall had recently left; Fritz had been left behind to turn over to the Allies the Luftwaffe archives.

While Heintges chatted, other "Cottonbalers" ascended the hill to Hitler's Berghof on Kehlstein Mountain. The house had been bombed by the British RAF, then set afire by the SS, but the pantries were still stuffed with food and the walls were lined with shelves of liquor. Isadore Valentini, a medic and former coal miner, sat in Hitler's great room and drank the Führer's wine with his friends. The Nazi flag flying over the Berghof was torn down, chopped into pieces, and distributed to the officers of the Third Infantry Division. In a nearby house, a soldier took the German Luger from the hand of Lieutenant General Gustav Kastner-Kirkdorf, who had committed suicide with it. Soon, the men of the Seventh Infantry Regiment were rolling giant wheels of cheese down the streets and helping themselves to Göring's personal collection of liquor from his nearby house, which numbered 16,000 bottles. There was, clearly, no Alpine Redoubt, as Eisenhower and his advisors had feared. The last bastion of Nazi resistance had withered with barely a shot.

––––––––

Neuschwanstein lay at the end of a long, treacherous hairpin drive through the dense mountains of the German-Austrian border, a perfect reflection, James Rorimer thought, of the course his search had taken since meeting Rose Valland in Paris. He had gone to the City of Light hoping to save its great monuments and buildings; now he was driving a Red Cross truck through the German countryside, hoping to find stuffed into a remote castle one of the largest collections of masterpieces ever assembled. Had it been moved or, worse, destroyed? Were the ERR documents, which would be essential to unraveling what had been stolen and from whom, still there? Was he even heading to the right place?

"Yes, there is art at Neuschwanstein," Martha Klein, the restorer he had met at Buxheim, told him. "But the salt mine at Altaussee, that is the richest of the caches by far."

He had hesitated upon hearing that, but only for a moment. The Allies had not yet taken the region near Altaussee, a rural valley high in the mountains and far from any military objective, so there was really no choice. And he had been dreaming of Neuschwanstein for months. There was no way he could turn away now; not when he was so close, and not after the promises he had made to Rose Valland. With a little luck, there might be time to reach the salt mine, too.

Any lingering doubts were wiped clear by the sight of the castle. "The fairy-like castle at Neuschwanstein near Füssen," Rorimer wrote, "had been built in a fantastic pseudo-Gothic style by the Mad Ludwig of Bavaria. As we approached it from the north through an open valley, it looked in its mountain setting like a prototype of all story-book castles. It was a castle in the air come to life for egocentric and mad thirsters after power; a picturesque, romantic and remote setting for a gangster crowd to carry on its art looting activities."[1]

The great iron doors were guarded by two cannons mounted on armored cars. Otherwise, the Germans had fled, leaving it completely defenseless. The American unit that had taken the castle reported no resistance, and the total arms confiscated from the Germans in residence amounted to a couple of shotguns. Thanks to Rose Valland's information and Rorimer's efforts, the unit had known the importance of the castle, and it had been sealed and placed off-limits immediately upon its capture. No one, of any rank, had entered the treasure rooms.

With the castle's long-serving custodian as his guide—the Nazis had retained the castle's prewar staff, trusting these servants more than their own men—James Rorimer, his new assistant, Monuments Man John Skilton, and a small complement of guards entered the castle. The interior was a labyrinth of stairs, designed not by an architect but by a theatrical stage designer Mad Ludwig had admired. The stairs were steep and precarious, each topped by a door unlocked by a German watchman with a comically large set of keys, then locked again behind them. Behind most of the doors were claustrophobic rooms, with foot-thick walls and tiny aperture windows. Others led to magnificent hallways, sometimes a balcony overlooking a mountain vista, followed by another set of precarious stairwells, this one on the outside of the building. The castle went up and up at seemingly impossible angles, room after bizarre room, and in each one Rorimer saw boxes and crates, racks and platforms, all containing the patrimony of France which had been shipped directly from Paris. Whole rooms housed nothing but gold decorations; others had paintings crammed tightly onto shelves or piles of crates with the ERR initials stenciled over the symbols of Parisian collectors. Rorimer could see that many of the crates had never been opened.

Other sections of the castle were stuffed with furniture. Some contained tapestries; others table services, goblets, candelabras, and various household goods. There were several rooms of books, with rare engravings and prints shoved haphazardly between them or dropped behind the shelves. Behind one steel door, locked with two keys, was the world-famous Rothschild jewelry collection and more than a thousand pieces of silver belonging to Pierre David-Weill. "I passed through the rooms as in a trance," Rorimer wrote, "hoping that the Germans had lived up to their reputation for being methodical and had photographs, catalogues and records of all these things. Without them it would take twenty years to identify the agglomeration of loot."[2]

In the Kemenate, a part of the castle containing
the fireplace room and reached by a separate door, the
Nazis had burned uniforms and documents. Rorimer
saw Hitler's signature, still visible on a curled corner of
burned paper, and feared the archives destroyed. But
the next room was lined with filing cabinets containing photographs, catalogues, and records. There was a
catalogue card for every confiscation undertaken by the
ERR in France—more than 21,000 confiscations in
all, including shipments that had gone to other repositories. It was evidence of much of what the Nazis had
stolen from Western Europe; and as Rose Valland had
understood when she told him about the importance of
Neuschwanstein, it was absolutely essential to identify-
ing and getting it all back home.

"No one comes in here," Rorimer told the sergeant
of the guard, who was trailing the inspection party.
"Not even the guards. This building is off-limits."

There was a trapdoor in the floor. Rorimer had it
nailed shut, then a steel trunk was placed over the top.
The heavy doors of the Kemenate were pulled shut and
locked. Then James Rorimer, with the flair of a show-
man, took an ancient Rothschild seal he had discovered
in the looted treasures—*SEMPER FIDELIS*, "always
faithful," it read—and emblazoned the crack between
the doors with sealing wax.

CHAPTER 47

Final Days

Berlin, Germany, and
Southern Germany
May 5–6, 1945

On May 2, Red Army troops entered the upper half of an area in the middle of Berlin that housed several famous German museums. German troops had fled the area, known as Museum Island, only hours before, after the curators responsible for the Pergamon Altar had persuaded them not to use pieces of the famous ancient Greek altar as a protective barricade for the fighting.

With the city's museums secure, Red Army art experts turned to the enormous flaktowers (anti-aircraft towers) that held many of the large paintings and other works of art that could not be evacuated to Merkers and other German repositories. The Zoo Flaktower, the largest of the three, was 135 feet high and went six stories underground. The concrete walls were eight feet thick, the windows covered with steel shutters. In addition to a hospital, military barracks, national radio station, ammunitions stores, and museum storage, it could shelter 30,000 people.[1]

On May 1, Soviet troops had overrun the Zoo Flaktower, looking for gold, Hitler's body, and other high-ranking Nazis. They had found only wounded soldiers and civilians, laid out by desperate doctors atop crates that contained carved reliefs from the Pergamon Altar, the treasures of ancient Troy (known collectively as Priam's Gold), and countless other masterpieces. By May 4, the wounded had been evacuated and the flaktower was under the control of Stalin's Trophy Brigades, which were in charge of transporting anything of value (from art to food and machinery) to the Soviet Union as unofficial restitutions in kind for the devastation incurred at the hands of the Nazis. The Trophy Brigades immediately began organizing the contents for transport east; within a month, the tower was largely empty.

The Friedrichshain Flaktower, which contained 434 large-scale and extremely important paintings, hundreds of sculptures, porcelain objects, and antiquities (treasures Rave had been unable to move to Merkers), met a different fate. Between May 3 and May 5 Soviet troops inspected the tower and noticed it had been broken into. There were 800,000 freed Eastern European slave laborers wandering throughout the city, and many more desperate Germans trying their best to survive in the void. Looting was rampant. The thieves at the flaktower had been drawn by the food stockpiled on the first floor; they hadn't touched the valuable paintings stored nearby. But the treasures were by no means safe, for on the night of May 5 a fire broke out in the tower. The remaining foodstocks and artworks stored on the first floor were destroyed.

Was the fire set by common thieves? Was it the result

of the burning torches so many carried since the city had no electricity? Or were Nazi fanatics and SS officials so desperate to keep the treasures of the German state out of Soviet hands that they extended the Nero Decree to these works of art?

The answer hardly mattered, at least not to those particular Soviet troops. They refused to post guards even though valuable artwork remained undamaged on the second and third floors. While the Trophy Brigades worked at the Zoo Flaktower, the Friedrichshain Flaktower was left to the usual assortment of desperate scavengers. It wasn't long before a second fire broke out, more extensive than the first. The contents—sculpture, porcelain, books, and the 434 paintings, including one by Botticelli, one by van Dyck, three by Caravaggio, ten by Rubens, and five by Hermann Göring's favorite artist, Lucas Cranach the Elder—were assumed destroyed, the latest victims of the void.

In Unterstein, the frantic and hungry townspeople, whipped up by rumors that the railcars contained schnapps, descended on Hermann Göring's personal train. Some left with bread and wine—the Reichsmarschall had added extra boxcars of supplies to his train to support himself in exile—while, as Allied investigator and Monuments Man Bernard Taper later discovered, "those who came later had to be satisfied with things like a school of Rogier van der Weyden painting, a thirteenth century Limoges reliquary, four late Gothic wood statues, and other such baubles— whatever they could grab. It was a real mob scene.

Three women laid hands on the same Aubusson carpet, and a heated struggle ensued until along came a local dignitary, who said to them, 'Women, be civilized, divide it among you.' So they did. Two of the women used their portions as bedspreads, but the third cut hers up to make window curtains."[2]

———

Each evening, Robert Posey and Lincoln Kirstein, the brilliantly matched Monuments Men for Third Army, looked at the big map tacked to the wall of their forward operating base. The map was covered in acetate, and each day's advance was marked in red crayon. Every night, the lines were adjusted as rumors were sifted for fact. The Soviets had been met at Torgau in late April. Italy had surrendered. A warrant officer claimed he had gone to Bohemia and back with no resistance. Posey and Kirstein noticed only one constant: The area of German control always got smaller, but the land still outside the grasp of the Western Allies always managed to contain the salt mine at Altaussee.

Nor was that their only disappointment. As the Allied armies closed in on the Austrian Alps, another truth was becoming increasingly apparent: Altaussee was not going to fall into U.S. Third Army territory, as Posey and Kirstein had always hoped and believed, but into that of U.S. Seventh Army. James Rorimer was going to be the Monuments Man tasked with the mine; Posey and Kirstein were going to be left with battered towns and minor castles.

Robert Posey was bothered by the injustice, not so much for himself—like all the Monuments Men, he had always shared information as soon as he received it—but for Third Army. It seemed absurd to him that another army group would receive the honors of a find like Altaussee when, in the last few months, Third Army had destroyed an entire German army east of the Moselle River, jumped the Rhine, and broken the enemy's spirit with its deep thrusts into the German heartland. Wasn't it Third Army that had led the charge across France? That had broken the unbreakable citadel at Metz? That had scoured the industrial regions of south-central Germany? And wasn't it he and Lincoln Kirstein, Third Army men, who had discovered not just the existence but the location of Hitler's treasure room?

"I am sorry that it was not our army who was supposed to meet the Russians if you were looking forward to it with so much anxiety," he wrote Alice, with typical Third Army pride. "I can assure you that this is the glamour army of all the Allied ones, and the part we are called upon to play is always the difficult one and so the important one. This outfit feels itself to be king pin pretty much as an ever winning football team does. The other armies are looked upon as all right but not brilliant and anyone back of the combat zone is simply too low to even be thought of. If they are as far back as England they are simply civilians in a sort of uniform. People who don't feel that way gradually go out into some other kind of organization. Generally it is their own choice for to be in a club that vociferously declares itself to be the outstanding thing of all time would be too much for soldiers of less strong convictions."[3]

Kirstein, far from motivated by perceived slights

or the camaraderie of Third Army, found this new world depressing. "If you work too long in the skeletons of fine buildings," he wrote, "estimating the love and care of their creation, the irrelevance of their destruction, the energy needed for their approximate restoration—wondering even about the possibility of their restoration—your confusion settles into gloom. After seeing the spectacular corpses of Mainz and Frankfurt, Würzburg, Nuremberg and Munich, it was always a relief to come upon some small, untouched market town."[4]

A few days deeper into the southern German countryside, he was beyond even the comfort of small untouched towns. The German people—and especially the German aristocracy—were grinding him down as much as the destruction. On May 6, he wrote:[5]

Recently mad activity has been given way to by mad activity. On our trail for loot we have uncovered the local aristocracy in a series of enormous castles spread all over this picturesque province filled with cases of the contents of all the museums, plus cases of personal belongings, books, and dealers who were invited into the schloss to save their lives from the advance of the russian-jewish-negro-american army. One lovely old countess received us in bed. She was ill, oh so ill and her house was a hospital for German (lightly) wounded. She only had one poor little room in this elegant old mansion, and almost broke her neck flying into bed no doubt, as we swept into the court. She was an ancient bitch, Italian, who married a great german name, and is harboring a whole slue of art dealers,

young "sick" counts and barons...and my, have they
had a terrible time. They almost didn't get out of Paris
in time, and them with their weak lungs....She so
hoped that her lovely boys (pictures brought out), and
they were wildly pretty, her two adorable SS officers
were privileged to surrender to the Americans all of
whom are perfectly charming (where have I been all
my life), rather than to the un-democratic and dirty
awful Russian-jewish-polacks, who we MUST fight
quickly, and besides she had only one little insignificant
request to make. It seems some displaced Russian jewish polack american negroes had taken to shooting the
deer in the animal-park, and it was not in season, and it
was giving the chief Forester NIGHTMARES....She
clacked her false teeth. Her sister the maiden ladied
princess about 58, was at least honest in her nastiness.
She said that she would shake hands if it was allowed.
Oh I laughed, you know in the war I don't care who I
shake hands with. Anyway the old countess was useful,
and we uncovered what we wanted to uncover, and she
gave us notes on her coronetted note paper to all her
cousins in all the other castles each of whom is harboring a nest of itching vipers....The [art] dealers were
another little knot of grimness....They had all gotten
rich at the point of a pistol, and they never had bought
stolen goods from expropriated jewish collections,
unless the collections had been purified by passing
through two or 3 intermediaries who took their cut.
Surely the Americans would not force them to surrender properties thus perfectly in good faith acquired. As
for what will ultimately happen to the materials, fine
porcelains, good uninteresting minor masters, stamps,

snuff boxes, furniture, etc. I do not in the slightest care of the original owners who are doubtless dead or the present owners who are doubtless charming people who love dogs and horses get them back or keep them or let them fade rot, or break in their cellars. I am interested in only one bit of art history. How do I get home.

It was the endlessness of the operation, the limitlessness of the robbery and the snobbery and the excuses. That's what depressed him, even as he and Posey pushed toward the Alpine region that was home to most of the great Nazi storehouses of stolen art. As he summarized the situation in a letter home, "As you can tell my temper improves and my hair falls out, as each nameless and numberless day passes one-footedly by. I have hit the don't care low of all time, as everything grows glamorouser and glamorouser.... I am not interested in lousy old Germany's lousy old future."[6]

CHAPTER 48

The Translator

Munich, Germany
May 7, 1945

While the Monuments Men in the field raced toward their destinations, Private Harry Ettlinger sat glumly in an enormous *Kaserne*, or German military barracks, on the outskirts of Munich. It was May 7, nearly four months since he'd been pulled off the troop truck in Belgium, and he hadn't done a thing but eat and sleep. Harry's thoughts drifted to an afternoon several weeks earlier at his last bivouac, a tent camp outside Worms, Germany, when he had climbed a nearby hill. The weather was finally warm, and the trees in bloom. Shadows fell over him, and Harry looked up expecting planes. It was only a flock of birds. Down on the road, he noticed a solitary figure. For twenty minutes, he watched the man climb. When he was a few steps away, Harry realized he had an artificial leg. Harry offered a hand, but the man shrugged him off. He was the priest of the chapel over the crest of the hill. He had lost his leg more than two years before on the Soviet front. They said little, but Harry left feeling he had, for the first time in months, had a real conversation with another human being. So far, it had been his only contact with the enemy.

"I hear you speak German." It was so unexpected, Harry looked up to see if the soldier was talking to him.

"Yes sir," Private Harry Ettlinger said, almost saluting before noticing the soldier was a private.

"I've been translating for the last two days," the man said. "It's interesting work, but it's not for me. I want to be in military intelligence. A German girl was raped by four American soldiers. I want to investigate it. Are you interested?"

"In the rape?"

"No, in the translation job."

"Yes sir," Harry said again, without even stopping to ask about the work.

The office the private directed him to was across the parade ground of the *Kaserne*, in what turned out to be the U.S. Seventh Army headquarters building. It was a small room on the second floor, full of desks and papers. Two men were working at the desks, while another stood in the middle giving orders.

"Are you the new translator?" the man snapped.

"Yes sir. Private Harry Ettlinger, sir."

"You sound German, Ettlinger."

"American, sir. But born a German Jew. From Karlsruhe."

"Are you assigned to a unit, Ettlinger?"

"Not that I know of, sir."

The man handed him a stack of papers. "Read these documents and tell us what's in them. Just the gist, and anything specific: names, locations, works of art."

"Works of art?"

Before Harry could even get the question out, the man had turned and left. *Now that's a man who gets things done*, Harry thought. He knew if he did a good job on the translations that man would get him assigned to this section, whatever section it was, and because of that man he couldn't imagine a better job. Only later did Harry Ettlinger discover that, before switching units, he had been assigned to the translation corps for the Nuremberg trials. That, apparently, was what he had been waiting for the past four months.

"What a wheeler-dealer," Harry said, turning to one of the men in the office.

"You don't know the half of it," the man replied. "He's trying to secure the two most sought-after buildings in Munich, Hitler's office and the former Nazi Party headquarters. Patton wants them for his regional headquarters, but knowing our lieutenant they'll soon be MFAA Collecting Points. We'll have the building all to ourselves. Ourselves and the hundreds of thousands of things you're going to read about in those documents, that is."

Harry looked at the paper. "What am I going to read about?"

The man laughed. "Welcome to Monuments work. I'm Lieutenant Charles Parkhurst, from Princeton."

"Harry Ettlinger, from Newark." He waited, expecting more. "And who was that?" he asked finally.

"That was Lieutenant James Rorimer. Your new boss."

New boss. Harry liked the sound of that. "Where's he gone?"

"Salzburg. He's going to mount an armed expedition to the salt mines at Altaussee."

CHAPTER 49

The Sound of Music

Bernterode, Germany
May 7, 1945

At Bernterode, George Stout was taking his time. More than twenty people had been assigned to remove the treasures from the mine—including the ordnance unit that had found the shrine, a small group of engineers, and fourteen former French slave laborers who had worked there for the last few years—and every one of them wanted to be done as quickly as possible. The mine was dark and musty, dripping with water, and plagued by frequent power outages that lasted for hours. Even Walker Hancock, who by now had vast experience with the handling of art in war zones, felt anxious to finish. After all, the whole operation was being conducted on top of 400,000 tons of explosives.

George Stout would have none of it. What mattered in the outside world, where rumors swirled about the end of the war, didn't have any bearing on what happened in the Thuringian forest eighteen hundred feet underground. Before anything was moved, a thorough inspection was needed. Fortunately, the ordnance unit had already checked most of the fifteen miles of tunnels. They didn't find any more treasure, but they did locate several stores of German military supplies. Stout had the gas-proof boots cut into rubber padding to keep objects from rubbing against one another; gas-proof mantles were perfect for wrapping the paintings, especially important in the dripping mine. With the packing materials taken care of, the contents of the shrine were inventoried and organized for removal. Walker Hancock looked up one afternoon—he assumed it was afternoon anyway, since he had existed for two days in perpetual blackness—and noticed Stout frowning at him. Hancock realized he had been thinking of home, of Saima and the house they would buy together and one day, maybe, even the children they would have, and had been coiling a rope with the exaggerated swinging motion of the Massachusetts fishermen he had so often observed back home. Stout, on the other hand, was deliberately coiling the rope over his hand and elbow in precise, measured loops.

As soon as Stout turned away, the man next to Hancock whispered, "How long does he think we're going to keep laying these ropes out in lengths of just twenty-three and one-half inches, all pointing one degree east of north?"[1]

The man was Steve Kovalyak, an infantry combat lieutenant who had been assigned to help after Walker Hancock delivered the coronation paraphernalia to the brass in Frankfurt. A jeepload of gold covered in jewels meant little to Hancock, who had seen so much already, but it was eye-popping for the boys back at headquarters. Hancock had simply borrowed Stout's jeep to drive the regalia to headquarters at Weimar, but General Hodges wasn't taking any chances. He ordered an escort of two motorcycles, three jeeps, two armored cars, a weapons carrier, and fifteen soldiers for Hancock and the treasures, even though the area between Weimar and Frankfurt had been cleared of enemy forces and was safer, Hancock felt, than the Merritt Parkway back in Connecticut. He wondered what the general would have thought of the first part of the journey, when Hancock had driven the jewels alone through the forests of Thuringia on a road where six convoys had been ambushed in the last week alone.

"Don't worry," Hancock told the young lieutenant, "George Stout knows what he's doing." He told Kovalyak and a few nearby ordnance officers about Büsbach, where Stout had taken the time to record everything about a painting even though shells were falling outside. "I've worked with that man a long time," he said, "and I can tell you this: We're all amateurs compared to George Stout."

A few hours later, the power went out, plunging the mine into darkness. Again. Hancock turned on his flashlight. His beam flashed over books, gold, paintings, coffins, and, so suddenly it made him jump, George Stout's face.

"I'll send Kovalyak," Hancock said. It was Stout's standard operating procedure in a blackout to send Lieutenant Kovalyak to cajole the local *Bürgermeister* into keeping his generators operational, even though Kovalyak was one of the few officers present who didn't speak a word of German. It was tedious work, more finesse than force, but years in the infantry had taught Kovalyak all the tricks of navigating local power plays, out-of-touch procedures, and bureaucratic red tape. Hancock had the impression he had skirted court-martial many times, sometimes for pleasure, but mostly to get the job done right.

Soon Hancock found himself alone in the darkness, and as he did in all his down moments, he thought of home. It all seemed so close now—the new house, the return to his sculpting, Saima's embrace—but at the same time it had never felt farther away. He was in a hole, in a forest in Germany, in the dark. Even daylight seemed forever away. To heck with saving his batteries. He turned on his flashlight, pulled a box out to the middle of the room, and, using the wooden backing of a four-hundred-year-old Cranach painting as a table, wrote Saima a letter.[2]

Precious Saima:

You could never imagine what strange circumstances this is being written under. I can't tell you now, but I do want you to have a line actually written in one of the most unbelievable places....Geo. Stout is working here to help me—and the rush of our work brought on by Germany's sudden collapse is so great that letters have been out of the question....No more till later— except that I love you more than I can ever say—but that's not news. Some day soon I'll be able to settle down to a room with a bed and a table and catch up on letter writing.

Devotedly,
Walker

The packing started on May 4, only to be interrupted again by a major power outage. Kovalyak left the mine to meet with the mayor of the nearest town; the 305th Combat Engineer Battalion rigged an emergency genera-tor eighteen hundred feet underground; the French workers, former slave laborers, slipped quietly away down side passages, something they had been doing with increasing frequency; Hancock pulled out his flashlight and, using Feldmarschall von Hindenburg's coffin as his table this time, wrote Saima that "these are very homesick days" despite the excitement of his work.[3] He loved the company of kindred souls, be they soldiers in the field or friends back in his sitting room in Massachusetts, and being on his own for months, without even an assistant to keep him company, had beaten him down. "Geo. Stout is here to give me an urgently needed boost," he wrote. "He is really a friend in need."[4]

By May 5, the packing crews were arranged in two shifts, one from 0800 to 1600 and the other from 1600 to 2200. This was no place for the claustrophobic, as the men and packing materials crowded the shrine and the corridor. By the end of the next day, most of the objects had been padded, wrapped, waterproofed, then loaded onto the elevator for the slow trip to the surface, where they were restacked in a shed at ground level—and where Steve Kovalyak had learned to appreciate the careful planning and his precise, pre-cut pieces of rope.

Another George Stout disciple, Hancock thought.

The next day, it was time for the coffins. Frau von Hindenburg, the lightest, went first. It was a quarter mile from the shrine to the mineshaft. A couple of soldiers crossed themselves as she rose slowly to the surface in the rickety elevator. "She will never be buried deeper," Stout said, by way of benediction.

Next went the Soldier King and then, with Walker Hancock riding on top of the coffin, Feldmarschall von Hindenburg. Now all that was left were the mortal remains of Frederick the Great and his massive steel coffin. The engineers had insisted the coffin wouldn't fit on the elevator, but Stout reminded them that if it could make it down into the shaft, it could also make it back up. They measured again; wedged precisely into the elevator, it would fit with half an inch to spare.

Unfortunately, the coffin weighed, by their estimate, twelve hundred to fourteen hundred pounds. First, it had to be shifted so that a series of slings could be run underneath it. Then the crew of fifteen men had to lift it, squeeze it through the door of the shrine, and maneuver it around the corner into the dark, uneven, dripping-wet mineshaft. The funeral procession went slowly, the pallbearers groaning at their straps. It took the better part of an hour to fit the great steel beast onto the elevator, working it into position inch by inch. Finally, just before 2300 hours, they were ready for the ascent to the surface. It had taken the men all day to disinter the four coffins.

The elevator rose slowly a few feet, then stopped. George Stout and six of the crew climbed onto the lower rigging of the cage and, slowly, the elevator started rising. It took fourteen minutes to climb eighteen hundred feet, the men thinking of nothing more than their hope that the old elevator really could hold a ton of weight, because that's nearly how much it was lifting. As they neared the top, the men began to hear music. Somewhere above them, a radio was playing "The Star-Spangled Banner." As the coffin emerged into the dark, clear night, another song followed: "God Save the King." It was May 7, 1945, the Germans had unconditionally surrendered at Reims. The Allies had officially won the war.

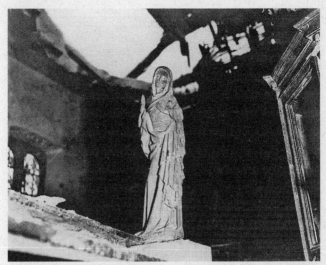

LA GLEIZE, BELGIUM, FEBRUARY 1, 1945: During the Battle of the Bulge, the church in La Gleize was severely damaged. This statue, known as the *Madonna of La Gleize*, was fully exposed to one of the harshest winters on record. Note the gaping hole in the roof overhead. *(Walker Hancock Collection)*

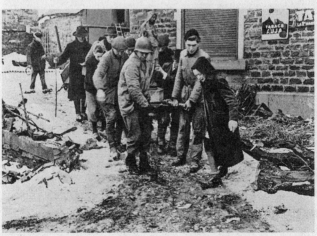

LA GLEIZE, BELGIUM, FEBRUARY 1, 1945: Monuments Man Walker Hancock (front left, in U.S. Army helmet) assisted residents of the town of La Gleize with the relocation of the *Madonna of La Gleize* to a more secure site. *(Walker Hancock Collection)*

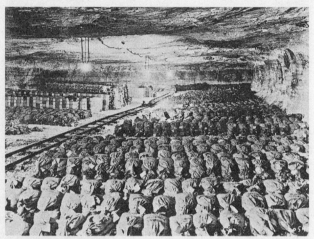

MERKERS, GERMANY, APRIL 1945: Hidden inside the Merkers salt mine was the majority of Nazi Germany's gold reserves and paper currency. All but the largest paintings from the Kaiser-Friedrich Museum in Berlin were also placed there for safekeeping. In today's dollars the value of the gold found in Merkers would be almost $5 billion. *(National Archives and Records Administration, College Park, MD)*

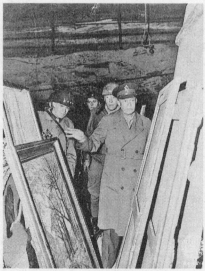

MERKERS, GERMANY, APRIL 12, 1945: Gen. Omar N. Bradley, Lt. Gen. George S. Patton Jr., and Gen. Dwight D. Eisenhower inspect the German museum treasures stored in the Merkers mine. Also pictured in the center is Maj. Irving Leonard Moskowitz. *(National Archives and Records Administration, College Park, MD)*

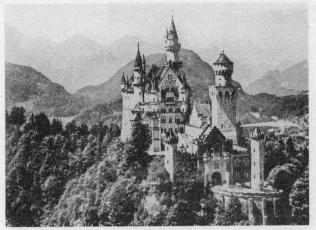

NEUSCHWANSTEIN, GERMANY: The castle of Neuschwanstein was the key Nazi repository for the greatest works of art stolen from France. Built by "Mad Ludwig" of Bavaria in the nineteenth century, it contained so many stolen works of art that it took the Monuments Men six weeks to empty it. The extreme vertical height and absence of elevators required most of the works to be carried down the innumerable flights of stairs. *(National Archives and Records Administration, College Park, MD)*

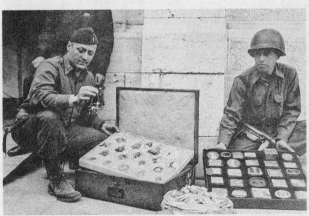

NEUSCHWANSTEIN, GERMANY, MAY 1945: Monuments Man James Rorimer (left) and Sgt. Antonio T. Valim examine valuable art objects stolen from the Rothschild collection in France by the ERR and found in the castle. *(National Archives and Records Administration, College Park, MD)*

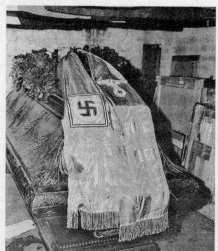

BERNTERODE, GERMANY, MAY 1945: The bronze coffin of Friedrich Wilhelm of Prussia was one of four enormous coffins found at the Bernterode repository by Monuments Man Walker Hancock. *(Walker Hancock Collection)*

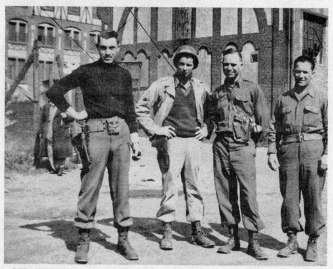

BERNTERODE, GERMANY, MAY 1945 Monuments Men George Stout (left), Walker Hancock (center right), and Steven Kovalyak (right) during the excavation of Bernterode. The soldier standing between Stout and Hancock is a Sgt. Traverse. *(Walker Hancock Collection)*

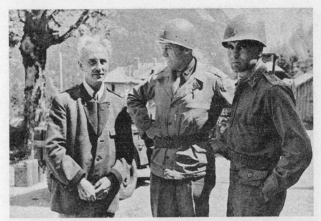

ALTAUSSEE, AUSTRIA, MAY 1945: Dr. Hermann Michel, Monuments Man Robert Posey, and an unidentified U.S. Army officer standing in front of the mine administration building during the confusing initial days after arriving at the Altaussee mine. *(Robert Posey Collection)*

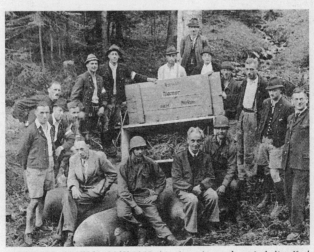

ALTAUSSEE, AUSTRIA, MAY 1945: Austrian mine workers, including Karl Sieber (seated at lower left, in suit) and Dr. Hermann Michel (seated between two U.S. Army soldiers), are sitting on two of the half-ton bombs that had been hidden in crates marked "Attention - Marble - Do Not Drop." *(Robert Posey Collection)*

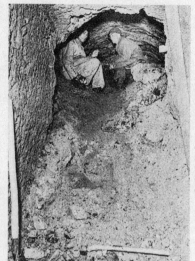

ALTAUSSEE, AUSTRIA, MAY 13, 1945: Monuments Men Robert Posey and Lincoln Kirstein were greeted by the terrifying scene of "palsied" tunnels upon their arrival on May 12, 1945. Within several days, however, they were able to inspect the mine's contents. Here, a mine worker and a GI sit atop the rubble, spades in the foreground, after having created enough space to pass over to the other side. *(Robert Posey Collection)*

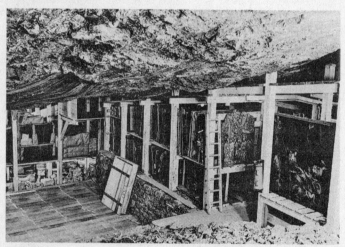

ALTAUSSEE, AUSTRIA, MAY 1945: One of the many mine chambers in which the Nazis had constructed wooden shelves to house the enormous number of stolen works of art. To understand the volume of space in this one chamber, note the nine-foot ladder in the center right portion of the photograph. *(Robert Posey Collection)*

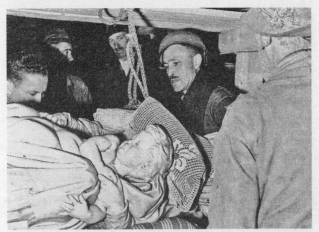

ALTAUSSEE, AUSTRIA, JULY 10, 1945: Removal of priceless works of art from the salt mine at Altaussee posed problems for Monuments Man George Stout unlike any ever contemplated. Stout constructed a pulley to lift Michelangelo's *Bruges Madonna* onto the salt cart to begin its long trip home to Belgium. Visible on the far left is Monuments Man Steve Kovalyak, an expert in packing art, who was a key assistant to Stout. *(National Gallery, Washington, D.C., Gallery Archives)*

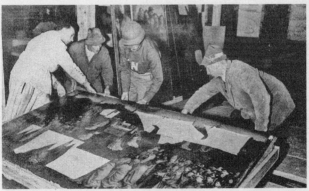

ALTAUSSEE, AUSTRIA, JULY 1945: The central panel of the Ghent Altarpiece, due to its size and weight, proved particularly challenging to move through the narrow passageways. Other panels of the altarpiece are visible in the background behind Stout. Note the tissue that has been applied to the painted surface to secure loose or flaking paint, a process known as "facing." Stout was proud of his U.S. Navy background and usually wore an "N" for "Navy" on his jacket or helmet. *(National Archives and Records Administration, College Park, MD)*

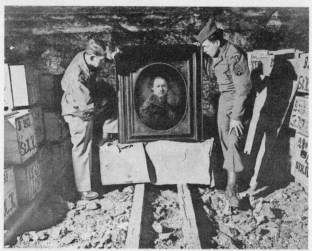

HEILBRONN, GERMANY, 1946: This *Self Portrait* by Rembrandt, inspected by Monuments Men Dale V. Ford and Harry Ettlinger (right), was stored for safekeeping by museum officials from Karlsruhe in the Heilbronn mine. The painting was ultimately returned to the Karlsruhe Museum. This was just one of thousands of paintings and other works of art that were found in Heilbronn, as can be seen by the crates stacked behind each man. *(National Archives and Records Administration, College Park, MD)*

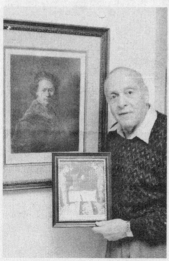

NEW JERSEY: Almost sixty-five years later, Harry Ettlinger reflects with pride on a life well-lived as a Monuments Man as he stands in front of his grandfather's print of the very painting he was never allowed to see as a Jewish boy growing up in Karlsruhe, Germany. *(Bill Stahl)*

CHAPTER 50

End of the Road

Altaussee, Austria
May 12, 1945

The news came unexpectedly: U.S. Third Army had turned south. They, not U.S. Seventh Army, were moving into the Alps near Altaussee. James Rorimer, who had been planning an armed expedition to the salt mine, was diverted to Berchtesgaden, where the rumors of looting by displaced persons were running as hot as the rumors of stockpiled treasures. Altaussee was now, suddenly, the responsibility of Robert Posey and Lincoln Kirstein. Unfortunately, they were more than two hundred miles away on another assignment.

For once it didn't take the Monuments Men long to obtain clearances and a vehicle, although information from the area was sketchy and reports from the mine itself nonexistent. Soon they were careening through the wasteland of southern Germany, where even the roads were bombed out and torn to bits. Lacking flags, German civilians hung white pillowcases from their houses in a sign of surrender, but despite the linens every window appeared sinister and black. There were numerous stories of soldiers gunned down in seemingly quiet villages; of Hitler Youth, fired by childish passion and ignorance, standing in the darkness of second-floor windows with their guns trained down on the narrow part of the street. The crowds of displaced persons were full of soldiers, mainly from the Eastern front, who had stripped off their uniforms to mix better with the civilians. Many crowds seemed filled both with despair and evil intention. At one point in their recent travels, Kirstein had made a wrong turn into the middle of a convoy of German soldiers. There was no place to turn around, so he and Posey spent a tense few minutes surrounded by the enemy, wondering if they had been taken prisoner or if it was the other way around. Eventually, they turned off without incident; the Germans simply kept going.

When the Monuments Men crossed the Austrian border, the horror seemed to lift, and for the first time they could breathe. Instead of pillowcases, the houses flew red-and-white flags, the sign of the Austrian Resistance. The roads began to wind, looping into the hills. In the distance rose snowcapped peaks, and the scattered Alpine villages were like gingerbread towns, with colorful chalets and candy-cut woodwork.

On the other side of Bad Ischl, they encountered the German Sixth Army, stretched out for what seemed like a mile "in charcoal burners, horse-drawn deadmotored ambulances and trucks. There were women and wounded, Hungarian Panzer units, on foot, without armor—thousands of beaten, home-going, and eminently cheerful soldiers."[1]

They stopped briefly at an inn near the town of Altaussee, a tidy village tucked in the woods near a pristine alpine lake. Outside, trimly uniformed SS officers were offering their services to the liberators, who they were sure would soon be at war with the Soviets. No? Then the SS officers were happy to surrender, as long as they could keep their sidearms. They feared their own troops would shoot them in the back.

Inside, American troops were celebrating. Guided by Austrian mountaineers, some of their fellow soldiers had tracked Ernst Kaltenbrunner, the notorious commander of the Nazi security police, through the mountains for most of the night, finally catching up to him at dawn. The wily Nazi had thrown his medals into a lake and successfully passed himself off as a doctor. But he was identified when his mistress screamed out his name and waved to him as he passed with a group of German prisoners through a nearby town.

Posey and Kirstein hurried on. There was only one steep, winding ascent left to the mine, but the bleak, empty road made them feel they had left the safety of numbers behind. To their surprise, the buildings outside the salt mine—a nondescript guardhouse and a low office bunker beneath towering mountains—were swarming with activity. Two jeeps and one truckload of troops from the 80th Infantry Division had taken the few buildings without a fight, but what exactly they had taken was still up for debate. None of the enemy groups—miners, art men, guards, Nazis—seemed to agree on what had happened. And especially on who had done what.

After a quick conversation with the commanding officer, Major Ralph Pearson, who assured them the main shaft was not booby-trapped, Posey and Kirstein grabbed some acetylene lamps and headed into the mine. The tunnel went straight back into the side of the mountain. Instinctively, the two men ducked their heads, although the tunnel entrance was seven or eight feet tall. The light of their lanterns swung side to side as they hurried along, the darkness opening before them and then closing again in their wake. Kirstein touched the wall and felt a mild electric shock—live demolition wires, either damaged or cut, he couldn't be sure. About a quarter of a mile down, or maybe a half mile— it was too hard to tell in the darkness—debris lay scattered on the floor. The men scrambled quickly over it. In the wall, Kirstein noticed a hole full of tubes, and he knew from his brief ordnance training that it was dynamite. Packed for destruction, but unlit. He scrambled over the slabs of rock and jumped down to the tamped-earth floor, following his captain deeper into the mountain. Their steps echoed now, rebounding off the scattered debris. Their lights swung forward and back. It was cold in the tunnel, but not nearly cold enough to produce the shiver Kirstein felt when Posey suddenly stopped and held up his acetylene torch. Before them, reflecting the lantern's dim glow, was a solid wall of fallen stone. The mine had been blown.

SECTION

V

The Aftermath

We do not want to destroy unnecessarily what men spent so much time and care and skill in making . . . [for] these examples of craftsmanship tell us so much about our ancestors. . . . If these things are lost or broken or destroyed, we lose a valuable part of our knowledge about our forefathers. No age lives entirely alone; every civilisation is formed not merely by its own achievements but by what it has inherited from the past. If these things are destroyed, we have lost a part of our past, and we shall be the poorer for it.

—BRITISH MONUMENTS MAN RONALD BALFOUR,
DRAFT LECTURE FOR SOLDIERS, 1944

All the works of art for whose fate we still tremble will return to us, bringing the light of their beauty to attract, as before, pilgrims from every country and to inspire thoughts of peace.

—DR. CESARE FASOLA, UFFIZI LIBRARIAN,
THE FLORENCE GALLERIES AND THE WAR

CHAPTER 51

Understanding Altaussee

Altaussee, Austria
March 30–May 5, 1945

Hitler's intentions for the treasure trove at Altaussee have long been debated. Yet it seems clear from his last will and testament, the last document he would sign, just hours before committing suicide, that he never intended for the artwork to be destroyed.

Somehow, the significance of his deliberate and clearly stated wish—that the "pictures" he collected for a great museum in Linz be given to the German state—has been all but ignored by historians examining that document. Seen in the full context of Adolf Hitler and his lifelong ambitions as an artist, the last will should quiet any discussion that he wanted the artwork destroyed. This does not redound to his credit, though, since it is equally clear his decisions while in power made the destruction of the mine at Altaussee nearly inevitable. By refusing to plan for defeat or to surrender when all was lost, he created a void in which rogue actors would determine the fate of tens of thousands of lives, buildings, and artistic treasures. He also failed to state, in no unequivocal terms, that the artwork was not to be destroyed.

But most importantly, his orders over the course of many years—including the burning of books; the destruction of "degenerate" art; the pillaging of personal property; the arrest, detention, and systematic annihilation of millions of human beings; and the willful and vengeful destruction of great cities—put the artwork, and everything else within reach of any Nazis anywhere in the world, at tremendous risk. Monuments Man S. Lane Faison Jr. once commented that Hitler "wrote a book called *Mein Kampf.* And if people had just read it carefully, every single thing that's happened was already predicted...the whole Jewish situation is there in clear writing in ink."[1] The same is true for most of his other actions. Hitler's Nero Decree of March 19, 1945, simply formalized everything he had preached and done over the previous two decades, empowering his followers to unleash the violence and fury of his reign. In the hands of a man like August Eigruber, it was a messianic calling.

But what exactly happened in those remote Austrian mountains during the void between Hitler's loss of control and the arrival of the Monuments Men? Who was ultimately responsible for the actions taken there? And who should bear the credit and the blame for how things turned out? The broad outlines have long been known, but it took decades to piece together the actual sequence of events and the roles played by the mine officials, the miners, Nazi officials, resistance fighters, and Western Allied forces. Even today, delving into the original German documents reveals new insights into one of the great (if largely unknown) turning points in the history of man's cultural achievements. As so often happens in life—and history—it's not just what happened, but what might have occurred that bears analysis.

The basic facts are not in dispute.

Had it not been for the heroic action of several individuals, the Altaussee art repository would have been destroyed by the bombs placed there on the orders of August Eigruber. But it wasn't destroyed, nor was any piece of artwork stored there irretrievably damaged. Instead, sometime between May 1 and May 7 (U.S. forces, led by Major Ralph Pearson, arrived on May 8), the eight massive bombs were removed and hidden alongside the road under a group of fir trees. The mine tunnels were packed with charges. The resulting explosions—the conspirators referred to them as a "palsy," another word for paralysis[2]—collapsed the tunnels and sealed the mine, placing the artwork beyond Eigruber's destructive intent. The question has always been: Who ordered and executed the palsy?

Writing in the magazine *Town and Country* in the fall of 1945, Lincoln Kirstein admitted that "so many witnesses told so many stories that the more information we accumulated the less truth it seemed to contain."[3] Nonetheless, he believed the heroes were the Austrian miners. In Kirstein's scenario, which became the unofficial MFAA explanation, the miners accidentally discovered Eigruber's crates containing bombs and secretly removed them from the chambers in the dead of night. They then sealed the mine entrances, knowing this was the best way to prevent more serious damage to the source of their livelihood. In a way, salt saved art. When Eigruber discovered the treason, he "ordered all the Austrians to be shot, but it was already too late; the Americans were on the other side of the mountain. It was May seventh."[4]

The miners confirmed this account in 1948, when in a report to the Austrian government signed "Freedom Fighters of Altaussee" they claimed to have acted alone to save the mine.[5] Their account overlooks the fact that, among other inconsistencies, the miners could never have prepared the complicated palsy (controlled explosions) without the technical expertise of engineers like Högler and Mayerhoffer. The government, however, never questioned their claims.

The Austrian government, in fact, was a most important source of misinformation about Altaussee. Kirstein's opinion had no doubt been influenced by a common misconception: that the Austrians were innocent victims of the Nazis, not their willing accomplices. This was not the case, as film footage and documents from the period prove. The Austrian government, however, was quick to buttress this aura of innocence, and even produced a defense of its actions known as the *Red-White-Red-Book* (mocked by many as "The Viennese Masquerade") in 1946.[6] In it, the self-described Austrian Resistance claimed it knew of the artistic treasures at Altaussee and had forced Kaltenbrunner at gunpoint to rescind Hitler's order to destroy them. The claim was absurd. While the Austrian Resistance was active in the Aussee area, they had no knowledge of the artwork and no influence on activities at the mine. Their only real role was, weeks later, to supplement the meager American guard. Nonetheless, by 1948 the Resistance, with the support of the Austrian government, was claiming primary responsibility for saving Altaussee. Later writers even claimed the miners were members of the Austrian Resistance; in fact, many were members of the Nazi Party.

Within this framework of trumped-up Austrian bravery, many individuals stepped forward to take credit for thwarting Eigruber. Sepp Plieseis, an actual Austrian Resistance leader (unlike the writers of the *Red-White-Red-Book*), claimed his group had saved the mine.[7] An Austrian named Albrecht Gaiswinkler claimed to have been parachuted into the area by the British to organize resistance.[8] Among his ridiculous stories: He had forced Kaltenbrunner to rescind Hitler's order, personally ordered the artwork moved to safer chambers, and in one night had overseen the setting and detonation of the palsy charges—a complicated procedure that actually took weeks. By 1946, he was even claiming Eigruber had ordered the artwork destroyed with flamethrowers. On the back of these lies, he was elected to the Austrian National Assembly. But as his stories became more fantastic, his support waned. He was kicked out of the assembly in 1950.

Far more effective were the efforts of Dr. Hermann Michel, head of the Mineralogical Department of the Natural History Museum, Vienna. Michel, supposedly, sent the message alerting Major Pearson, who was leading an infantry unit in the spearhead of the U.S. Third Army advance, to the treasures hidden at Altaussee, including the Hungarian crown jewels. (The crown jewels were not in the mine. They were found in an oil barrel sunk in marshland near the village of Mattsee in Bavaria.) Despite Posey's and Kirstein's best efforts to alert the most forward U.S. troops to Hitler's hoard, this was the first Pearson had heard of Altaussee. The message was real, but it is unclear if Michel was the person who sent it.

When Pearson arrived on May 8 with two jeeps and a truckload of infantrymen, Michel was there to greet him. Passing himself off as an expert, he gave the American commander a tour of the area, explaining that half a billion dollars' worth of cultural treasures were inside the collapsed mine. He also implied, and later backed up with documents bullied from other participants, that he had been intimately involved in the plot to remove Eigruber's bombs. Pearson believed Michel's account for a simple reason: He was the only person at the mine who spoke English. In fact, Michel at best had a tangential role in what happened at Altaussee.

In 1938, Dr. Michel had been deposed from his position as director of the Natural History Museum Vienna, despite strenuous efforts to cozy up to the Nazi elite.[9] Under its new director, the museum became a propaganda tool for racial ideology. The chastened Michel, now head of the Mineralogy Department, vociferously supported its exhibits focusing on racial divisions among humans, the "racial and emotional" appearance of Jews, and the "ideal" man and woman—Nordic, of course.[10] He often spoke at public functions in support of Hitler, joined the Rotary Club "to weaken the Jewish influence,"[11] and was the public relations official for the local branch of the Nazi Party.

Michel was less a racist, though, than an amoral opportunist.[12] For years, he had cozied up to history's worst murderers and racists, but he realized sooner than most that the new powers would be the liberators of places like Altaussee. The void of April to May 1945 was a period where past deeds could quickly be buried or mischaracterized, and today's lie could become tomorrow's truth. Those who stepped forward, Michel knew, could not only save their own necks, but become invaluable to the Allied conquerors.

This was happening all over Germany and Austria, as people from all walks of life—hardened Nazis and brave resisters alike—angled for the best possible position in the new world order. George Stout saw through their acts. "I am sick of all schemers," he wrote, "of all the vain crawling toads who now edge into positions of advantage and look for selfish gain or selfish glory from all this suffering."[13] Posey was equally suspicious, having most of the obvious Nazis at Altaussee arrested, but Michel's story stuck. Soon, the mineralogist was being featured in American newspapers as the hero of Altaussee.

And then things went quiet. The story of Altaussee, so monumental in the world of art and culture, was quickly subsumed by larger stories—Auschwitz, the atomic bomb, and disintegrating relations with the Soviet Union that would define the new world order as the cold war. Kirstein had anticipated this when he wrote on May 13, 1945, that "by the time you get this you may have read about it [the find at Altaussee], but most of the correspondents are celebrating in Paris, and due to its unusual nature this may get no coverage at all." Still, he had added, "Although I doubt it."[14] After all, how could one of the most important and unbelievable moments in art history—not to mention the history of a world war—simply become a forgotten footnote?

But that's exactly what happened. A few articles and books were written over the years, but soon even the art community forgot about the dramatic events at Altaussee. It wasn't until the 1980s that an Austrian historian named Ernst Kubin located the source material—letters, orders, interviews, and first-person accounts—to determine what really happened at Altaussee. That source material, viewed again for this book, provides a surprising story with even more surprising heroes. It is also a near-perfect summary of what happens in the void of war and how history is more often than not a messy combination of intention, courage, preparation, and chance.

If Hitler's orders created the momentum and opportunity to destroy history's greatest works of art, as I believe, it was his loyal retainer Albert Speer who created the countermomentum to stop it. On March 30, 1945, Speer convinced Hitler to change his Nero Decree from the "total destruction" of nonindustrial sites to "crippling them lastingly." Speer then issued secret orders on his own to scale back and undermine those guidelines. These orders gave mining officials at Altaussee the cover and courage they needed to stand up to Eigruber's plan.

They had not learned of that plan by chance, as Kirstein believed. They were informed of it on April 13, 1945, by Dr. Helmut von Hummel who, as Martin Bormann's secretary in the bunker with Hitler, was privy to most communiqués in the Third Reich.[15] Von Hummel's intention was to stop Eigruber's actions, but he would not publicly acknowledge his role—the last days of the Third Reich were dangerous, and von Hummel was a typical Nazi coward—leaving the mine director, Dr. Emmerich Pöchmüller, to confront Eigruber without high party backing. When Eigruber refused to accept Pöchmüller's phone call, the mine director drove to Linz on April 17 in hopes of a face-to-face meeting. His plan, if he could not talk sense into the gauleiter, was to trick him. With the help of the mine's technical director, Eberhard Mayerhoffer, Pöchmüller had devised a plan to blow up the mine entrances and seal the bombs inside, leaving Eigruber with no way to detonate them. They would sell the plan to the gauleiter as a way to strengthen the bomb blasts and guarantee destruction of the mine.

The busy Eigruber (his office, you'll recall, was full of petitioners) agreed to the lesser explosions. But his assertion that he would "stay bullheaded"[16] on total destruction and a claim that he would "personally come and throw grenades into the mine"[17] if the Nazis lost the war, shocked Pöchmüller into an understanding of the seriousness of the situation. By April 19, he had worked out the specifics of the plan with his mining counselor (foreman) Otto Högler. It was a difficult and complicated job, necessitating hundreds of moving parts and careful planning to ensure, as much as possible, that the blasts wouldn't cause unintended collapses inside the various mine chambers where the art was stored. On April 20, work began. Högler believed the job would take at least twelve days—until May 2—to complete.

On April 28, 1945, Pöchmüller signed what could

have been his own death warrant when he ordered Högler to remove the bombs. The "agreed palsy" that would take place at a time "presented to you by myself personally" (see page 414 for the whole text) referred to the explosions that would collapse the entrances to the mine.[18] Pöchmüller must have been horrified when, two days later, Eigruber's adjunct District Inspector Glinz overheard Högler discussing trucks for the removal of the bombs and discovered the order. By the end of the day, six armed guards loyal to Eigruber were stationed at the entrance to the mine.

By May 3, the situation was desperate. The Americans were stuck in Innsbruck, 150 miles away; Eigruber's guards controlled entry into the mine; the bombs were still inside; and a demolition team had been spotted in a nearby valley. But all was not lost. The "palsy" charges were almost set and Karl Sieber, the art restorer and Pöchmüller confidant, had convinced two of Eigruber's guards of the barbarity of the gauleiter's plan.[19] Meanwhile, word was spreading among the miners that the crates contained bombs, not the sculpture advertised on the crate exteriors. A miner named Alois Raudaschl, an active Nazi, knew that Ernst Kaltenbrunner, a local boy who had risen to the top tier of the Nazi Party, was on his way to the area and suggested contacting the notorious SS deputy and leader of the Gestapo.

At 2:00 p.m. on May 3, 1945, Raudaschl met with Kaltenbrunner in the home of a mutual friend. Soon after, Kaltenbrunner met with Högler and agreed neither the great artwork stolen by Hitler nor the livelihood of the miners should be needlessly destroyed.

When Högler asked if he had Kaltenbrunner's permission to remove the bombs, the SS officer replied, "Yes, do it."[20]

That night, the bombs were removed by the miners, with the implicit sanction of Eigruber's guards. The work took four hours. The miners knew nothing of the three weeks of planning and courage that had created this opportunity; they thought they were sneaking the bombs out on their own initiative. This honest mistake, taken as fact, caused the Americans and history to misunderstand the situation entirely.

Around midnight, another of Eigruber's loyal adjuncts, Tank Staff Sergeant Haider, arrived at Altaussee. If the bombs were removed, Haider warned, Högler would be held responsible and "ruthlessly eliminated."[21] The bombs would stay in the mines at all costs. If this was not done the gauleiter would "come himself to Altaussee the following morning and hang each single one of them."[22] (Thus the subsequent rumors the miners were threatened, when it was really the plotters who were in danger.) Kaltenbrunner was alerted to the threat and reached Eigruber by phone at 1:30 a.m. on the morning of May 4. After a vicious tongue-lashing, the gauleiter backed down.[23] He asked only that the bombs be left beside the road for his men to pick up, not dumped into a lake as Högler had intended.

One day later, at the crack of dawn on May 5, 1945, Emmerich Pöchmüller and Otto Högler, two of the true heroes of Altaussee, stood outside the entrance to the mine. The miners had worked twenty hours straight to finish the preparations for the palsy, which included not only the six tons of explosives but 386 detonators and 502 timing switches. On Pöchmüller's orders, the switches were thrown and seventy-six bomb blasts echoed out of the mountain, sealing 137 tunnels in the ancient salt mines at Altaussee.[24]

CHAPTER 52

Evacuation

Altaussee, Austria
May 1–July 10, 1945

When Monuments Men Robert Posey and Lincoln Kirstein arrived at Altaussee on May 12, 1945, the small mining village was being held by a handful of American infantry soldiers. There were also dozens of miners and several Austrian and German officials, and almost as many conflicting stories. According to Kirstein, "A hive of wild rumors buzzed about the entrance: the mine had been blown; we could see nothing; there was no use trying to enter."[1] But enter the Monuments Men did, pushing through the cold mine to the huge sloping wall of dirt and rock brought down on Pöchmüller's order. The blast was intended to create a barrier forty feet deep, but nobody was sure if that was actually the case. And nobody knew what they would find on the other side.

The miners estimated it would take two weeks to clear a space through the bomb-blasted rocks. Posey, with an architect's training, felt sure combat engineers could clear it in less than a week. The miners, now under orders from the Americans, set to work with old-fashioned picks and shovels. By the next morning, they had cleared a small crevice at the top of the tunnel large enough for a man to squeeze through.

Robert Posey went through first, followed by Lincoln Kirstein. Another world awaited them beyond the wall: dusty, dark, and eerily silent. Their old-fashioned acetylene torches threw light a few yards down a main corridor filled with debris. The iron security doors, blasted apart by the force of the detonations, hung wildly from their hinges. The air was damp, suggesting broken sluices and flooded chambers. The first door they approached sheltered a dynamite magazine. Past the door, a narrow side passage branched off into the mountain. The second door was solid iron, and took two keys to open. Inside, silently reading a book, was Van Eyck's Virgin Mary. Next to her, on four empty cardboard boxes, were seven more panels of the Ghent Altarpiece. "The miraculous jewels of the Crowned Virgin seemed to attract the light from our flickering acetylene lamps," Kirstein later wrote. "Calm and beautiful, the altarpiece was, quite simply, there."[2]

The Monuments Men backtracked and, by way of half-hidden, pitch-black tunnels, were able to maneuver around the bomb blast. A guide led them deep into the cold heart of the mountain, past branching passageways, to a large rock-vaulted chamber. Their torchlight, swinging into the gloom, illuminated rack after rack of plain pine boxes filled with some of the world's great artistic masterpieces before falling, finally, on the milky white surface of Michelangelo's *Bruges Madonna*. She was lying on her side on a filthy brown-and-white-striped mattress, almost assuredly the very same mattress onto which she had been pushed just days before

British Monuments Man Ronald Balfour had arrived in Bruges eight months earlier. Monuments Man Thomas Carr Howe Jr. (who arrived in June) would later write, "the light of our lamps played over the soft folds of the Madonna's robe, the delicate modeling of her face. Her grave eyes looked down, seemed only half aware of the sturdy Child nestling close against her, one hand firmly held in hers."[3] A few days later, in a deep chamber, the Monuments Men discovered the remaining four panels of the Ghent Altarpiece, Vermeer's *The Artist's Studio*, and, farther into the dark recesses of the chamber, the Rothschild family's Vermeer, *The Astronomer*.

On May 18, with the size of the find slowly coming into focus, Lincoln Kirstein was sent back to headquarters to pick up "an expert in air, humidity and paint chemistry so we could see what the pictures have been in for. The expert," he wrote, "is always George Stout, who is perhaps the nicest man in the world."[4]

The indispensable Stout arrived at Altaussee on May 21. His first action was to dutifully record the known contents of the mine, which had been summarized in a report by mine personnel staff Karl Sieber and Max Eder and handed over to Stout by the solicitous Dr. Michel:[5]

6577 paintings
230 drawings or watercolors
954 prints
137 pieces sculpture
129 pieces arms and armor
79 baskets of objects
484 cases objects thought to be archives

78 pieces furniture

122 tapestries

181 cases books

1200–1700 cases apparently books or similar

283 cases contents completely unknown

He then set about interviewing the mine personnel and inspecting the chambers. "It was fascinating," Kirstein wrote, "to hear him compare American methods of determining absolute, or relative, or some kind of humidity with the Austrian methods used by the Professor of Mineralogy from the University of Vienna [the notorious Dr. Michel], who had always been at the depot, and who showed us his credentials from the Austrian Resistance Movement."[6] After three days of study, Stout declared the artwork in the mine safe for another year. Then, leaving the mine in Posey's command, he traveled to Third Army rear to press for a war crimes investigation of what had happened in the remote salt mine in the Austrian Alps. No investigation ever took place.

On June 14, George Stout returned to Altaussee with Lieutenant Steve Kovalyak, his new disciple from Bernterode. The mine passageways were finally cleared the next day and all "palsied" tunnels reopened. The effort had taken 253 work shifts by the miners, who had removed 879 cartloads of debris.

Ten days later, on June 25, Stout received grave news. President Harry Truman had knuckled under to Stalin. The Western Allies would not be holding their conquered territory, but instead falling back to the postwar boundaries determined by the Big Three (Roosevelt, Churchill, and Stalin) at the Yalta Conference in February. American military officials feared that numerous repositories would end up in the Soviet Zone of Occupation. Everything at Altaussee, Stout realized, could be handed over to Stalin. The Monuments Men would not have a year to remove the treasures from Altaussee, as Stout had assumed. They had until July 1. Four days.

Stout cracked the whip. Karl Sieber and Stout's two new assistants, Monuments Men Thomas Carr Howe Jr. and Lamont Moore, were sent deep into the mine to select the most important pieces for priority removal. Stout had brought with him the German sheepskin coats he had used to wrap artwork at Merkers; they were now used for the same purpose at Altaussee. Once wrapped and crated, the artwork was placed on the small trolley carts (referred to as "mine dogs") that wound on narrow tracks throughout the mine. The miners walked beside the mine dogs as a small engine pulled them toward the surface. Outside, the artwork was loaded onto trucks and, accompanied by two half-tracks, driven down the hazardous mountain roads to an MFAA art collecting center, known as the Munich Collecting Point, established by James Rorimer. There, the trucks were unloaded and the sheepskin coats—as well as any crates or other packing material available—driven back to Altaussee to be used for the next shipment.

Conditions deteriorated quickly. Behind schedule, Stout implemented a sixteen-hour workday, from 4:00 a.m. to 8:00 p.m. Outside, it rained incessantly, complicating the loading of trucks and making even walking to the bunkhouse miserable. Inside, the mine's electrical and lighting systems, knocked out by Pöchmüller's explosions, still didn't work. There weren't enough places to sleep; food was scarce; communication with the outside world almost nonexistent. Stout scraped his knuckles on the salty mine walls and got an infection; every night, he had to soak his fingers for hours in a helmet filled with hot water to keep the swelling down. "All hands grumbling," he wrote in his diary, in typical understated fashion.[7]

They missed their July 1 deadline. Fortunately, there was disagreement in high political circles over whether the deadline applied only to Germany, or to Austria as well. The men kept working. At breakfast on July 10, George Stout announced, "This looks like a good day for the gold-seal products."[8] He had spent several days with Steve Kovalyak wrapping the *Bruges Madonna* with coats, paper, and rope until it looked, in the words of Stout's assistant Thomas Carr Howe Jr., "like a trussed ham."[9] A one-ton trussed ham, that is, on which even a tiny scratch would be forever noticed by the world. But Stout was confident. Using a specially devised rope and pulley system, he carefully lifted the statue onto a waiting mine dog, declaring, "I think we could bounce her from Alp to Alp, all the way to Munich, without doing her any harm."[10] He then proceeded to personally walk the mine dog and statue to the mine entrance.

The Ghent Altarpiece, each panel already carefully loaded into its own crate, came next. The truck was prepared in a similar manner to the dozens that had already carried other priceless cultural artifacts from the mine. First, the bed was lined with waterproof paper, which had been intended as protection for the Wehrmacht against gas attacks. A strip of felt was laid over the paper, then "sausages" placed on the felt. These were essentially eighteen-inch-wide pillows fashioned by George Stout from ecru curtain material found in the mine. In the case of the altarpiece, the crates were then lashed upright on the sausages, with stowing cases on either side for balance and shock absorption. When all twelve panels were standing parallel to each other on the truck, more felt and waterproof paper were layered over the top, and the whole load lashed firmly to the sides.

The packing of the *Bruges Madonna* and the Ghent Altarpiece, undertaken with extraordinary care, consumed an entire day. The next morning, with George Stout in the lead and half-tracks following behind, two of Europe's great masterpieces wound their way 150 miles down the steep Alpine mountains to Munich. Their journey home had begun.

Less than a month later, on August 6, 1945, George Stout left Europe. He too was on his way home: forty-seven years old, tired, but none the worse for wear. In a little more than thirteen months, he had discovered, analyzed, and packed tens of thousands of pieces of artwork, including eighty truckloads from Altaussee alone. He had organized the MFAA field officers at Normandy, pushed SHAEF to expand and support the monuments effort, mentored the other Monuments Men across France and Germany, interrogated many of the important Nazi art officials, and inspected most of the Nazi repositories south of Berlin and east of the Rhine. It would be no exaggeration to guess he put 50,000 miles on his old captured VW and visited nearly every area of action in U.S. Twelfth Army Group territory. And during his entire tour of duty on the continent, he had taken exactly one and a half days off.[11]

Letter from James Rorimer
To his wife, Katherine
May 17, 1945

You may indeed complain about not having heard
from me these past days. I have never in my life
worked at a more exciting pace and with more
results than during these past two or three
weeks where I have covered our area which has
taken me to Salzburg and Füssen [the closest town
to Neuschwanstein Castle] twice each, battered
Munich, Worms, Frankfurt, Darmstadt, Mannheim,
Heidelberg, and dozens of smaller places. By now
you will guess that we are permitted to mention
locations as has not been possible since I left
home over a year ago, and more. I am stationed
at Augsburg for the moment, but have scarcely
had a chance to see the town as I have been
very much on the run when I was not actually
doing things at Headquarters. I have run down
the most exciting Information and documents on
the wholesale looting of art in Europe by the
Nazis and have been working with the Nazi big-
wigs of the past and checking clues and finding
art treasures such as I have rarely expected to
find. [Monuments Men] Kuhn and Lt. Col. McDonnell
were here again to see some of the things I
have discovered. I have found some of the key
culprits in the racket, and information which is
making the headlines of the world press if I am
not mistaken. Go to the News Reels and see for
yourself. My contact with the world press will
have to be through you.

Göring's art collector, his private train, his
house in Berchtesgaden as well as Hitler's and
the Braunhaus in Munich and the castles at Füssen
[Neuschwanstein] and the Monasteries which were
used for hiding things have been the scenes of
my work. I am way behind in my reporting, but my
diary is up to date. What exciting stories I can
now write in the book I hope to publish. Now I
really can say that I have played my part in the
war effort. I had a pleasant interview with Maj-
Gen. Taylor of the 101 Airborne who sent for me
the other day. I go to see him again on Sunday.
Harry Anderson of the Amer. Institute is taking
charge of the Göring things under my supervision
so to speak. He is a captain. I expect to
have another officer to help me in a few days.
[Monuments Man] Calvin Hathaway is still here
and he is a great help. Skilton is also here
and certain enlisted personnel will no doubt
help—what a life for a first Lt. I think that I
was finally released from Paris after the non-
concurrence of 2 generals. I am glad indeed to be
here. Train loads of art are being reported all
the time. I just cannot collect my thoughts these
days. . . .

I have not as yet seen news announcements
of my activity which has included getting the
backbone people, information and works of art of
the Einsatzstab Rosenberg. That was my personal
ambition when I joined the army, when I went
into Civil Affairs, when I told the board at the

American School Center at Shrivenham and when I worked at other matters during eight months in Paris. I almost didn't get to Germany. I cannot explain how I was so lucky as to have our army go to these places which with two important exceptions are the most important....Now my fervent desires are to finish up my military career and get back to civilian life.

Do not bother to send me anything....At the moment nothing is much use to me as I am living out of a barracks bag. Where we go next I do not know, but I have to keep on the move all the time.

Now I must go back to work. Love and more when things quiet down.

Jim

CHAPTER 53

The Journey Home

Heilbronn, Germany
September–November 1945

The end of active hostilities was not the end of the Monuments Men's work. Not by far. As the situation at Altaussee demonstrated, finding looted Nazi treasures was just the first step of a very long process. The treasures had to be inspected and catalogued, then packed and shipped out of the mines, castles, monasteries, or simple holes in the ground where they had been stored. Almost every site contained Nazi archives, which also had to be transported so that researchers could determine where the artwork had come from and who was the rightful owner. The archives inevitably led to the discovery of other repositories, as did interviews with the Nazis now being rounded up in the collapsed German-Austrian state. And almost every day, army units stumbled upon unfathomable treasures hidden in basements, traincars, food caches, and oil barrels.

By June 4, less than a month since the end of hostilities, 175 repositories had been found in U.S. Seventh Army territory alone. The MFAA was adding officers and enlisted men as quickly as possible—a vast majority of the almost 350 men and women who served in the multinational MFAA effort would join after the end of combat—but still only a handful of those mines and castles had been emptied. And every piece that was brought out of a hole had to be taken somewhere. Fortunately, the industrious and insightful James Rorimer had managed to secure the most coveted buildings in Munich: the former Nazi Party headquarters complex. Soon, artwork and other stolen cultural items were pouring into the buildings, now known as the Munich Collecting Point, from all over southern Germany and Austria. By July, the usable space was almost full, so Rorimer secured another building of almost equal size in Wiesbaden. A few weeks later, a building at Marburg University was requisitioned for the collection of archives. Walker Hancock, the optimistic Monuments Man for U.S. First Army, was placed in charge.

James Rorimer, meanwhile, never stayed in one place long. And soon he was bringing along Harry Ettlinger, the German-Jewish-American private from Karlsruhe who had wandered into his office the day before Germany's surrender, as his personal translator. Suddenly, Harry's tour of duty was as breakneck and interesting as his previous four months of service had been plodding and dull.

In mid-May, Rorimer took him to a Munich jail for a four-hour interrogation of a German national. Rorimer had been working on the man for days: befriending him, giving him cigarettes, feigning sympathy. The Nazi had finally opened up, and now Rorimer needed Harry to take down specific information on his art collection. The man was Heinrich Hoffman, Adolf Hitler's close friend and personal photographer. How must it have felt for a persecuted German Jew to stand that close to a man who had dined regularly with the Führer, and had been his staunch supporter and confidant for more than twenty years? Hoffman, of course, insisted he was a bystander. He had taken propaganda photographs of Hitler only because he received royalties every time one was reprinted, even on German stamps. He had bought artwork of dubious origin from "reputable" dealers only so he could make reproduction photographs. He had grown rich off Nazism, but he had never been a... believer, only an economic opportunist. Wasn't this the American way?

Soon after, Harry accompanied Rorimer to Berchtesgaden. While Rorimer dealt with the art treasures in the village—the Reichsmarschall wasn't the only high Nazi official who had hidden his stolen loot near the former Nazi stronghold—Harry went up the mountain to Hitler's chalet, known as the Berghof. He stood alone in the Führer's living room and stared through the enormous window (the glass long gone) out of which Adolf Hitler had so often surveyed his empire. How did it feel for a German Jew, whose friends and relatives had died in the Holocaust, to stand among the conquerors in the halls of the defeated dictator? It felt good. The house had been picked over by visiting troops, but Harry managed to scrounge a few epaulettes and some paper bearing the letterhead of a high SS general. He looked out over Germany, now free, and thought those three simple words. "It feels good."

Near the end of May, Captain Rorimer took Private Ettlinger to Neuschwanstein. Neuschwanstein! Harry

Ettlinger saw it rise before him out of the alpine valley almost exactly as James Rorimer had seen it weeks
before, with its towers soaring against an enormous sky.
Only Altaussee could rival it both in setting and quality of stolen artwork. But Altaussee didn't have the history. Like many German children, Ettlinger had grown
up with stories of this castle and its vast riches; passing
through its gates was like stepping into a fairy tale from
his childhood. Here was the Germany of legend, with
its famous golden throne room. But it was also the Germany of the present, filled room after room with stolen
artwork. At the entrance, Ettlinger had watched Rorimer turn away a British two-star general. The American captain was adamant: no one allowed inside. But
here was Harry Ettlinger, a buck private, gazing at the
kind of art and gold and treasure—Rothschild treasure!—not even dreamed of during his days growing
up in Karlsruhe. He had been translating documents
for weeks, but those were simply words and numbers.
To see actual paintings by artists like Rembrandt piled
up as booty was another thing entirely. "My knowledge
of the Holocaust," Harry would later say, "started really
with the realization that it was not only the taking of
lives—that I learned much later in my experience—
but the taking of all of their belongings.... [For me]
Neuschwanstein was the start of really opening up that
part of history that should never be forgotten."[1]

In September 1945, James Rorimer sent Harry
Ettlinger to Heilbronn, to the mine he had saved from
flooding back in April. The sounds of war had retreated
into the past, but the echoes had not. The Kronprinz
Hotel where Harry lived with twenty other enlisted

men was the only building standing on a block formerly full of stone buildings. The streets were empty of people, but full of rubble, and nothing had been done to clear them. The devastated center of town showed little sign of life. Harry's main landmark as he walked to the salt mine was the Bockingen railroad station, also completely destroyed. Across from the station a large concrete block marked the site of an air raid shelter. The entrance had been sealed after the devastating Allied bombing runs of December 4, 1944. The air raid shelter had somehow caught fire; inside were the remains of the two thousand Germans who had sought safety there. If he needed a more personal reminder of the horrors of war, Harry need only look at Ike, a seventy-pound survivor of Auschwitz and Dachau who had been "adopted" by their detachment.

But thanks to James Rorimer, the Heilbronn mine had been brought back into production, seemingly the only beast awake in that slumbering land. The pumps had been repaired and were cycling the seepage from the Neckar River out of the underground chambers. The skips were carrying large quantities of salty rocks to the surface. From there, the rocks were transferred to a massive furnace, where they were liquefied at 1200 degrees Fahrenheit so the salt crystals could be skimmed off. The furnace was powered by coke, a coal product, and since there was an excess of coke at the mine, the nearby glass factory was up and running, too. Amid all the destruction and sorrow, where even a scrap of food or decent bed was difficult for most people to come by, the factory was churning out thousands of Coca-Cola bottles.

At Heilbronn, Private Harry Ettlinger felt for the first time the immensity of the MFAA task. There were only two Monuments Men in Heilbronn, but they were expected to remove from underground literally tons of artwork. At the surface worked the operation's commander, Monuments Man Lieutenant Dale Ford, an interior designer recently pulled by the Roberts Commission from a camouflage unit in North Africa. Ford and three Germans—an art historian, an administrator, and a former junior ERR staff member assigned during the war to Paris (and possibly the Jeu de Paume, it was never clear)—spent their days in a small office next to the mine elevator, searching the ERR archives. Their primary job was to find the world-class pieces hidden in the dross.

Harry's job was to transport them to the surface. Each morning, after passing the air raid crypt and the Coca-Cola bottle plant, he was handed a list of objects and their location. He would then descend seven hundred feet into the darkness with two German miners. Two mines had actually been used (the second, located nearby, was known as Kochendorf) and together they had miles of chambers. Inside those chambers were more than 40,000 cases, from which Harry was supposed to pluck dozens of pieces a day. It was a daunting task, but Harry had two things working to his advantage. First, the ERR records were excellent, describing down to the number of the crate on the shelf of the wall bin exactly where each piece was located. Second, as the mine's chief engineer had assured Rorimer in April, the artwork was all stored in a series of smaller chambers on the upper level of the mine. The larger bottom levels, many flooded during or shortly after the battle for Heilbronn, contained factory equipment.

Still, the mine was dark and cold. Tunnels branched off in numerous directions, and once out of the main shaft it was easy to get lost. The number of chambers was intimidating, but nothing compared to the fact that each chamber held hundreds of similar-looking brown crates, any of which could contain cultural treasures, gold coins, bombs, booby traps...or something as common as personal photographs. The task was unpredictable. Harry had learned this a few weeks into the job when he noticed a chamber walled up with bricks. No one knew what was behind it, so he ordered the wall taken down. Inside were long tables piled with bottles. Each bottle contained a thin liquid separated from a thicker sludge. The miners recognized it immediately: nitroglycerin. The alarm was sounded, and everyone raced from the mine. Then experts were sent to very carefully bring the bottles to the surface. The separating of the liquids, the miners told Harry, made the solution volatile. One more month and the thinner liquid would have exploded. There seemed little doubt that this "accident" was exactly what the person who built the wall had in mind.

Despite the danger, the recovery effort plowed forward. As the fighting neared its conclusion, there had been some discussion of what exactly to do with the treasures discovered in Germany and Austria. Eventually, the decision was made that all cultural objects, *even those that belonged to Germany*, would be returned to their country of origin. Once that decision was made, the Western Allies were determined to return the treasures as quickly as possible. The army couldn't afford the manpower, for one thing. And restitution on this scale was unprecedented; the world was rightfully dubious. The Western Allies had sacrificed their national fortunes and a generation of young men; would they really hand back the spoils of their victory?

In late summer, General Eisenhower answered that question in resounding fashion. Ever mindful of the importance of his Western Allies, Ike ordered the immediate return of the most important works of art to each respective country until the more systematic process of returns could be implemented. First to be returned was the Ghent Altarpiece. Soon others followed, including the famous stained-glass windows from Strasbourg Cathedral, which the French considered a national treasure. The message went down the line from commander to commander and, finally, seven hundred feet underground to Private Harry Ettlinger. The windows weren't difficult to find, even in Heilbronn—they were very large—but extracting such delicate masterpieces from a working salt mine was nerve-jangling work. Then came the packing: seventy-three cases in all. By mid-October, the windows were inventoried, packed, and ready for transport. Instead of traveling to an MFAA collecting point, the stained-glass windows were taken by convoy directly from the mine to Strasbourg. On November 4, 1945, their return was celebrated in an elaborate ceremony, during which James Rorimer received the French Legion of Honor, becoming the first Monuments Man bestowed with such a high honor.

Meanwhile, Harry had received another important

assignment. The story of Nazi looting, after all, wasn't merely the robbing of nations of their treasures and the human race of its historical and cultural touchstones. More than anything, the Nazis robbed families: of their livelihoods, their opportunities, their heirlooms, their mementos, of the things that identified them and defined them as human beings. This was brought home to Harry Ettlinger in the form of a letter from his grandfather, Opa Oppenheimer, in October 1945. Just before he fled Germany in 1939, Opa had been forced to stash in a storage facility near Baden-Baden his beloved collection of ex libris bookplates and art prints. He kept with him the name of the facility, the warehouse number, the combination to the locks, and the hope that his personal treasure would survive the war and somehow find its way back into his hands. Now, six years later, his grandson was stationed in central Germany, as a Monuments Man recovering art. Opa Oppenheimer hoped Harry could facilitate the return of his collection—if it still existed.

An opportunity didn't present itself until November, when the personal valet of the governor of the French Occupied Zone came to stay at the Kronprinz Hotel. The valet, Jacques, was an automobile repair expert, and he had come to study the Mercedes motorworks in the nearby town of Stuttgart. Harry asked if he could facilitate a trip to Baden-Baden, which was in the French Zone. The valet readily agreed.

So on a sunny day in November 1945, Jacques, Private Harry Ettlinger, and his detachment's "adopted" member Ike, the Holocaust survivor, set out in a jeep to find a collection of prints and bookplates representing the mementos of a common life well lived. The trip took just over an hour. They found the facility without difficulty. Pulling open the warehouse doors, Harry Ettlinger's heart leapt almost like it had on that long-ago day in Belgium when the sergeant had called him off the convoy headed to the front. Here in this dark and dusty room were the wonders Harry had known since childhood—thousands of signed, original book-plates; hundreds of prints from turn-of-the-century German Impressionists; and the beautiful autographed print of an etching of the Rembrandt of Karlsruhe. They were just as Opa Oppenheimer had left them.

Clapping Harry on the back, the valet suggested they go out for a celebratory meal. He took them to a rural valley, where they dined on trout fished right out of a brook and drank toasts with the local specialty: cherry schnapps. By the time they dropped off the valet in Baden-Baden, Harry and Ike were feeling fine. Maybe too fine. Ike, who liked his liquor, missed a turn on the mountainous road back to Heilbronn and went into a ditch. It took ten men to lift the jeep back onto the road, at which point they discovered the brake line was snapped. Ike turned around and coasted three precarious miles back into Baden-Baden.

Harry was now AWOL (absent without leave, punishable by an army prison sentence), since he hadn't bothered with an overnight pass. And even worse, at least at the moment, the two men had no place to sleep. They tracked down the only person they knew in town, Jacques the valet, who fortunately had a girlfriend who worked in the city's finest hotel. She met them at the back door and slipped them up the backstairs to the one place no one at the front desk would think to look: the penthouse suite. That night, a Holocaust survivor from Auschwitz and a buck private in the U.S. Army— a former German Jew who had been forced out of his homeland by the ruthless Nazi purges—slept in beds reserved for the Kaiser of Germany. Even Adolf Hitler and Eva Braun were never afforded such a luxury.

A few weeks later, while the public streamed into Strasbourg by the thousands to marvel at the newly reinstalled stained-glass windows of its world-famous cathedral, another shipment of precious objects arrived by truck at the Heilbronn mine. There, Harry Ettlinger and the two German miners carefully packed them in exactly the same way they had packaged the great cathedral windows and the Old Master paintings. These precious objects, however, went not to a European government or a great collector, but to an apartment on the third floor of an old house at 410 Clinton Avenue in Newark, New Jersey. The Oppenheimer-Ettlinger family treasure had come home from the war.

CHAPTER 54

Heroes of Civilization

Germany, Britain, France, America, and the World
Then, Now, and Forever

The reconstruction of Europe after World War II was one of the most complicated and comprehensive international efforts of modern times. The identity and infrastructure of the nations of Europe had to be rebuilt, and the restitution of artwork was a vital component. To say the war was the greatest upheaval of cultural items in history would be a grave understatement. In the end, the Western Allies discovered more than one thousand repositories in southern Germany alone, containing millions of works of art and other cultural treasures, including church bells, stained glass, religious items, municipal records, manuscripts, books, libraries, wine, gold, diamonds, and even insect collections. The job of packing, transporting, cataloguing, photographing, archiving, and returning this plunder to its country of origin—the respective countries were then responsible for returning it to the individual owners—fell almost exclusively to the MFAA section. The job would take six long years.

Despite the best efforts of the men and women of the MFAA, hundreds of thousands of works of art, documents, and books have yet to be found. The most famous is perhaps Raphael's *Portrait of a Young Man*, stolen from the Czartoryski Collection in Cracow, Poland, and last known to have been in the possession of the notorious Nazi governor-general Hans Frank. Tens of thousands were no doubt destroyed. These include the personal collection of SS chief Heinrich Himmler, which was burned by SS stormtroopers before British troops could intervene. The famed Amber Panels of Peter the Great, looted by the Nazis from Catherine Palace outside St. Petersburg (formerly Leningrad), are likely another cultural victim of the war, in all probability destroyed during an artillery battle that took place at Königsberg but for the small portable mosaics, one of which surfaced in Bremen in 1997. Thousands of paintings and other works of art have never been claimed, either because their provenance could not be determined or their owners were among the millions who died or were murdered in Hitler's military and racial crusades. Sadly, not all museums, the interim custodians of some of these works of art, have demonstrated the determination of the Monuments Men to locate their rightful owner or heirs.

More than sixty years after the death of Adolf Hitler, we still live in a world altered by his legacy. His personal belongings are scattered, although many have made their way into public museums and collections. Most of his library books are in the U.S. Library of Congress Rare Book and Special Collections Division, and eighty volumes may be found at Brown University in the John Hay Library's Rare Book collection. Many of his paintings and watercolors are stored at the

National Museum of the U.S. Army, Army Art Collection. The original duplicates of his last will and political testament are at the National Archives in College Park, Maryland, and the Imperial War Museum in London. His beloved Haus der Deutschen Kunst (House of German Art) still stands in Munich, although today as the Haus der Kunst, home to temporary exhibits of contemporary art. But the lasting impact of his bitter reign is best measured in more ephemeral ways: fifty million loved ones who never returned home from the war to rejoin their families or start one of their own; brilliant, creative contributions never made to our world because scientists, artists, and inventors lost their lives too early or were never born; cultures built over generations reduced to ashes and rubble because one human being judged groups of other human beings less worthy than his own.

The highest officials in Hitler's government were prosecuted for crimes against humanity at the Nuremberg trials beginning in October 1945. Hitler's would-be successor and rival for the cultural treasures of Europe, Reichsmarschall Hermann Göring, was arrested by American soldiers on May 9, 1945. Dressed in his most resplendent uniform and carrying his baton of state, he had been attempting to secure an audience with Allied Supreme Commander Eisenhower. He was taken to a prison cell in Augsburg instead. Like the other party leaders at Nuremberg, he at first denied his role in the Holocaust, proclaiming, "I revere women and I think it unsportsmanlike to kill children....For myself I feel quite free of responsibility for the mass murders."[1] In the end, however, he was one of the few to acknowledge personal participation in the worst aspects of the Third Reich.

Göring saved his denials for accusations about his collection of art. "Of all the charges which have been leveled against me," he is quoted as saying in the *Nuremberg Interviews*, "the so-called looting of art treasures by me has caused me the most anguish."[2]

In another section of the *Nuremberg Interviews*, he explained his thinking: "They tried to paint a picture of me as a looter of art treasures. In the first place, during a war everybody loots a little bit. However, none of my so-called looting was illegal.... I always paid for them or they were delivered through the Hermann Göring Division, which, together with the Rosenberg Commission supplied me with my art collection. Perhaps one of my weaknesses has been that I love to be surrounded by luxury and that I am so artistic in my temperament that masterpieces make me feel alive and glowing inside. But always my intention was to contribute these art treasures...to a state museum after I had died or before, for the greater glory of German culture. Looking at it from that standpoint I can't see that it was ethically wrong."[3]

The harshest blow for the Reichsmarschall came when he was confronted in his jail cell by the fact that one of his prized possessions, Jan Vermeer's *Christ with the Woman Taken in Adultery*, for which he had traded 150 paintings, was a forgery. (The forger, Han van Meegeren, had been arrested in Holland for collaboration with the Nazis and plundering Dutch culture. When it was revealed he had duped the hated Reichsmarschall, he was hailed by some as a national hero.) Monuments Man Stewart Leonard delivered the news to Göring and said afterward that he "looked as if for the first time he had discovered there was evil in the world."[4] The Reichsmarschall had fancied himself a Renaissance man; in the end, he was revealed to be nothing more than an unsophisticated and greedy fool.

Hermann Göring did not appeal his death sentence at Nuremberg. He asked only to be executed with dignity, by firing squad, rather than hanged like a common criminal. His request was denied. On October 15, 1946, the night before his scheduled hanging, the broken-down Reichsmarschall committed suicide with a potassium cyanide capsule. It is still unclear how the poison found its way into his prison cell.

Alfred Rosenberg, leader of the ERR and Hitler's chief racial theorist, proved completely unrepentant and denied complicity in any wrongdoing. He was found guilty and executed by hanging on October 16, 1946.

Ernst Kaltenbrunner, the Gestapo leader, was found guilty at Nuremberg of the mass murder of civilians, selecting and executing racial and political undesirables, establishing concentration camps, the forced labor and execution of prisoners of war, and many other heinous and unfathomable crimes. He also was executed by hanging on October 16, 1946. Interceding to help save the artistic treasures at Altaussee turned out to be the only positive deed in an otherwise thoroughly miserable and rotten life.

Hans Frank, the notorious Nazi governor-general caught with stolen masterpieces near the end of the war, renewed his faith in Catholicism and expressed some remorse for his reign of terror in Poland. He expressed relief at being hanged with his fellow Nazi leaders, but never revealed the location of the missing Raphael painting.

Albert Speer, Hitler's personal architect and friend who had almost managed to take a stand against the Führer's Nero Decree, was the only other high-ranking Nazi to express remorse for his actions. He was found guilty of war crimes and crimes against humanity and, after a bitter split among the jurors, sentenced to twenty years in prison. After his release in 1966, he became an author. His three memoirs of life in Hitler's government, and most notably his first book *Inside the Third Reich*, have become invaluable to historians. Albert Speer died of a stroke in 1981.

August Eigruber was arrested in May 1945 and prosecuted at the Mauthausen Trial in March 1946. He was found guilty of war crimes committed at the Mauthausen concentration camp, including the execution of prisoners of war. Much of the evidence used to convict him was from archives found in the salt mine at Altaussee, probably another reason he was so keen to destroy the mine. He went unrepentant to the gallows on May 28, 1947. His last words, just before the trapdoor opened, were *"Heil Hitler!"*

Hermann Bunjes, the art scholar who had sold his soul in Paris and tried to buy it back by telling Monuments Men Posey and Kirstein about Altaussee, hanged himself from the window of his prison cell on July 25, 1945. It was later reported by Lincoln Kirstein, and repeated in numerous history books, that Bunjes had not only killed himself, but shot his wife and children to death as well. That was not true. He left his family penniless, starving, and terrified in a broken Germany, but very much alive. His wife, Hildegard, in fact, lived until August 2005. She went to her grave declaring, "My husband was not an active Nazi; he was an idealist."[5]

Bruno Lohse, Göring's representative to the ERR in Paris, was arrested by James Rorimer on May 4, 1945. Rorimer had found his name in the registration book at Neuschwanstein and had been informed he was staying at a nursing home in the nearby village. When confronted, Lohse tried to pass himself off as a simple corporal in the Luftwaffe (which was his technical rank). Rorimer, warned by Valland that Lohse was "a most untrustworthy, double-crossing scoundrel," wasn't fooled.[6] The "corporal" was placed under arrest.

Lohse admitted he had been involved with the ERR operation at the Jeu de Paume, but insisted he had done nothing wrong. He was a servant of Göring, he said, and thus his actions were legitimate. He became increasingly disillusioned as the interrogators described Göring's dealings, especially the fact that the Reichsmarschall had never bothered to pay his debt to the ERR. Lohse had been a fervent admirer of Göring, and he was disconsolate to learn his boss was so cheap that he hadn't even paid the absurdly low prices assigned to his looted art by the intimidated assessors of Paris.

In exchange for leniency, Bruno Lohse testified against his fellow looters and helped the French locate several caches of stolen art. (It helped that his coconspirators, Kurt von Behr and Hermann Bunjes, had both committed suicide.) He was released from prison in 1950, and soon after became a "legitimate" art dealer in Munich. By the mid-1950s, he was publicly denying having committed any crimes and was working diligently to rehabilitate his reputation. Much of this effort involved the intimidation and harassment of his chief accuser, Rose Valland. In a 1957 letter, Valland warned James Rorimer, with whom she had remained close friends, that "Lohse, who appears before you as a victim, assumes an entirely different personality when in Munich, judging from the conversations reported to me, and once again becomes the Nazi eager to avenge himself and to discredit the restitutions. For example, he regrets that he did not follow von Behr's orders and did not order my disappearance (deportation and execution) according to von Behr's plans. In Germany, he has become the champion of all these pitiful people who had been forced to obey the orders of the Nazi police and whose feelings we have hurt by asking them to be accountable for their actions."[7]

Lohse died in March 2007 at age ninety-five, having lived his final decades in relative quiet and anonymity. In May 2007, a safety deposit box he controlled was discovered at a bank in Zurich, Switzerland. Inside was a Camille Pissarro painting stolen by the Gestapo in 1938, as well as paintings by Monet and Renoir. Records showed that at least fourteen other paintings had been removed from the box since 1983. An international investigation continues.

Then there were the lesser figures of Altaussee. These ordinary men, unknown to higher authorities, had to find their own way through the disorder of postwar Austria and Germany. This task was complicated by the fact that, to a man, they had been members of the Nazi Party. None, however, were active party members. In Austria and Germany in the 1930s, a person had to become a Nazi Party member to hold a professional position. Along with the scoundrels and villains, the "de-Nazification" of Germany in the postwar years swept up many innocent, even on occasion heroic, men.

One such man was Otto Högler, the mine foreman whose support and knowledge made possible Pöchmüller's palsy at Altaussee. Högler was arrested on May 9, 1945, the day after the arrival of the Americans. Interestingly, a copy of the arrest report was sent to Dr. Michel, with a note assuring him that "the report was only signed by those clearly devoted to the cause." Was Högler sent away so Michel could take credit for the rescue at Altaussee? Impossible to say. Nonetheless, Högler spent eight months in detention. He was released in December 1945, but rearrested three months later. Fired from the mine, he was working as a rat exterminator.

Högler was released from prison in 1947 and, after years of petitions, rehired by the mining company in 1951 on the condition he never mention anything about the rescue of the art treasures. After his retirement in 1963, however, he worked to set the record straight. He did not succeed. In 1971, he summarized the situation in a letter to a magazine that had recently run an erroneous account of the rescue. "One thing in your article is true—there was no gratitude toward the savior of the art treasures (possibly only for one or two impostors) and this might possibly be the reason why this thankworthy achievement had been misused for all sorts of gangster novels." In 1972, he made one final attempt, compiling a report with the support of several miners on what had actually happened in April and May 1945. The report was politely accepted by the Austrian government but never examined. Otto Högler died in 1973.[8]

Dr. Herbert Seiberl, the Austrian art official who had been an early conspirator with Pöchmüller, lost his job and was banned from working in his field because of his registration in the Nazi Party. He tried working as a Christmas card maker, painter, restorer, and author, but without success. He died in 1952 at the age of forty-eight, leaving behind a widow and four children. His family was saved from destitution by gifts from a Mrs. Bondi and a Mr. Oppenheimer, both of whom had artwork rescued from Altaussee.[9]

Karl Sieber, the restorer, remained at the mine and became a valuable source of information for the Americans. Although he never spoke publicly of his role, his descriptions of the preparations at the mine were related by George Stout's assistant, Monuments officer Thomas Carr Howe Jr., in his book *Salt Mines and Castles*. The book became the source of later theories ascribing the rescue to the quiet restorer. The Americans helped him return home to Germany, and later got him released from house arrest, but Sieber never worked as a restorer again. He died in 1953.[10]

The worst fate, unfortunately, was meted out to the unknown hero of Altaussee, mine director Dr. Emmerich Pöchmüller. He was arrested there on June 17, 1945, and charged with trying to blow up the treasures at Altaussee. During his interrogation, he was beaten so mercilessly by an American officer that he lost six teeth and was unable to stand for a day. In November 1945, his sister obtained an audience with the Austrian Ministry of Education. She showed them her brother's diary, which detailed his actions at the mine. The answer from the court counselor was that "what your brother writes is all correct. We have checked it. But we cannot influence his discharge."[11]

Pöchmüller was finally released from detention in July 1947, and immediately began the fight to rehabilitate his reputation. In the fall of 1947, he confronted Dr. Michel about his false claims, which had been in the press for two years. On December 15, 1947, Michel wrote to the Austrian ministry, detailing Pöchmüller's true role at Altaussee. (Michel later recanted this statement, the only true one he ever made about Altaussee.)[12] Mayerhoffer, the engineer with whom he'd planned the palsy, confirmed Pöchmüller was a patriot and hero. A police investigation at the mine found no abuse of power or Nazi activity by its director. The archbishop of Vienna appealed for clemency on his behalf, and his official file in the Austrian government acknowledged that he had "taken an invaluable part in saving the art treasures."[13] Nonetheless, Pöchmüller's petition for an Act of Mercy (dismissal of charges for illegal Nazi activity) was turned down in 1949. It had been supported all the way to the office of the president, where it was summarily dismissed. Those who had benefited from the false stories of Altaussee had been working behind the scenes to defeat the petition.

Without the Act of Mercy, Pöchmüller was unable to work. He had joined the Nazi Party in 1932 and in

1934 was named an honorary member of the National Socialist Motor Corps, a division of mostly apolitical industrialists and businessmen. Because of this membership, he was barred from employment in Austria and Germany. In 1950, the German courts ruled that those bearing this honorary position were to be taken off the rolls of ex-Nazis, freeing Pöchmüller to seek employment. The stigma remained, however, and he was unable to find steady work. Unemployed, vilified, and impoverished, his health deteriorated.

Finally, a small publisher agreed to publish his book, *World Art Treasures in Danger*, which he had unsuccessfully self-published in 1948. Karl Sieber supported him, writing that "all facts described in this report are, as far as I have been present, true. Because the events which I have not been present at, but which correspond with the reports of different people I am aware of, I come to the conclusion that Engineer Dr. E. Pöchmüller has tried his utmost to write an absolutely objective, truthful report."[14] Nobody cared. Hardly any copies of the book were printed, and today it is very difficult to find (but not impossible, as we eventually discovered).

Devastated and bitter, Pöchmüller filed a lawsuit under an Austrian law that anyone who had saved artwork for a third party could claim 10 percent of its value as a reward. Although he publicly stated he did not want the money, only an Act of Mercy and public recognition of his role in rescuing the art treasures, he was castigated by the press and other interested parties—like Dr. Michel—as greedy and selfish.

Throughout the 1950s, he continued to lodge lawsuits in an attempt to clear his name, with limited success. In 1954, he was categorized as "less guilty," making him eligible for employment in his former profession. He finally found a job in 1955, but in Germany, not his beloved Austria. He made a last attempt to clear his name in 1959, writing to the Austrian government that "I would like my efforts for rescuing the art treasures to be officially recognized so that my wish (for family reasons) of being able to work in an appropriate position in Austria again is met. For this I am prepared to waive everything else." He never heard back.

Dr. Emmerich Pöchmüller died of a heart attack in 1963, having never received recognition of his accomplishments or freedom from suspicion and censor. His long fight for justice had broken him, body and soul.

Dr. Hermann Michel, meanwhile, did not escape unscathed. Although he was restored to his old job as director of the Natural History Museum Vienna, he was always viewed with suspicion. In 1945, he had convinced the Ministry of Education that he had joined the Nazi Party "to be able to easily carry out his work for the resistance movement at the museum."[15] The Ministry of the Interior was not convinced, and placed him on the ex-Nazi list in 1947.

In 1948, after the accounts by Pöchmüller surfaced, Michel was ordered to explain in writing his actions at Altaussee. Michel delayed writing the account until 1950, and then only turned in a partial draft. When asked why, he claimed that Pöchmüller, who he said greedily wanted the reward money from the rescue for himself, was threatening him.

The report was never filed with the government, but the effort to maintain his vast complex of lies finally wore Michel down. He began to lash out at his acquaintances, and even sued a fellow curator claiming he had stolen from the museum. The judge, in finding the man not guilty, said that "regarding the witness, Court Counselor Dr. Michel, one thing has to be clearly stated. This witness has evidentially made false statements. He also tried to influence another witness and is therefore guilty of incitement to perjury."

Michel was placed on administrative leave in December 1951 while the accusations were investigated. In May 1952, he was forced into early retirement. He died in October 1965. Although he had left in disgrace, the Natural History Museum—trying desperately to clear the shame of its racist Nazi past—claimed in 1987 that "Dr. Michel together with the freedom fighters prevented the destruction of the art treasures [at Altaussee]."[16]

Meanwhile, in France, Jacques Jaujard was hailed as a national hero for his role in protecting the state collections from the Nazis. He was named a Commander of the Legion of Honor, received the Medal of Resistance and was promoted to the secretary-general of cultural affairs in the post-occupation French government of André Malraux. When he retired to the Académie des Beaux-Arts in 1955, his predecessor praised him as a defender of the arts, saying, "He faces the future with the marvelous trail of all the masterpieces he has preserved."[17]

In contrast to many other prominent museum figures in France, Jaujard never wrote about his service as director of the French National Museums during World War II, or of his role in saving the French patrimony. He was firm in his discretion and his belief that those who remained silent probably did more than those who spoke publicly of their actions. His only known written account of the war was a seven-page description of the service performed by Rose Valland during the German occupation of Paris. Whether it was written at her request or to counter questions about her heroism or actions is unclear. But clearly, he remained her advocate.

Jacques Jaujard died unexpectedly of a heart attack in 1967. He was seventy-two years old. Friend and famed historian André Chamson said in his memorium, "[His] transcendental moment took place during the years of occupation, [an] interminable moment of truth, when everything depended, in a heads or tails fashion, on courage and lucidity.... [He] fought like a soldier, with a clear mind, with a skillful persuasion, a servant of the duties he had added to the responsibilities of his position, already responsible in front of the liberated fatherland of the Republic that would be reborn."[18] In 1974, a book of Jaujard's philosophies was published in a limited printing. One was, "It matters little that you are afraid if you manage to hide it. You are then at the edge of courage." Another: "There are fights that you may lose without losing your honor; what makes you lose your honor is not to fight them."[19] His friend Albert Henraux, the French Resistance leader, cited Jaujard's elegantly self-effacing motto for all Louvre employees: "*Maintenir*." To Preserve.[20]

Count Franz von Wolff-Metternich, the German Kunstschutz official who aided Jaujard in thwarting the Nazis, was also hailed as a hero by the French. After the war, he helped the Western Allies restitute German art. He then worked in the Foreign Office of West Germany tracking looted works. In 1952, Metternich became director of the esteemed Hertziana Library in Rome, a German library once confiscated by Hitler. He died in 1978.

Rose Valland, Jaujard's collaborator, continued her forceful advocacy on behalf of the French cultural patrimony long after James Rorimer's departure from Paris. On May 4, 1945, nearly a month after Rorimer's assignment to U.S. Seventh Army, Valland received a commission in the French First Army. "Along the [German] roads," she wrote, "I witnessed the heart-wrenching processions of refugees passing by like five year old ghosts from the [evacuation of Paris in 1940]....It was the same kind of misery....Seeing them, I lost the very clear notion of the enemy that had sustained me until then. I learned that we are only truly able to savor victory after having left the horrors of war."[21]

She arrived at Neuschwanstein sometime between May 14 and 16, 1945, only a week and a half after Rorimer. Here, seemingly, was the endpoint of her journey, a place that had seemed so inaccessible as to be almost mythical during her years at the Jeu de Paume, but for which she had risked her life countless times. She got as far as the gate, where the American sentry, having no idea who she was, denied her admission. Rorimer had declared no one was to enter; no exceptions. Since the energetic Monuments Man was away on other business, there was no way to argue. Rose Valland was turned away from her own greatest achievement.

But only on this day. She remained in Germany for several years as a fine arts officer attached to French First Army. She loved the company of men, and there are numerous pictures of her at the MFAA collecting points in her captain's uniform blending in with the male officers. She usually had a smile on her face and cigarette in hand.

Far from being the "shy, timid curator" depicted by history, Rose Valland was a tireless and vocal advocate for the restitution of artwork. She was able to blend into the background when necessary, but as when she challenged Bruno Lohse after he told her "you could be shot for any indiscretion,"[22] she was not afraid to question the methods and actions of anyone at any time. Upon returning home from Germany in 1951, Valland continued searching for looted French-owned works of art. Her success in this and other endeavors proved she was not a wilting flower, but a bold, strong-minded, courageous, and intelligent woman fired by a passion to fulfill the destiny fate and Jaujard had provided her in 1940.

For her efforts, Rose Valland received the French Legion of Honor and the Medal of Resistance. She was made a Commander of the Order of Arts and Letters, making her one of the most decorated women in France. She also received a Medal of Freedom from the United States in 1948, and an Officer's Cross of the Order of Merit from the Federal Republic of Germany. In 1953, after twenty years of service to the French cultural establishment, she was finally awarded the position of "curator." Her 1961 book *Le Front de L'Art* (The Battle for Art) was made into a 1965 movie entitled *The Train*, starring Burt Lancaster. The movie was a fictionalized account of the rescue of the art train; the Jeu de Paume and a character named "Mlle. Villard," who was meant to portray Rose Valland, were only briefly mentioned.

Despite her decorations and medals, Rose Valland's accomplishments were never widely known or admired in France. Partly this can be attributed to her background: She was a woman of little means from a small country town working in a field dominated by aristocratic men. The fact that, in Jaujard's words, "Miss Valland took the calculated risk, in order to save from the war and then to recuperate tens of thousands of works of art, to give this information directly to an American,"[23] was for some French citizens a severe breach of protocol bordering on unpatriotic. Finally, many of her contemporaries came to resent her relentless pursuit of information about the Nazis and restitutions of stolen art. There was a period when many wanted to forget the horrible events of the war; Valland would never forget and never let it rest. Perhaps, despite Jaujard's support, she was always doomed to be an outsider.

Rose Valland spent the last two decades of her life in relative quiet and died on September 18, 1980. After a viewing at Les Invalides in Paris, she was buried in a simple grave in her home village of Saint-Etienne-de-Saint-Geoirs. Her fellow Louvre curator Magdeleine Hours would later comment:[24]

> She received little understanding from her colleagues; she unleashed envy and passions, and we were few to show our admiration. On the day of her funeral at

Les Invalides, the Director of the Musées de France administration, the Chief Curator of the drawing department and myself, with a few museum attendants, were practically the only ones present to show the respects that were due to her. This woman, who had risked her life so often and with such persistence, who had brought honor to the corps of curators and saved the property of so many collectors, was treated by many with indifference, if not hostility.

On April 27, 2005, fifty years after the end of the war, a plaque was finally placed on the south wall of the Jeu de Paume to commemorate Rose Valland's extraordinary service and her commitment "to save a little bit of the beauty of the world."[25]

But if history and the people of France never truly understood and acknowledged her heroism, her fellow Monuments Men did. In the years to come, they would repeatedly describe Rose Valland as a great hero of the war and one of the few indispensable persons in the monuments preservation effort. Without her, they believed, the MFAA effort to locate not only the thousands of stolen works of art from France, but also the critically important ERR records, might never have succeeded.

Like Valland, the other Monuments Men continued to work for the preservation of art after the end of active hostilities, but their tours of duty were for the most part short-lived.

On August 21, 1945, the Ghent Altarpiece left the Munich Collecting Point for Belgium. It was the most important piece of artwork stolen by the Germans, and therefore the first returned. A special airplane was chartered, and the twelve panels of the altarpiece strapped down in the passenger compartment. There was only room for one other passenger: Monuments Man Robert Posey.

At 2:00 a.m. on August 22, the plane arrived at a British airfield in Belgium. It was supposed to land hours earlier at the Brussels airport, but a violent storm caused a change of plans. Instead of the grand reception the Belgian government had planned, the airfield was deserted. Posey telephoned an American officer, who shanghaied about twenty soldiers out of Belgian bars. The panels were unloaded in the driving rain and arrived at the Royal Palace in Brussels at 3:30 a.m. Posey left a few hours later, with a receipt for delivery. When he arrived back at U.S. Third Army headquarters after a brief stay in Paris, the commanding officer gave him his reward: the Order of Leopold, one of Belgium's highest honors. The Belgian government had intended to give it to him at the arrival ceremony, but never got the chance. He was later awarded the French Legion of Honor.

That was Posey's final lasting military achievement, however, for he found the post-combat work tedious and clashed with the newly arriving Monuments Men. In early May, before the end of fighting, he had scoffed at those back of the combat zone as "too low to even be thought of. If they are as far back as England they are simply civilians in a sort of uniform." Now that Germany had become a "civilian" world, he felt lost. He agreed with the rigid discipline of his boss, General Patton, who insisted that breakfast for all the men of Third Army, including the Monuments Men, occur early in the morning during a narrow period of time, just as it had during combat. The newly arriving Monuments Men wanted to sleep late. Even worse, they hired a busty German secretary, when it was forbidden to hire German nationals (even buxom blondes); Posey fired her.

Posey left Europe in September 1945, a month after the return of the Ghent Altarpiece and three months before his mentor and idol General George S. Patton Jr. died of injuries suffered in an automobile accident near Mannheim, Germany, in December. By 1946, Posey had resumed his work as an architect, and began his career at the prominent firm Skidmore, Owings & Merrill. As a senior associate, he worked on such notable projects as the Union Carbide Building and Lever House in New York, and the Sears Tower in Chicago. He retired in 1974 and died in 1977.

His partner, Lincoln Kirstein, who had despaired of leaving "before my retirement pay starts,"[26] returned to America in September 1945 on a hardship waiver after his mother was diagnosed with cancer. In 1946, he and his business partner, the choreographer George Balanchine, established a new dance troupe, the Ballet Society (renamed the New York City Ballet in 1948), one of the most influential dance companies of the twentieth century. Kirstein served as its general director until 1989. The poems he composed while in the army were published in 1964 as *Rhymes of a PFC*. Otherwise, he rarely spoke of his tour of duty in Europe, although he corresponded with Posey for several years and even entertained writing a book with him. He even encouraged George Stout to coauthor a book about the Monuments Men, stating, "It's not a picture book, but a story."[27] Far from viewing his role as glamorous, though, Kirstein often felt guilty that he had not faced more danger. He was the kind of man who struggled to find contentment in his many considerable achievements.

By the end of his life, Lincoln Kirstein was widely considered one of the major cultural figures of his generation, and perhaps its greatest patron of the arts. "He was one of those rare talents who touch the entire artistic life of their time," wrote critic Clement Crisp. "Ballet, film, literature, theatre, painting, sculpture, photography all occupied his attention."[28] In 1984, he was presented with the Presidential Medal of Freedom by Ronald Reagan. He also received the National Medal of Arts (1985), and, with Balanchine, the National Gold Medal of Merit Award from the National Society of Arts and Letters. Lincoln Kirstein died in 1996 at the age of eighty-eight.

Walker Hancock left Europe in late 1945, after establishing the Marburg Collecting Point. He returned home and built the house that he had spent so many months dreaming of while at war, and he and his new wife Saima lived and worked in Gloucester, Massachusetts, for the rest of their lives. He resumed teaching at the Pennsylvania Academy of Fine Arts, remaining there until 1967. He also continued to be a sought-after sculptor, and his works include such monumental pieces as the famous carving of Confederate generals on the side of Stone Mountain outside Atlanta, Georgia. His most enduring work may be the Pennsylvania

War Memorial, located in the 30th Street train station in Philadelphia. Completed in 1952, the piece is a tribute to the thirteen hundred railroad employees who died in World War II, and depicts a soldier lifted up by Michael, the archangel of resurrection. One of his last pieces was the official bust of President George H. W. Bush.

Hancock received the National Medal of Arts (bestowed by the first President Bush) in 1989, and the Presidential Medal of Freedom in 1990. His precious Saima died in 1984; Walker Hancock outlived her by fourteen years, dying in 1998 at the age of ninety-seven, beloved to his last day by all who knew him. He maintained his positive attitude until the end, writing in 1997 at the age of ninety-six, "Although I have lived an exceptionally happy life, continually accompanied by good fortune, I possess, of course, my share of painful memories—some of these tragic ones, indeed. However I have clung to the prerogative—perhaps, in old age, the necessity—of dwelling as little as possible on such subjects."[29]

James Rorimer stayed in Europe until early 1946 as the chief of U.S. Seventh Army/Western Military District MFAA. He then returned to the Metropolitan Museum in New York City, becoming director of the Cloisters, home of the Met's medieval art collection which as a young curator he had helped establish and build, in 1949. His letters home during the war indicated he was interested in writing a book; after many false starts, *Survival*, a memoir of his MFAA experiences, was published in 1950. By then the country had been flooded with war memoirs, and the book did not prove popular with the public. It was one of the few disappointments in a life of almost constant achievement. In 1955, James Rorimer, tenacious and hardworking as ever, succeeded Roberts Commission member Francis Henry Taylor to one of the highest positions in the American museum world: director of the Metropolitan Museum of Art.

In many ways James Rorimer was the right man at the right time—although this was hardly an accident, as men with the energy, ambition, and intelligence of James Rorimer usually find their place in the world. In the late 1940s and early 1950s, the United States was transformed from a cultural backwater to the center stage of world culture and the arts. World War II had exposed millions of young American men and women to the art and architecture of Europe and Asia and almost overnight created an interest in and appreciation for the arts that would normally require generations to nurture. The "new" nation of America for the first time—and suddenly—had a broad audience that wanted to learn, to be exposed and thrilled, and to simply enjoy painting, music, and sculpture. The Monuments Men, themselves enlightened by their experiences overseas, were at the forefront of providing their fellow citizens that opportunity. Using the same farsighted vision and diplomatic skills he had showcased during the war, James Rorimer harnessed the nation's enthusiasm to build on the Met's world-class reputation, developing its Watson Library into one of the largest art libraries in the country and acquiring some of the most famous pieces in the museum's collection, such as *Aristotle Contemplating the Bust of Homer* by

Rembrandt and the *Annunciation* (also known as the Mérode Altarpiece) by the early Netherlandish master Robert Campin. During his tenure, the Met saw an extraordinary surge in attendance from two million to six million annual visitors.

Extremely proud of his service in the MFAA, Rorimer wore his army combat boots almost every day, even to work, and even with tuxedos and suits. It was a terrible loss both to the memory of the Monuments Men and to the art world when he died unexpectedly of a heart attack in his sleep in 1966. He was only sixty years old.

Appropriately, his memorial service was held at his beloved Cloisters, the first such service ever held there. It was attended by more than a thousand of his many friends and admirers, for James Rorimer was renowned around the world. "Steeped in history," eulogized his friend and fellow Monuments Man Sherman Lee, "he cultivated the virtues of patience and direction. Possessed by the grasp of quality and connoisseurship, he knew and measured the worth of man's visible heritage and determined, in the midst of constant change, to preserve and enhance that heritage so that it might be visible to anyone with eyes to see."[30]

Rorimer's own words, however, may summarize his life best. When asked his formula for success, he replied, "A good start, a willingness—even eagerness—to work beyond the call of duty, a sense of fair play, and a recognition of opportunities before and when they arrive. In other words, it is important to find a course and steer it."[31] He might as well have been describing the MFAA and his role within it.

By the summer of 1946, only two of the original group of Monuments Men remained on the continent: the two who had died there.

Walter "Hutch" Huchthausen, killed in western Germany, was buried in the U.S. military cemetery at Margraten, Holland. In October of 1945, his alma mater of Harvard received a letter from Frieda van Schaïk, who had befriended Hutch while he was stationed with U.S. Ninth Army in Maastricht and was tending to his grave. "After we first met him, several times he visited our home and so he became a very good friend of ours...we have been deeply saddened by the message of his sudden death....I'd be very pleased if I could come in touch with his family. He is buried at the large U.S. military cemetery at Margraten, Holland (a place 6 miles from where I live) and I have been taking care for his grave....If you know the address of Walter Huchthausen's mother, I'll be much obliged to you if you'd let me know."[32] One of his bosses at SHAEF wrote his mother saying, "He was so happy in his work when I visited him at Maastricht last February and so proud of what he was able to do. You—as well as the rest of us—can be proud of him. He is a great loss."[33] Walker Hancock's observation that "the few people who saw him at his job—friend and enemy— must think more of the human race because of him" had proved true.[34]

Ronald Balfour was buried in the British cemetery outside Cleves, Germany. In 1954, his photograph was placed in the city's restored archives building beside a plaque reading, "Major Ronald E. Balfour, Lector in King's College of the University of Cambridge, died

in action March 1945 near Kloster Spyck. This gentleman saved as British Monument Officer precious medieval archives and items of lower Rhine towns. Honor to
his memory."[35] When Balfour's mother visited Cleves
a year later on the tenth anniversary of his death, the
town leaders assured her they kept "the memory of
such a man in high esteem"[36] and promised to "do our
utmost to take permanent special care of his grave."[37]
It was, no doubt, small comfort for the loss of her son.

The last of the original Monuments Men on active
duty in a combat theater was, of course, George Stout.
He left Europe for the United States in late July 1945,
but only for a two-month leave. He had requested and
received a transfer to the Pacific theater. He arrived in
Japan in October 1945, where he served as chief of the
Arts and Monuments Division at Headquarters of the
Supreme Command for the Allied Powers, Tokyo. He
left Japan in mid-1946. For his years of service, Stout
received the Bronze Star and Army Commendation
Medal.

After his tour in Japan, Stout returned briefly to
Harvard's Fogg Museum. In 1947, he became director of the Worcester Art Museum in Massachusetts,
where he served until becoming director of the Isabella
Stewart Gardner Museum in Boston. The Gardner
Museum, which had a static collection, was the ideal
job for George Stout.

By the time Stout retired in 1970, he was considered
one of the giants in the field of art conservation. He
published an article on his early years at the Fogg—
heralded by then as "America's first department of art
conservation"—in 1977. In 1978, he was hailed in the

trade journals, along with his friend the chemist John Gettens, as one of the "two significant Fogg Founding Fathers" who had ushered in the modern era of conservation.[38] His legacy, another journal proclaimed, was his reconciliation of new technologies with "the aesthetic sensibilities of traditional art restoration and historical scholarship."[39] He was a modernizer, in other words, who never forgot the importance of the individual people behind the machines.

His service in World War II, meanwhile, remained almost completely unknown. One major reason was that Stout rarely discussed it. When the Smithsonian came to interview him in early 1978 for its Archives of American Art interview collection, Stout simply told the interviewer, in typical understated fashion, that he was drafted for Monuments work and fulfilled his duty like any soldier. He made no mention of the fact that he had, more than any other person, created and shaped the Monuments mission. When George Stout died in Menlo Park, California, in July 1978, his obituary mentioned only that he was "known internationally as an expert and author on art restoration" and that, during World War II, he had helped develop camouflage techniques and "later was assigned to Gen. Dwight D. Eisenhower's command as a member of the General's staff on monuments, fine arts and archives."[40]

Those who knew him, though, were unequivocal about the significance of his contribution to the MFAA and the preservation of European culture. The military, in its official report, noted that "motivated by the urgency of his task, he spent almost all of his time alone in the field, disregarding comfort and personal convenience...

his relationship with the many tactical units with whom he worked were managed with unfailing tact and skillful staff work."[41] It's also worth repeating the assessment of Monuments Man Craig Hugh Smyth, who worked with Stout near the end of his tour of duty in Europe: "Stout was a leader—quiet, unselfish, modest, yet very strong, very thoughtful and remarkably innovative. Whether speaking or writing, he was economical with words, precise, vivid. One believed what he said; one wanted to do what he proposed."

Neither really gets to the truth of Stout's contributions, or to the esteem and love his fellow Monuments Men felt for him. Their letters and memoirs were full of praise for this tireless, efficient, and likable officer, but Lincoln Kirstein put it best because he put it most bluntly. "[George Stout] was the greatest war hero of all time—he actually saved all the art that everybody else talked about."[42]

Nonetheless, it is not surprising that George Stout's contribution to the MFAA was never truly appreciated because, in the decades following the war, the MFAA section and its work was itself lost in the fog of history. Part of this was circumstance. The Monuments Men were typical of "the Greatest Generation" and tended to downplay their roles in the war. Since they did not serve as a unit, there was no official history. A few of the men developed and maintained strong ties, but most didn't know each other well or at all. There turned out to be no single leader who would become emblematic of these self-effacing cultural experts, much less speak of their accomplishments.

Perhaps because of this, the army essentially forgot

about the monuments conservation effort. In 1957, Robert Posey volunteered to reenter the army so that he could serve as a Monuments Man in the Korean War. It's not surprising the army turned him down since he was fifty-three years old and retired from the reserves. But the fact remained that, even if he had been accepted, there was no place for him. There was no dedicated unit equivalent to the Monuments, Fine Arts, and Archives section in the Korean War, and there hasn't been one in any war since.

The Monuments, Fine Arts, and Archives legacy was immortalized by the words of Monuments officer Edith Standen, who stated that "it is not enough to be virtuous, we must also appear to be so."[43] Standen understood, just as President Roosevelt and General Eisenhower before her, that first impressions carry lasting significance. All countries ignore the Monuments Men's legacy at their own peril. For example, several years ago I spoke with one of the key officers in charge of tracking down some of the 15,000 works of art looted from the National Museum of Iraq in Baghdad during and following the U.S.-led invasion in 2003. He acknowledged that he had never heard of the Monuments Men.

Today, dedicated Civil Affairs officers and soldiers along with civilian experts, including Colonel Matthew Bogdanos (ret.), Major Corine Wegener (ret.), and Professor John Russell, have gallantly and tirelessly attempted to repair the damage to this great museum, including finding and returning about half of the missing items to date. They also conduct training seminars for troops serving in the Civil Affairs section. But despite their efforts the first impressions of the United States' experience with handling the aftermath of the looting of the National Museum of Iraq remain indelibly etched in the minds of the public worldwide.

More remarkable, perhaps, even the art community has for decades overlooked the achievements of these extraordinary men and women. After the war, the Monuments Men returned to their home countries and assumed leading roles in major cultural institutions. In the United States, these included the Metropolitan Museum of Art, MoMA, National Gallery of Art, Toledo Museum of Art, Cleveland Museum of Art, Frick Collection, Fogg Art Museum, Brooklyn Museum, Nelson-Atkins Museum of Art, Isabella Stewart Gardner Museum, Legion of Honor Museum in San Francisco, Yale University Art Gallery, Worcester Art Museum, Baltimore Museum of Art, Philadelphia Museum of Art, Dallas Museum of Art, Amon Carter Museum, and Library of Congress, among others. Monuments Men and their wartime advisors were integral to the creation of two of the most powerful cultural organizations in the nation: the National Endowment for the Humanities and the National Endowment for the Arts. In fact, search the leadership rolls of any major U.S. cultural institution during the 1950s and 1960s and you are almost sure to find a former member of the Monuments, Fine Arts, and Archives section of the U.S. Army. And yet when I speak to these organizations, few of them are aware that one of their former directors or curators helped to preserve the world's cultural heritage during and after the Second World War.

Even when the quest to discover and repatriate Nazi-stolen works of art began anew in the 1990s, the Monuments Men and their incredible achievements were mostly overlooked. Occasionally, one was asked to attend a conference, but only if their specific experience was sought. To paraphrase a major player in the restitution movement who attended these conferences, even his dedicated and knowledgeable colleagues failed to notice the treasures standing before them: not the billions of dollars of unrecovered works of art, not the hundreds of thousands of still missing items, but the 350 or so stoop-shouldered veterans of the MFAA section. Even today, news accounts about the recovery or restitution of major works of art almost without exception focus on the dollar value and include the token line "returned after the war by Allied Forces." In fact, it was the work of the Monuments Men that, time and time again, enabled these restitutions to occur.

In 2007, the Monuments Men finally began to receive a small portion of the recognition they deserve. On June 6, 2007, the sixty-third anniversary of the D-Day landings in Normandy, resolutions in both houses of the United States Congress officially acknowledged for the first time the contributions of the Monuments Men and women of thirteen nations. The resolutions, sponsored by both conservative and liberal members of the House and Senate, passed unanimously.

Soon after, the Monuments Men and their primary advocacy group, the Monuments Men Foundation for the Preservation of Art, were awarded the 2007 National Humanities Medal, which some say is the

United States' equivalent of "knighthood." Four of the twelve living Monuments Men were able to travel to Washington, D.C., to attend the ceremony, including a spry, eighty-one-year-old Harry Ettlinger. As an enlisted private just out of high school, Harry was twenty years younger than most of the other Monuments Men who served in the war zone.

Unlike almost all the other Monuments Men, Harry Ettlinger did not pursue a career in the arts after the war. He was discharged in August 1946, and upon returning to New Jersey attended college on the GI Bill. He received a bachelor's degree in mechanical engineering and took a job overseeing the manufacture of Singer sewing machine motors. In the mid-1950s, he switched to the defense industry, eventually working on flight indicators, portable radar systems, sonars, and finally as a deputy program director in the development and production of the guidance system for the submarine-launched Trident missile.

He was also active in veterans groups and Jewish causes. It was from fellow members of the Jewish War Veterans of the USA, in fact, that Harry learned about the work of Raoul Wallenberg, the wealthy Swedish diplomat of Lutheran faith. In 1944, Wallenberg inspired others to help him save the lives of 100,000 Hungarian Jews. In January 1945, he and his chauffeur were taken by the Soviets and were never seen again. After retiring in 1992, Harry co-led a committee raising funds for a sculpture honoring Wallenberg and then cofounded the Wallenberg Foundation of New Jersey to recognize students who emulate his character, thus leading to a better, more compassionate world. It was in this capacity that Harry learned another story about the mines in Heilbronn and Kochendorf.

The lower levels of the mine, Harry knew, had been used as factories. The sixty-foot-wide by forty-foot-high chambers had been lined with concrete floors and electric lines to power the machinery. In the Kochendorf mine, one or more chambers had been designed as secret manufacturing centers for the mass production of a crucial Nazi invention: the jet engine. If the Nazis could have gotten the factory at Heilbronn running—they were supposedly just weeks away when the Americans arrived—it might have radically changed the war. This may have been the reason for the defiant stand of the Wehrmacht in the hills above Heilbronn.

In 2001, Harry learned what took place in that Kochendorf mine from two of the few survivors of those terrible days. The physical work at the mine, such as the expansion of the underground chambers, had been performed by fifteen hundred Hungarian Jewish slave laborers sent from Auschwitz to Germany. In September 1944, the British bombed Heilbronn to smithereens, knocking out the power plant and plunging the region into silence and darkness. As the roar of the planes retreated, a chant rose mysteriously from the black belly of the mine. First, it was barely audible. Then it was repeated louder, then a third time louder still, clearly audible this time in the surface world beyond the mine. It was Yom Kippur, the Day of Atonement, and the Hungarian Jews were chanting the prayer of Kol Nidre. For almost all of them, it was the last time. In March 1945, less than a month before the arrival of the Americans, the slave laborers were shipped to Dachau. Most froze to death during the five-day journey. The others were sent directly to the gas chamber.

Today, Monuments Man Harry Ettlinger lives in a condominium in northwest New Jersey. He remains active in Wallenberg Foundation activities; veterans' organizations on local, state, and national levels; and Holocaust and other Jewish-related affairs. His grandfather's beloved art collection has been scattered among his descendants, but Harry still owns the largest share. He admits most of it is in his closet. Even the print of the Rembrandt is hung inconspicuously, although he'll move it to the place of honor above the sofa if requested.

The only visible memento of Harry's war years is a small photograph on a nearby end table. Taken in the Heilbronn mine in early 1946, it shows Monuments officer Lieutenant Dale Ford and (recently promoted) Sergeant Harry Ettlinger staring down at a self-portrait by Rembrandt. The painting is perched on a mine cart, with the rock walls and steel rails of the mine clearly visible. In 1946, the photograph was used by the army for promotional purposes and reprinted around the world. The caption simply said, "American soldiers with a Rembrandt." No one seemed interested in the fact that the painting was the Rembrandt from the museum in Karlsruhe, and that the nineteen-year-old soldier standing next to it was a German Jew who had grown up three blocks from that museum, and by chance had descended seven hundred feet into a mine to behold, for the first time, a painting he had always heard about, but never had the right to see.

CAST OF CHARACTERS

Secondary Figures

John Edward Dixon-Spain: World War I Veteran; British Monuments Man assigned to U.S. First Army with George Stout

S. Lane Faison Jr.: Served in the OSS, precursor to the CIA; interrogated many Nazis involved in artistic and cultural looting

Dale V. Ford: Interior designer; Monuments Man assigned to U.S. Seventh Army after the end of active hostilities; worked with Harry Ettlinger at the Heilbronn mine

Ralph Hammett: Architect; Monuments Man assigned to Communications Zone

Mason Hammond: Classics scholar; advisor on fine arts and monuments, Sicily, and the unofficial first Monuments Man

Albert Henraux: President of the French Commission de Récupération Artistique

Thomas Carr Howe Jr.: Director of the California Palace of the Legion of Honor in San Francisco; Monuments officer assigned to Altaussee

Sheldon Keck: Conservator; assistant Monuments officer assigned to Walter "Hutch" Huchthausen in U.S. Ninth Army

Stephen Kovalyak: Athletic coach; Monuments officer assigned to various repository evacuations

Bancel LaFarge: Architect; first Monuments Man ashore in Normandy, when attached to British Second Army; promoted to SHAEF headquarters in France in early 1945

Everett "Bill" Lesley: Professor; Monuments Man for U.S. First Army with Walker Hancock and later U.S. Fifteenth Army

Lord Methuen: British Monuments Man assigned to Comm Zone

Lamont Moore: Curator of Education at the National Gallery of Art, Washington, D.C.; assistant Monuments officer for U.S. Twelfth Army Group, U.S. First Army, and U.S. Ninth Army

Paul Sachs: Founder of Harvard's "Museum Course" and George Stout's boss at the Fogg Museum; head of the Harvard Group that created monuments maps and guidebooks for use in the field; instrumental, as a member of the Roberts Commission, in recruiting the core of the Monuments officers in northern Europe

Francis Henry Taylor: Director of the Metropolitan Museum of Art; president of the American Association of Museum Directors; prominent member of the Roberts Commission

John Bryan Ward-Perkins: Archaeology scholar; British artillery officer in North Africa who assisted with conservation efforts; later deputy director of MFAA in Italy

Geoffrey Webb: Architectural historian; British MFAA advisor at SHAEF (Supreme Headquarters Allied Expeditionary Force) and the lead MFAA officer in northern Europe

Sir Eric Mortimer Wheeler: British artillery officer and archeologist for the London Museum; his conservation of Roman and Greek ruins in North Africa in 1942 were the first such Allied efforts

Sir Charles Leonard Woolley: British archeological advisor to the War Office and civilian leader of the MFAA; ran the MFAA under the motto "We protect the arts at the lowest possible cost," often to its detriment

Germans and Nazis

Colonel Baron Kurt von Behr: Head of the Dienststelle Westen in the Einsatzstab Reichsleiter Rosenberg (ERR); overseer of the Nazi looting operation in France headquarters at the Jeu de Paume museum

Martin Bormann: Reichsminister; private secretary to Hitler

Dr. Hermann Bunjes: Former employee of the Kunstschutz in France who became a key participant in the ERR in Paris; loyal to Von Behr and Reichsmarschall Göring

August Eigruber: Fanatical Nazi and gauleiter (district leader) of Oberdonau, which included Hitler's boyhood hometown of Linz, Austria, and the salt mine at Altaussee

Dr. Hans Frank: Reichsleiter; governor-general of Poland

Hermann Giesler: Architect for Linz

Hermann Göring: Reichsmarschall of Nazi Germany; head of the Luftwaffe; the Nazis' second in command and Hitler's chief rival in the looting of Europe

Heinrich Himmler: Reichsführer SS; head of Waffen-SS and Gestapo

Adolf Hitler: Führer of the Reich; "purifier" of Germany who destroyed modern art; "glorifier" of Germany who thought the Reich should own Europe's cultural treasures, many to be displayed at his Führermuseum at Linz

Walter Andreas Hofer: Art dealer; director of Göring's art collection and central figure in the looting operation at the Jeu de Paume in Paris

Dr. Helmut von Hummel: Personal assistant of Martin Bormann, Hitler's private secretary, and primary conduit for information to and from Berlin in the last days of the Reich

Ernst Kaltenbrunner: High-ranking Nazi from Austria; chief of the Reich Security Main Office (RSHA, or Reichssicherheitshauptamt); SS *Obergruppenführer* (senior group leader); chief of the Security Police (Gestapo) and the SD

Prof. Dr. Otto Kümmel: Director of Berlin State Museums who compiled a list of all "Germanic" art in Europe and the justification for repatriating it to the Fatherland

Dr. Bruno Lohse: Hermann Göring's representative to the ERR looting operation at Jeu de Paume museum

Dr. Hans Posse: original director of the Führermuseum in Linz; died of cancer in 1943

Alfred Rosenberg: Head of the Einsatzstab Reichsleiter Rosenberg (ERR), a racist organization that became the primary "legal" avenue for Nazi looting in Western Europe

Prof. Dr. Albert Speer: Hitler's personal architect and close confidant; Reichsminister for Armaments and War Production

Prof. Dr. Count Franz von Wolff-Metternich: Head of Kunstschutz in Paris, the German arts and monuments protection program

Key Figures at Altaussee

Max Eder: Engineer

Glinz: *Gauinspektor* (district inspector) working for Eigruber

Otto Högler: Engineer and mining counselor (*Oberbergrat*)

Eberhard Mayerhoffer: Engineer; technical director of the salt mines (*Oberbergrat DI*)

Prof. Dr. Hermann Michel: Ex-director of the Natural History Museum Vienna and head of the Mineralogical Department of the museum

Ralph E. Pearson: U.S. Army colonel with the 318th Infantry; led "Task Force Pearson" to the salt mine at Altaussee

Dr. Emmerich Pöchmüller: General director of the salt mines at Altaussee

Alois Raudaschl: Miner and Nazi Party member

Dr. Herbert Seiberl: Austrian official; Institute of Monuments Preservation, Vienna

Karl Sieber: Restorer from Berlin who worked inside the salt mine

Abbreviations

Ad Sec—Advance Section

CAO—Civil Affairs officer

Comm Zone—Communications Zone

CO—Commanding officer

ERR—Einsatzstab Reichsleiter Rosenberg

HQ—Headquarters

MFAA—Monuments, Fine Arts, and Archives

MP—Military Police

ROTC—Reserve Officers' Training Corps

SHAEF—Supreme Headquarters Allied Expeditionary Force

NOTES

Abbreviations

AAA   Smithsonian Archives of American Art, Washington, DC

DÖW   Dokumentationsarchiv des Österreichischen Widerstandes, Wien, Austria

NHM   Naturhistorisches Museum, Wien

NARA   National Archives and Records Administration, College Park, MD

NGA   National Gallery of Art, Washington, DC

RG   Record Group

The book's epigraphs are drawn from: President Franklin D. Roosevelt, "Remarks made at the dedication ceremony of the National Gallery of Art, March 17, 1941," Gallery Archives, NGA; and Robert Edwin Herzstein, *World War II: The Nazis* (Alexandria, VA: Time-Life Books, 1980), 107.

Section 1

The epigraphs to this section are drawn from Eisenhower, *At Ease*, 254; and Stout, "Our Early Years at the Fogg," 13.

  1. Stout to Margie, June 16, 1994, roll 1421, Stout Papers.

Chapter 1: Out of Germany

1. Ettlinger, "Ein Amerikaner," 18.
2. Ibid., 19.

Chapter 2: Hitler's Dream

1. Spotts, *Hitler and the Power of Aesthetics*, 323.
2. Tutaev, *The Consul of Florence*, 11.

The document on p. 20 is reproduced from Aksenov, *Favorite Museum of the Führer*, photo pg. 3; the caption is drawn from Art Looting Investigation Unit, "Consolidated Interrogation Report #4: Linz," attachment 1, NARA.

Chapter 3: The Call to Arms

1. Godwin letter to Finley, December 5, 1940, RG 7, Box 77, Museum Correspondence, Conservation of Cultural Resources, Defense, Gallery Archives, NGA.
2. "Minutes of a Special Meeting of the Association of Museum Directors on the Problems of Protection and Defense held at the Metropolitan Museum of Art," pp. 134–135, RG 7, Box 77, Publications, Metropolitan Museum, Conservation of Cultural Resources, Defense, Gallery Archives, NGA.
3. Stout to Taylor and Constable, "General Museum Conservation," December 31, 1942, Section 6a, W. G. Constable Papers, Smithsonian AAA.
4. Stout, *Protection of Monuments: A Proposal for Consideration During War and Rehabilitation*, 6a, Constable Papers.

The document on pp. 31–32 is drawn from *Nazi Conspiracy and Aggression*, Vol. III, 186.

Chapter 4: A Dull and Empty World

1. Stout, "Our Early Years at the Fogg," 11.
2. Ibid., 13.

3. Hancock, "Experiences of a Monuments Officer in Germany," 279.
4. Stout to Warner, October 4, 1944, roll 1421, Stout Papers.
5. Nicholas, *The Rape of Europa*, 214.
6. Stout to Margie, March 20, 1943, roll 1420, Stout Papers.
7. Stout to Margie, March 16, 1943, roll 1420, Stout Papers.
8. Constable to Stout, June 1, 1943, 6a, Constable Papers.
9. Stout to Constable, April 3, 1943, 6a, Constable Papers.
10. Stout to Constable, March 28, 1943, 6a, Constable Papers.
11. Stout to Margie, July 12, 1943, roll 1420, Stout Papers.

The document on pp. 40–41 is drawn from *Nazi Conspiracy and Aggression*, Vol. III, 188–189.

Chapter 5: Leptis Magna

1. The collection of the former London Museum is today part of the Museum of London.
2. Woolley, *The Protection of the Treasures of Art and History in War Areas*, 14.

Chapter 6: The First Campaign

1. Woolley, *The Protection of Treasures*, 18.
2. Hammond letter to Reber, July 24, 1943, RG 165, NM-84, Entry 463, NARA.
3. Smyth, *Repatriation of Art from the Collecting Point in Munich after World War II*, 77.
4. Stout letter to Sachs, Sept 13, 1943, RG 239, M1944, roll 57, Frame 180, NARA.

The document on pp. 55–56 is drawn from *Nazi Conspiracy and Aggression*, Vol. III, 40–41.

Chapter 7: Monte Cassino

1. *Report of the American Commission for the Protection and Salvage of Artistic and Historic Monuments in War Areas*, 68.

2. Ibid., 48.
3. Majdalany, *Cassino*, 122.
4. Ibid., 121–122.
5. Hapgood and Richardson, *Monte Cassino*, 227.

The document on pp. 63–64 is drawn from *Nazi Conspiracy and Aggression*, Vol. III, 1.

Chapter 8: Monuments, Fine Arts, and Archives

1. Ambrose, *Eisenhower*, 177.
2. Stout to Margie, October 31, 1943, roll 1420, Stout Papers.
3. Stout to Margie, January 17, 1944, roll 1421, Stout Papers.
4. Piña, *Louis Rorimer*, 123.
5. Woolley, *The Protection of Treasures*, 6.

Chapter 9: The Task

1. *Report of the American Commission*, 102.
2. Ambrose, *Eisenhower*, 301.

Section II

The letter on p. 87 is from the James J. Rorimer Papers, New York, NY.

Chapter 10: Winning Respect

1. D'Este, *Eisenhower*, 534.
2. Ambrose, *Citizen Soldiers*, 43.
3. Rorimer, *Survival*, 3–4.
4. Skilton, *Defense de l'art Européen*, 19.
5. Rorimer, *Survival*, 2.
6. Rorimer letter, February 4, 1944, Rorimer Papers.
7. Rorimer letter, March 10, 1944, Rorimer Papers.
8. Rorimer letter, June 6, 1944, Rorimer Papers.
9. Rorimer letter, April 30, 1944, Rorimer Papers.
10. Ibid.

11. Ibid.
12. Rorimer letter, May 7, 1944, Rorimer Papers.
13. Rorimer letter, April 6, 1944, Rorimer Papers.
14. Rorimer, *Survival*, 4.
15. Ibid., 8.
16. Ibid., 14.

The letter on pp. 105–106 is from roll 1421, Stout Papers.

Chapter 11: A Meeting in the Field

1. Ambrose, *Citizen Soldiers*, 75.
2. Rorimer, *Survival*, 15.
3. "The Capital of the Ruins" was the title of a short report by Samuel Beckett, 1946.
4. Rorimer letter, undated, Rorimer Papers.
5. Ibid.
6. Smyth, *Repatriation of Art*, 16.
7. Rorimer, *Survival*, 19.
8. Ibid., 37.
9. Ibid.
10. Ibid., 39.

The letter on pp. 122–123 is from roll 1421, Stout Papers.

Chapter 12: Michelangelo's Madonna

Details of this chapter are drawn from "Removal of Works of Art from the Church of Notre-Dame at Bruges," Sept. 24, 1944. King's College Archive Centre, Cambridge, The Papers of Ronald Edmond Balfour, Misc. 5.

Chapter 13: The Cathedral and the Masterpiece

1. Hancock to Saima, September 20, 1944, Walker Hancock Papers, Gloucester, MA.
2. Rorimer, *Survival*, 47.
3. Hancock to Saima, October 30, 1943.
4. Hancock, *A Sculptor's Fortunes*, 129.
5. Hancock to Saima, October 31, 1943, Hancock Papers.

6. Hancock to Saima, October 30, 1943, Hancock Papers.
7. Hancock to Saima, January 28, 1944, Hancock Papers.
8. Hancock to Saima, April 11, 1944, Hancock Papers.
9. Ambrose, *Citizen Soldiers*, 110.
10. Hancock to Saima, October 6, 1944, Hancock Papers.
11. Interview with Bernard Taper.
12. Hancock, *A Sculptor's Fortunes*, 136.
13. Hancock to Saima, October 6, 1944, Hancock Papers.
14. Hancock to Saima, October 10, 1944, Hancock Papers.

Chapter 14: Van Eyck's Mystic Lamb

1. Interview with Robert Posey.
2. Posey to Alice, September 23, 1944, Robert Posey Papers, Scarsdale, NY.

Chapter 15: James Rorimer Visits the Louvre

1. Rorimer letter, September 8, 1944, Rorimer Papers.
2. Ibid.
3. Taylor, "The Rape of Europa," 52.
4. Rorimer journal, September 27, 1944 entry, 28MFAA-J:1-1, James J. Rorimer Papers, Gallery Archives, National Gallery of Art, Washington, DC.
5. Simon, *The Battle of the Louvre*, 26.
6. Chamson, "In Memoriam, Jacques Jaujard," 151.
7. Franz Graf Wolff-Metternich, "Concerning My Activities as Adviser on the Protection of Works of Art to O.K.H. from 1940–1942 (Kunstschutz)," p. 3, RG 239, M1944, Roll 89, frames 352–372, NARA.
8. Ibid.
9. Ibid., p. 12.
10. Ibid., attachment "Re: Professor Dr. Graf Franz Wolff-Metternich, born 31.12.99 in Felkingen, Catholic, married, Provinzialkonservator for the Rhine, living in Bonn, Blücherstrasse 2."
11. Rayssac, *L'Exode des Musées*, 853.
12. Ibid., 706.

13. Von Choltitz, "Pourquoi en 1944 je n'ai pas détruit Paris."

The letter on pp. 175–177 comes from the Rorimer Papers.

Chapter 16: Entering Germany

1. Hancock to Saima, October 25, 1944, Hancock Papers.
2. Photo no. 00060179, Ullstein Bild.
3. Hancock to Saima, October 25, 1944, Hancock Papers.
4. Hancock, "Experiences of a Monuments Officer in Germany," 273.
5. Hancock, *A Sculptor's Fortunes*, 139.
6. Ibid., 140.
7. Ibid.
8. Hancock journal, Hancock Papers.

Chapter 17: A Field Trip

1. Hancock, "Experiences of a Monuments Officer in Germany," 277.
2. Ibid.
3. Ibid., 279.
4. Ibid.
5. The analysis notes are drawn from Hancock journal, November 18, 1944, Hancock Papers.

The letter on pp. 196–198 is from roll 1421, Stout Papers.

Chapter 18: Tapestry

1. Canady, "James Rorimer Left Cloisters to Excel in a Bigger Job."
2. Rayssac, *L'Exode des Musées*, 695.
3. Rorimer, *Survival*, 93.
4. Ibid.
5. Rorimer notes on Valland, 28MFAA-J:2-11, Rorimer Papers, NGA.
6. Ibid.

Chapter 19: Christmas Wishes

1. Sasser, *Patton's Panthers*, 127.
2. D'Este, *Patton*, 685.
3. Posey to Alice, July 9, 1944, Posey Papers.
4. Posey to Dennis, March 1, 1945, Posey Papers.
5. Nicholas, *The Rape of Europa*, 224.

The letter on pp. 220–221 is from the Posey Papers.

Chapter 20: The Madonna of La Gleize

The letter on pp. 225–226 is from the Hancock Papers.

Chapter 21: The Train

1. *Nazi Conspiracy and Aggression*, Vol. III, 186.
2. Rose Valland note, July 28, 1944, R32-1, Archives des Musées Nationaux.
3. Rose Valland note, August 16, 1944, R32-1, Archives des Musées Nationaux.
4. Rose Valland note, February 1944, R32-1, Archives des Musées Nationaux.
5. Rose Valland note, August 20, 1944, R32-1, Archives des Musées Nationaux.
6. Michel Rayssac, *Historail*, January 2008.
7. Rorimer, *Survival*, 112.
8. Valland, *Le Front de L'Art*, 218.
9. Rorimer letter, April 23, 1944, Rorimer Papers.
10. Rorimer letter, October 22, 1944, Rorimer Papers.
11. Rorimer letter, June 6, 1944, Rorimer Papers.
12. Rose Valland letter, October 21, 1944, Archives des Musées Nationaux.
13. Rorimer Manuscript, 28MFAA-J:3-14, Rorimer Papers, NGA.

Chapter 22: The Bulge

1. Posey to Alice, December 16, 1944, Posey Papers.
2. Ibid.

3. Stout to Margie, January 10, 1945, roll 1421, Stout Papers.
4. Author's interview with Robert Posey.

Chapter 23: Champagne

1. The details on the arrival of the Germans at the Jeu de Paume are drawn from Valland, *Le Front de l'Art*, chapter 7.
2. Ibid., 67.
3. Ibid., 68.
4. Ibid., 59.
5. The details on the liberation of Paris are drawn from Valland, *Le Front de l'Art*, chapter 23.
6. Valland letter, October 27, 1944, Archives des Musées Nationaux.

Chapter 24: A German Jew in the U.S. Army

The material in this chapter is drawn from the author's interview with Harry Ettlinger, 2008; and Ettlinger, "Ein Amerikaner."

Chapter 25: Coming Through the Battle

1. Hancock, "Experiences of a Monuments Officer in Germany," 285.
2. Ibid.
3. Ibid.
4. Ibid.

Chapter 26: The New Monuments Man

1. Duberman, *The Worlds of Lincoln Kirstein*, 373.
2. Ibid., 387.
3. Ibid.
4. Rorimer letter, June 27, 1944, Rorimer Papers.
5. Kirstein letter to Cairns, October 13, 1944, box 13-202, MGZMD, 97, Lincoln Kirstein Papers, ca. 1914–1991,

New York Public Library for the Performing Arts, Jerome Robbins Dance Division, Archives.
6. Adolf Hitler, *Mein Kampf,* as cited in Martin Gray and A. Norman Jeffares, eds., *A Dictionary of Quotations* (New York: Barnes and Noble Books, 1995), 323.

Chapter 27: George Stout with His Maps

1. Stout to Margie, undated letter, January 30–February 8, 1945, roll 1421, Stout Papers.
2. Journal entry, January 29, 1945, roll 1378, Stout Papers.
3. Stout to Margie, March 6, 1945, roll 1421, Stout Papers.
4. Stout to Margie, April 6, 1945, roll 1421, Stout Papers.
5. Stout to Margie, March 6, 1945, roll 1421, Stout Papers.

Chapter 28: Art on the Move

1. Yeide, *Beyond the Dreams of Avarice,* 17.
2. Sigmund, *Die Frauen der Nazis,* 65.

Chapter 29: Two Turning Points

The details of Ronald Balfour's death are drawn from "Translation of Article in Rheinpost 12th September 1985, Hachmann, The Sexton, Eyewitness of Major Balfour's Death," King's College Archive Centre, Cambridge, The Papers of Ronald Edmond Balfour, Misc. 5.

1. Hobbs, "A Michelangelo in Belgium?"
2. Rorimer letter, February 18, 1945, Rorimer Papers.
3. From Rorimer Manuscript, ERR 20, box 3-9, Rorimer Papers.
4. The details on the Nazis' burning of art in 1943 are taken from notes made by Rose Valland and Jacqueline Bouchot-Saupique based on Valland's eyewitness account, July 20, 1943, and July 23, 1943, Archives des Musées Nationaux. This story has been challenged by some historians, including Matila Simon in *The Battle of the Louvre.*
5. Rorimer, *Survival,* 114.

Chapter 30: Hitler's Nero Decree

1. Speer, *Inside the Third Reich*, 437.
2. Ibid., 562.

Chapter 31: First Army Across the Rhine

1. Hancock to Saima, March 12, 1945, Hancock Papers.
2. Ibid.
3. Stout to Margie, March 19, 1945, roll 1421, Stout Papers.

Chapter 32: Treasure Map

1. Posey to Alice, March 18, 1945, Posey Papers.
2. Kirstein to Groozle, March 24, 1945, box 2-25, MGZMD 97, Kirstein Papers. Kirstein used a variety of nicknames for those in his inner circle, most of them a variation of "Goosie"; for this reason it is difficult to determine with certainty the recipient of a letter so addressed.
3. "St. Lô to Alt Aussee," Posey Papers.
4. Kirstein to Groozle, March 24, 1945, box 2-25, MGZMD 97, Kirstein Papers.
5. Ibid.
6. Posey to Dennis, March 23, 1945, Posey Papers.
7. Posey, "Protection of Cultural Monuments During Combat," 130.
8. Kirstein, "Arts and Monuments," *The Poems of Lincoln Kirstein*, 264.
9. Kirstein, "Quest for the Golden Lamb," 183.
10. Kirstein, "Arts and Monuments," 265.
11. Bunjes letter presented at Nuremberg trials, *Nuremberg Trials*, Volume 9, 547–549.
12. Kirstein, "Quest for the Golden Lamb," 183.

Chapter 33: Frustration

1. Rorimer letter, undated, Rorimer Papers.
2. Speer, *Inside the Third Reich*, 452–453.
3. Ibid., 453.

4. Ibid., 453–454.
5. Ibid., 455.

The letter on pp. 346–347 is from the Hancock Papers.
The letter on pp. 348–351 is from roll 1421, Stout Papers.

Chapter 34: Inside the Mountain

1. Hancock to Saima, April 4, 1945, Hancock Papers.

Chapter 35: Lost

1. Nicholas, *The Rape of Europa*, 332.
2. Hancock to Saima, November 25, 1945, Hancock Papers.

Chapter 36: A Week to Remember

1. Kirstein, "The Mine at Merkers," box 13-206, MGZMD 97, Kirstein Papers.
2. Bradsher, "Nazi Gold: The Merkers Mine Treasure," 8.
3. Posey to Alice, April 9, 1945, Posey Papers.
4. Kirstein, "The Mine at Merkers."
5. Kirstein, "Hymn," *The Poems of Lincoln Kirstein*, 274.
6. Stout journal, April 11, 1945, roll 1378, Stout Papers.
7. Bradsher, "Nazi Gold: The Merkers Mine Treasure," 8.
8. D'Este, *Eisenhower*, 686.
9. David Eisenhower, *Eisenhower at War*, 763.
10. Bradley, *A General's Life*, 428.
11. D'Este, *Eisenhower*, 720.
12. Ibid.
13. Kirstein, "The Mine at Merkers."
14. Kirstein to Ma and Goosie, April 13, 1945, box 2-24, MGZMD, Kirstein Papers.
15. Stout journal, April 13, 1945, roll 1378, Stout Papers.
16. Ibid.
17. Stout journal, April 15, 1945, roll 1378, Stout Papers.
18. Stout journal, April 16, 1945, roll 1378, Stout Papers.
19. Ibid.
20. Stout journal, April 17, 1945, roll 1378, Stout Papers.

21. Kirstein, "The Mine at Merkers."
22. Stout to Margie, April 19, 1945, roll 1421, Stout Papers.
23. Posey to Alice, April 20, 1945, Posey Papers.

Chapter 37: Salt

1. Photograph, Posey Papers. The word *stürtzen* was misspelled on the crate; *stürzen* would be the correct spelling.
2. Ambrose, *Eisenhower*, 392.
3. Ibid., 391.
4. Hobbs, *Dear General*, 223.
5. Ambrose, *Eisenhower*, 400.
6. Hirshon, *General Patton*, 628.
7. Ambrose, *Eisenhower*, 393.

Chapter 38: Horror

1. Hancock to Saima, April 9, 1945, Hancock Papers.
2. Hancock to Saima, April 12, 1945, Hancock Papers.
3. Hancock, *A Sculptor's Fortunes*, 157.
4. Ibid., 158.
5. Hancock to Saima, April 20, 1945, Hancock Papers.
6. Hancock to Saima, April 15, 1945, Hancock Papers.
7. Kirstein to Goosie, April 20, 1945, box 2-24, MGZMD 97, Kirstein Papers.
8. Ibid.
9. Kirstein to Miss Marshall, April 24, 1945, box 8-90, MGZMD 123, Kirstein Papers.

Chapter 39: The Gauleiter

1. Pöchmüller, *Welt-Kunstschätze in Gefahr*, 57.
2. Kubin, *Sonderauftrag Linz*, 100.
3. Pöchmüller, *Welt-Kunstschätze in Gefahr*, 58.

Chapter 40: The Battered Mine

The details of the scene at Heilbronn are drawn from Rorimer, *Survival*, 135–143.

1. Rorimer, *Survival*, 137.
2. Rorimer letter, April 25, 1945, Rorimer Papers.

Chapter 41: Last Birthday

1. Joachimsthaler, *The Last Days of Hitler*, 105–106.
2. Ibid., 97.
3. Wheelock, ed., *Johannes Vermeer*, 168.

Chapter 42: Plans

1. Stout journal, May 1, 1945, Stout Papers.
2. Pöchmüller, *Welt-Kunstschätze in Gefahr*, 68.
3. Rorimer, *Survival*, 160–161.

Chapter 43: The Noose

The details on Hitler's will writing, marriage, and suicide are drawn from Joachimsthaler, *The Last Days of Hitler*, 128–130.

1. Adolf Hitler, "Last Will and Testament," April 30, 1945, RG 238 Entry 1 NM—66, U.S. Counsel for the Prosecution of Axis Criminality, Box 189, F: 3569—PS, NARA.
2. Hitler dictated a "political testament" and a "private will" on April 29, 1945. The following day he committed suicide. At least three, but probably four, copies were signed and witnessed. Three copies were dispatched from the underground shelter in the Reichschancellery after Hitler's death; the top copy to Grand Admiral Dönitz (courier Zander); another (without the "private will") to Field Marshal Schörner (courier Johannmayer); and the third to the Nazi Party archives in Munich (courier Lorenz). None of the three couriers carrying these documents reached their destination, and the testaments and wills were later discovered in different hiding places. The set intended for Dönitz is now in the National Archives in College Park, Md. and the others are held

by the Imperial War Museum in London. It is possible that Bormann carried the third "private will" with him when he left the bunker on the evening of May 1, 1945. It seems that a fourth set was likely handed over to the Soviet lieutenant general Vasily Ivanovich Chuikov during German general Hans Krebs's fruitless cease-fire negotiations on May 1, 1945. It is unlikely that Hitler intended a fourth copy to be transmitted to the Russians. This was most probably a maneuver arranged by Goebbels and Bormann during the evening of April 30, 1945. Depending on whether Hitler's signature on the fourth set can be determined as fake, he would either not have known of this fourth set (all witnesses would have still been in the bunker, though, to sign themselves and Bormann or Göbbels could have arranged that Frau Junge had slipped a fourth carbon in the typewriter), or it could have been that the fourth set was intended to be for Generalfeldmarschall Kesselring, who on April 29, 1945, was still involved in an independent surrender to the Allies in Italy and yet retained Hitler's confidence. There is no evidence that at the time when Hitler was making his will he had withdrawn his confidence in Kesselring. Therefore Kesselring as a potential recipient of a fourth set of "political testament" and "private will" is not improbable.

3. Högler, *Bericht über die Verhinderung der von Gauleiter Eigruber geplanten Vernichtung der Kunstschätze im Salzbergwerk Altaussee*, 30 December 1945, Archiv Linz, Sch 0018, Högler Papers, 4.

4. Ibid.

5. Kubin, *Sonderauftrag Linz*, 115.

6. Interview with Robert Posey, 2008.

7. Posey to Alice, April 18, 1945, Posey Papers.

Chapter 44: Discoveries

1. The details on the coffins in Bernterode are drawn from Hancock, *A Sculptor's Fortunes*, 159–160.

2. Ibid., 160.
3. Rorimer, *Survival*, 181–182.

Chapter 45: The Noose Tightens

1. Davidson, *The Trial of the Germans*, 439.
2. Rayssac, *L'Exode des Musées*, 758–760, 803.

Chapter 46: The Race

The details of the capture of Berchtesgaden are drawn from McManus, "The Last Great Prize," 51–56.

1. Rorimer, *Survival*, 183.
2. Ibid., 185.

Chapter 47: Final Days

1. The details on Berlin's flaktowers are drawn from Akinsha and Kozlov, *Beautiful Loot*, 52–95.
2. Bernard Taper, "Investigating Art Looting for the MFAA," in Simpson, ed., *Spoils of War*, 137.
3. Posey to Alice, May 2, 1945, Posey Papers.
4. Kirstein, "Quest for the Golden Lamb," 183.
5. Kirstein to Grooslie, May 6, 1945, box 2-25, MGZMD 97, Kirstein Papers.
6. Ibid.

Chapter 48: The Translator

This material in this chapter draws on the author's interview with Harry Ettlinger, 2008, and Ettlinger, "Ein Amerikaner."

Chapter 49: The Sound of Music

1. Hancock, "Experiences of a Monuments Officer in Germany," 299.
2. Hancock to Saima, May 4, 1945, Hancock Papers.
3. Hancock to Saima, undated letter #151, Hancock Papers.
4. Hancock to Saima, undated letter #150, Hancock Papers.

Chapter 50: End of the Road

1. Kirstein, "Quest for the Golden Lamb," 184.

Section V

The epigraphs to this section are drawn from Balfour, "Draft Lecture," 9, Balfour Papers; and Fasola, *The Florence Galleries and the War*, 75.

Chapter 51: Understanding Altaussee

1. Interview with S. Lane Faison Jr., courtesy of Actual Films.
2. Pöchmüller, *Welt-Kunstschätze in Gefahr*, 57–59.
3. Kirstein, "Quest for the Golden Lamb," 184.
4. Ibid., 185.
5. Freiheitskämpfer von Altaussee, *Bericht über die Aktion zur Rettung und Sicherstellung der im Salzbergwerk verlagerten Wert- und Kunstgegenständen Europas in den April- und ersten Maitagen des Jahres 1945*, February 1948, Archiv Linz, Sch 0042–0046, Michel Papers.
6. Kubin, *Sonderauftrag Linz*, 231–238.
7. Plieseis, Letter to the Editor of the Magazine "Neuer Mahnruf," 27 October 1960, Kubin Estate, Linz Archive.
8. Kubin, *Sonderauftrag Linz*, 211–225.
9. Michel, *Bergungsmassnahmen und Widerstandsbewegung*, Annalen des Naturhistorischen Museums in Wien, 56. Band, 1948. AuW, NHM, 3–6.
10. Riedl-Dorn, *Das Haus der Wunder*, 220.
11. Kubin, *Sonderauftrag Linz*, 196.
12. Michel, *Bericht über die ereignisreiche und denkwürdige Bewahrung unschätzbarer Kunstwerke in den Salzberg-Anlagen in Alt Aussee vor nazistischer Zertörung durch die Eigruber-Bande*, undated report, Archiv Linz, Sch 0042–0046, Michel Papers.
13. Roll 1421, Stout Papers.
14. Kirstein to Goosie, May 13, 1945, box 13-206, MGZMD 97, Kirstein Papers.

15. Kubin, *Sonderauftrag Linz*, 99.
16. Pöchmüller, *Welt-Kunstschätze in Gefahr*, 58.
17. Ibid., 51.
18. Ibid., 68.
19. Sieber, *Bericht über die Verlagerung von Gemälden innerhalb des Salzberges*, Altaussee, 12 May 1945, DÖW 3296a/b.
20. Högler, *Bericht über die Verhinderung der von Gauleiter Eigruber geplanten Vernichtung der Kunstschätze im Salzbergwerk Altaussee*, Archiv Linz, Sch 0018, Högler Papers, 11.
21. Ibid., 12.
22. Pöchmüller, *Welt-Kunstschätze in Gefahr*, 82–83.
23. Kubin, *Sonderauftrag Linz*, 128.
24. Ibid., 85.

Chapter 52: Evacuation

1. Kirstein, "Quest for the Golden Lamb," 184.
2. Ibid., 186.
3. Howe, *Salt Mines and Castles*, 183.
4. Kirstein to Grooslie, May 22, 1945, box 13-206, MGZMD 97, Kirstein Papers.
5. Eder, *Zusammenfassung der mir bekannten Einlagerungen im Salzbergwerk Altaussee*, DÖW 10610, 4.
6. Kirstein, "Quest for the Golden Lamb," 190.
7. Stout journal, July 3, 1945, Stout Papers.
8. Howe, *Salt Mines and Castles*, 159.
9. Ibid.
10. Ibid.
11. Nicholas, *The Rape of Europa*, 373.

The letter on pp. 486–488 is from the Rorimer Papers.

Chapter 53: The Journey Home

The details on Harry Ettlinger and Heilbronn are draw from the author's interview with Harry Ettlinger, 2008, and Ettlinger, "Ein Amerikaner."

1. Interview with Harry Ettlinger, courtesy of Actual Films.

Chapter 54: Heroes of Civilization

1. Goldensohn, *Nuremberg Interviews*, 132.
2. Ibid., 129.
3. Ibid., 128.
4. Bernard Taper, "Investigating Art Looting for the MFAA," in Simpson, ed., *Spoils of War*, 138.
5. Rayssac, *L'Exode des Musées*, 955.
6. Rorimer, *Survival*, 187.
7. Valland to Rorimer, June 25, 1957, Rorimer Papers, NGA.
8. Kubin, *Sonderauftrag Linz*, 189–191.
9. Ibid., 191–192.
10. Ibid., 193–194.
11. Ibid., 172–189.
12. Michel, Letter to the Bundesministerium für Unterricht, 1947, Archiv Linz, Sch 0042–0046, Michel Papers.
13. Kubin, *Sonderauftrag Linz*, 175.
14. Ibid., 194.
15. Michel, *Bergungsmassnahmen und Widerstandsbewegung*, Annalen des Naturhistorischen Museums in Wien, 56. Band, 1948. AuW, NHM, 3–6.
16. Kubin, *Sonderauftrag Linz*, 195–204.
17. Rayssac, *L'Exode des Musées*, 847.
18. Chamson, "In Memoriam, Jacques Jaujard," 152.
19. "A l'Institut: Gaston Palewski fait l'éloge d'un grand défenseur des Beaux-Arts Jacques Jaujard," *Le Figaro*, November 21, 1968.
20. "Albert Henraux (1881–1953)," p. XXII, Archives des Musées Nationaux.
21. Valland, *Le Front de l'Art*, 221.
22. Rose Valland note, February 1944, R32-1, Archives des Musées Nationaux.
23. Jacques Jaujard, "Activités dans la Résistance de Mademoiselle Rose Valland Conservateur des Musées Nationaux," R32-1, Archives des Musées Nationaux.
24. Rayssac, *L'Exode des Musées*, 850.
25. Ibid.

26. Kirstein to Goosie, April 20, 1945, box 2-24, MGZMD 97, Kirstein Papers.

27. Kirstein letter to Stout, March 16, 1947, Stout Papers.

28. See wikipedia.org/wiki/Kirstein.

29. Hancock, *A Sculptor's Fortunes*, vii.

30. "1,000 Pay Tribute at Rorimer Rites," *New York Times*, May 17, 1966.

31. Houghton, "James J. Rorimer," 39.

32. Letter to Harvard from Frieda van Schaïk, November 1945, Huchthausen Papers, Harvard University.

33. Letter from Marvin Ross, Huchthausen Papers.

34. Hancock to Saima, November 25, 1945, Hancock Papers.

35. Letter to Mr. Kenneth Balfour, October 1, 1954, Balfour Papers.

36. Letter to Mr. and Mrs. Balfour, November 17, 1955, Balfour Papers.

37. Letter to Mr. Kenneth Balfour, October 1, 1954, Balfour Papers.

38. Stoner, "Changing Approaches in Art Conservation," 41.

39. Cohn, "George Stout's Legacy," 8.

40. "George L. Stout, at 80; Expert on Restoration of Works of Art," *New York Times*, July 3, 1978.

41. "Report on Lieutenant George L. Stout, USNR, by Damon M. Gunn," November 19, 1944, roll 1420, Stout Papers.

42. Duberman, *The Worlds of Lincoln Kirstein*, 403.

43. Standen, "Report on Germany," 213.

BIBLIOGRAPHY

Books

Akinsha, Konstantin, and Grigorii Kozlov. *Beautiful Loot: The Soviet Plunder of Europe's Art Treasures.* New York: Random House, 1995.

Aksenov, Vitali. *Favorite Museum of the Führer, Stolen Discoveries.* St. Petersburg: Publishing House Neva, 2003.

Ambrose, Stephen. *Citizen Soldiers: The U.S. Army from the Normandy Beaches to the Bulge to the Surrender of Germany, June 7, 1944, to May 7, 1945.* New York: Simon and Schuster, 1997.

———. *D-Day: June 6, 1944; The Battle for the Normandy Beaches.* London: Pocket Books, 2002.

———. *Eisenhower: Soldier, General of the Army, President-Elect 1890–1952.* Norwalk, CT: Easton Press.

Bouchoux, Corinne. *Rose Valland: La Résistance au Musée.* France: Geste Editions, 2006.

Bradley, Omar N., and Clay Blair. *A General's Life: An Autobiography by General of the Army Omar N. Bradley.* New York: Simon and Schuster, 1983.

Bull, George. *Michelangelo: A Biography.* New York: St. Martin's Press, 1995.

Busterud, John A. *Below the Salt: How the Fighting 90th Division Struck Gold and Art Treasure in a Salt Mine.* United States: Xlibris Corporation, 2001.

Butcher, Capt. Harry C. *My Three Years with Eisenhower: The Personal Diary of Captain Harry C. Butcher, USNR, Naval*

Aide to General Eisenhower, 1942–1945. New York: Simon and Schuster, 1946.

Che cosa hanno fatto gli Inglesi in Cirenaica. Rome: Ministero Della Cultura Popolare, 1941.

Davidson, Eugene. *The Trial of the Germans: An Account of the Twenty-two Defendants Before the International Military Tribunal at Nuremberg.* New York: Macmillan, 1996.

D'Este, Carlo. *Patton: A Genius for War.* New York: HarperCollins, 1995.

———. *Eisenhower: A Soldier's Life.* New York: Henry Holt, 2002.

Duberman, Martin. *The Worlds of Lincoln Kirstein.* New York: Alfred A. Knopf, 2007.

Dulles, Allen W. *Secret Surrender: The Classic Insider's Account of the Secret Plot to Surrender Northern Italy During WWII.* Guilford, CT: Lyons Press, 2006.

Edsel, Robert M. *Rescuing Da Vinci: Hitler and the Nazis Stole Europe's Great Art, America and Her Allies Recovered It.* Dallas: Laurel Publishing, 2006.

Eisenhower, David. *Eisenhower at War, 1943–1945.* New York: Random House, 1986.

Eisenhower, Dwight D. *At Ease: Stories I Tell to Friends.* New York: McGraw-Hill, 1988.

Esterow, Milton. *The Art Stealers.* New York: Macmillan, 1966.

Fasola, Cesare. *The Florence Galleries and the War.* Florence: Casa Editrice Monsalvato, 1945.

Feliciano, Hector. *The Lost Museum: The Nazi Conspiracy to Steal the World's Greatest Works of Art.* New York: Basic Books, 1995.

Fest, Joachim. *Inside Hitler's Bunker: The Last Days of the Third Reich.* New York: Farrar, Straus and Giroux, 2002.

Flanner, Janet. *Men and Monuments.* New York: Harper & Brothers, 1957.

Friemuth, Cay. *Die Geraubte Kunst.* Berlin: Westermann, 1989.

Goldensohn, Leon. *Nuremberg Interviews.* New York: Knopf, 2004.

Gray, Martin, and A. Norman Jeffares, eds. *A Dictionary of Quotations.* New York: Barnes and Noble Books, 1995.

Hammer, Katharina. *Glanz im Dunkel: Die Bergung von Kunstschätzen im Salzkammergut am Ende des 2. Weltkrieges.* Wien: Österreichischer Bundesverlag, 1986.

Hancock, Walker, with Edward Connery Lathem. *A Sculptor's Fortunes.* Gloucester, MA: Cape Ann Historical Association, 1997.

Hapgood, David, and David Richardson. *Monte Cassino: The Story of the Most Controversial Battle of World War II*. Cambridge, MA: Da Capo, 2002.

Hastings, Max. *Victory in Europe: D-Day to VE Day in Full Color*. Boston: Little, Brown, 1985.

Hirshon, Stanley P. *General Patton: A Soldier's Life*. New York: Perennial, 2003.

Hitler, Adolf. *Mein Kampf*. Translated by Ralph Manheim. New York: Houghton Mifflin, 1943.

Hobbs, Joseph. *Dear General: Eisenhower's Wartime Letters to Marshall*. Baltimore: Johns Hopkins University Press, 1999.

Howe, Thomas Carr, Jr. *Salt Mines and Castles*. New York: Bobbs-Merrill, 1946.

Hughes, Anthony. *Michelangelo*. London: Phaidon, 1997.

Joachimsthaler, Anton. *The Last Days of Hitler: The Legends— The Evidence—The Truth*. Translated by Helmut Bögler. London: Arms and Armour Press, 1996.

Kirstein, Lincoln. *The Poems of Lincoln Kirstein*. New York: Atheneum, 1987.

Kubin, Dr. Ernst. *Sonderauftrag Linz: Die Kunstsammlung Adolf Hitler, Aufbau, Vernichtungsplan, Rettung. Ein Thriller der Kulturgeschichte*. Wien, Austria: ORAC Buchund Zeitschriftenverlag, 1989.

Kurtz, Michael J. *America and the Return of Nazi Contraband: The Recovery of Europe's Cultural Treasures*. Cambridge, UK: Cambridge University Press, 2006.

Linklater, Eric. *The Art of Adventure*. London: Macmillan & Co., Ltd., 1947.

Löhr, Hanns Christian. *Das Braune Haus der Kunst: Hitler und der "Sonderauftrag Linz."* Berlin: Akademie Verlag, 2005.

Majdalany, Fred. *Cassino: Portrait of a Battle*. London: Cassell & Co., 1999.

Methuen, Lord. *Normandy Diary: Being a Record of Survivals and Losses of Historical Monuments in North-Western France, Together with Those in the Island of Walcheren and in That part of Belgium Traversed by 21st Army Group in 1944–45*. London: Robert Hale Limited, 1952.

Nazi Conspiracy and Aggression, Vol. III. Washington, DC: U.S. Government Printing Office, 1946.

Nicholas, Lynn. *The Rape of Europa*. New York: Vintage, 1995.

Petropoulos, Jonathan. *Art as Politics in the Third Reich*. Chapel Hill: University of North Carolina Press, 1996.

————. *The Faustian Bargain: The Art World in Nazi Germany.* Oxford University Press, 2000.

Piña, Leslie A. *Louis Rorimer: A Man of Style.* Kent, OH: Kent State University Press, 1990.

Pöchmüller, Dr. Ing. Emmerich. *Welt-Kunstschätze in Gefahr.* Salzburg: Pallas-Verlag, 1948.

Puyvelde, Leo van. *Van Eyck: The Holy Lamb.* London: Collins, 1947.

Rayssac, Michel. *L'Exode des Musées: Histoire des Oeuvres d'Art Sous l'Occupation.* Paris: Editions Payot & Rivages, 2007.

Report of the American Commission for the Protection and Salvage of Artistic and Historic Monuments in War Areas. Washington, DC: U.S. Government Printing Office, 1946.

Riedl-Dorn, Christa. *Das Haus der Wunder: Zur Geschichte des Naturhistorischen Museums in Wien.* Wien, Austria: Holzhausen, 1998.

Rorimer, James J. *Survival: The Salvage and Protection of Art in War.* New York: Abelard Press, 1950.

Roxan, David, and Ken Wanstall. *The Rape of Art.* New York: Coward-McCann, 1964.

Sasser, Charles W. *Patton's Panthers: The African-American 761st Tank Battalion in World War II.* New York: Pocket Books, 2005.

Schrenk, Christhard. *Schatzkammer Salzbergwerk: Kulturgüter überdauern in Heilbronn und Kockendorf den Zweiten Weltkrieg.* Heilbronn, Germany: Stadtarchiv, 1997.

Schwarz, Birgit. *Hitlers Museum: Die Fotoalben Gemäldegalerie Linz.* Vienna: Böhlau Verlag, 2004.

Sereny, Gitta. *Albert Speer: His Battle with Truth.* New York: Alfred A. Knopf, 1995.

Shirer, William L. *Berlin Diary: The Journal of a Foreign Correspondent: 1934–1941.* Norwalk, CT: The Easton Press, 1991.

————. *The Rise and Fall of the Third Reich: A History of Nazi Germany,* Volumes I and II. Norwalk, CT: The Easton Press, 1991.

Sigmund, Anna Maria. *Die Frauen der Nazis.* Munich: Wilhelm Heyne Verlag, 2000.

Simon, Matila. *The Battle of the Louvre: The Struggle to Save French Art in World War II.* New York: Hawthorne Books, 1971.

Simpson, Elizabeth, ed. *Spoils of War*. New York: Harry N. Abrams, 1997.

Skilton, John D., Jr. *Defense de l'art Européen: Souvenirs d'un officier américain "Spécialiste des Monuments."* Paris: Les Editions Internationales, 1948.

Smyth, Craig Hugh. *Repatriation of Art from the Collecting Point in Munich after World War II*. New Jersey: Abner Schram Ltd., 1988.

Speer, Albert. *Inside the Third Reich*. New York: Macmillan, 1970.

Spotts, Frederic. *Hitler and the Power of Aesthetics*. Woodstock and New York: Overlook Press, 2002.

Trial of the Major War Criminals before the International Military Tribunal: Nuremberg 14 November 1945 – 1 October 1946. Nuremberg: International Military Tribunal, 1947.

Tutaev, David. *The Consul of Florence*. London: Secker and Warburg, 1966.

Valland, Rose. *Le Front de l'Art: 1939–1945*. Paris: Librarie Plon, 1961.

Vasari, Giorgio. *Lives of the Artists: Volume I*. Translated by George Bull. London: Penguin 1987.

Wheelock, Arthur K., ed. *Johannes Vermeer*. The Hague: Royal Cabinet of Paintings, Mauritshuis and the Board of Trustees, National Gallery of Art, Washington, 1995. Published in conjunction with the exhibit "Johannes Vermeer" shown at the National Gallery of Art, Washington, and the Royal Cabinet of Paintings Mauritshuis, The Hague.

Whiting, Charles. *Bloody Aachen*. New York: Stein and Day, 1976.

Woolley, Lt. Col. Sir Leonard. *The Protection of the Treasures of Art and History in War Areas*. London: His Majesty's Stationery Office, 1947.

Yeide, Nancy. *Beyond the Dreams of Avarice: The Hermann Goering Collection*. Dallas: Laurel Publishing, 2009.

Articles

"A l'Institut: Gaston Palewski fait l'éloge d'un grand défenseur des Beaux-Arts Jacques Jaujard." *Le Figaro*, November 21, 1968.

Bradsher, Greg. "Nazi Gold: The Merkers Mine Treasure." *Prologue Magazine* 31, no. 1 (Spring 1999).

Canady, John. "James Rorimer Left Cloisters to Excel in a Bigger Job." *New York Times*, May 12, 1966.

Chamson, André. "In Memoriam, Jascques Jaujard." *Musees et Collections Publiques* (1967): 151–153.

Cohn, Marjorie B. "George Stout's Legacy." *Journal of the American Institute for Conservation* 18, no. 1 (1978).

Esterow, Milton. "Europe is Still Hunting its Plundered Art." *New York Times*, November 16, 1964.

Gibson, Michael. "How a Timid Curator with a Deadpan Expression Outwitted the Nazis." *ARTnews* 80 (Summer 1981): 105–111

Hammett, Ralph. "Comzone and the Protection of Monuments in North-West Europe." *College Art Journal* 5, no. 2 (Jan. 1946): 123–126.

Hammond, Mason. "The War and Art Treasures in Germany." *College Art Journal* 5, no. 3 (March 1946): 205–218.

Hancock, Walker. "Experiences of a Monuments Officer in Germany." *College Art Journal* 5, no. 4 (May 1946): 271–311.

Houghton, Arthur A., Jr. "James J. Rorimer." *The Metropolitan Museum of Art Bulletin* (Summer 1966, Part Two).

Kirstein, Lincoln. "Quest for the Golden Lamb." *Town and Country* 100, no. 428 (Sept. 1945): 115.

McGregor, Neil. "How Titian Helped the War Effort." *The Times* (London), June 5, 2004.

McManus, John C. "The Last Great Prize." *World War II Magazine* (May 2005): 51–56.

Norris, Christopher. "The Disaster at Flakturm Friedrichshain; A Chronicle and List of Paintings." *The Burlington Magazine* 94, no. 597 (Dec. 1952): 337–347.

"1,000 Pay Tribute at Rorimer Rites." *New York Times*, May 17, 1966.

Plaut, James S. "Loot for the Master Race." *Atlantic Monthly* 178, no. 3 (Sept. 1946): 57–63.

———. "Hitler's Capital." *Atlantic Monthly* 178, no. 4 (Oct. 1946): 73–78.

Posey, Robert. "Protection of Cultural Monuments During Combat." *College Art Journal* 5, no. 2 (Jan. 1946): 127–131.

Rayssac, Michel. "Extrait de Historail: Janvier 2008." http://www.rosevalland.eu/hist-train.htm.

Standen, Edith. "Report on Germany." *College Art Journal* 7, no. 3 (Spring 1948): 209–215.

Stoner, Joyce Hill. "Changing Approaches in Art Conservation: 1925 to the Present," in *Scientific Examination of Art: Modern Techniques in Conservation and Analysis* (Washington, DC: National Academies Press, 2003).

Stout, George. "Our Early Years at the Fogg." *Art Dealer & Framer* (June 1977): 10–13, 16, 92–93, 96–97.

Taylor, Francis Henry. "The Rape of Europa." *Atlantic Monthly* 175 (Jan. 1945): 52.

Von Choltitz, Dietrich. "Pourquoi en 1944 je n'ai pas détruit Paris—IX: Hitler: Vous réduirez paris en un tas de décombres." *Le Figaro*, October 12, 1949.

Unpublished Materials

Duncan, Sally Anne. "Paul J. Sachs and the Institutionalization of Museum Culture Between the World Wars." PhD diss., Tufts University, 2001.

Ettlinger, Harry. "Ein Amerikaner: A Collection of Anecdotes in the Life of Harry Ettlinger" (New Jersey, 2002).

Hobbs, Jerry R. "A Michelangelo in Belgium? The Bruges Madonna" (Menlo Park, CA, 2004).

Films

Berge, Richard, and Bonni Cohen. *The Rape of Europa Collector's Edition*. Dallas: Agon Arts & Entertainment, 2008.

Bricken, Jules, and John Frankenheimer. *The Train*. Santa Monica, CA: MGM Home Entertainment, 1964.

Eichinger, Bernd, and Oliver Hirschbiegel. *Downfall*. Culver City, CA: Sony Pictures with Newmarket Films and Constantin Film, 2005.

Heller, André, and Othmar Schmiderer. *Blindspot: Hitler's Secretary*. Culver City, CA: Sony Pictures Classics Release DOR Film, 2002.

Public Collections

Archives des Musées Nationaux, France:
Rose Valland Papers

Archiv der Stadt Linz, Austria:
Nachlass Dr. Ernst Kubin
Högler, Otto. Papers, Sch 0018

Michel, Prof. Dr. Hermann. Papers, Sch 0008, Sch 0011, Sch 0042–0046
Plieseis, Sepp. Papers, Sch 0042–0046
Pöchmüller, Dr. Ing. Emmerich. Papers, Sch 0016, Sch 0032

Archiv und Wissenschaftsgeschichte des Naturhistorischen Museums Wien, Austria:
Annalen, 56. Band, 1948

Dokumentationsarchiv des Österreichischen Widerstandes, Wien, Austria:
Eder, Max. Papers, DÖW 10610
Michel, Prof. Dr. Hermann. Papers, DÖW 8378
Seiberl, Dr. Herbert. Papers, DÖW 3296a 1–2, DÖW 3296b
Sieber, Karl. Papers, DÖW 3296a 1–2, DÖW 3296b

King's College Archive Centre, Cambridge:
The Papers of Ronald Edmond Balfour, Misc. 5

Metropolitan Museum of Art, New York City, The Cloisters Archives:
James J. Rorimer Papers

National Gallery of Art, Washington, DC:
Gallery Central Files
Walter Farmer Papers
James J. Rorimer Papers
Edith Standen Papers

National Archives and Records Administration, Washington, DC:
RG 165, 238, 239, and 331
OSS Art Looting Investigation Unit Reports, 1945–46 M1782

New York Public Library for the Performing Arts, Jerome Robbins Dance Division, Archives:
Lincoln Kirstein Papers, ca 1913–1994 MGZMD 123
Lincoln Kirstein Papers, ca 1914–1991 MGZMD 97
[Writing by Lincoln Kirstein is © 2009 by the New York Public Library (Astor, Lenox and Tilden Foundations) and may not be reproduced without written permission.]

Smithsonian Archives of American Art, Washington, DC:
W. G. Constable Papers
James J. Rorimer Papers
George Stout Papers

Smithsonian Archives of American Art, Oral History Interviews:
George Stout

Private Collections

Dale V. Ford Papers, East Grand Rapids, MI
Walker Hancock Papers, Gloucester, MA
Robert Posey Papers, Scarsdale, NY
James J. Rorimer Papers, New York City, NY

Author Interviews and Conversations

Horace Apgar
Daniel Altshuler
Richard Barancik
Anne Olivier Bell
Corinne Bouchoux
Dr. Bruce Cole
Jill Croft-Murray
Harry Ettlinger
S. Lane Faison Jr.
Betsy Ford
Dorothy Ford
Deanie Hancock French
Thomas Hoving
William Keller
Kenneth Lindsay
Jim Mullen
Lynn Nicholas
Alessandro Olschki
Charles Parkhurst
Dr. Edmund Pillsbury
Emmanuelle Polack
Col. Seymour Pomrenze
Dennis Posey
Robert Posey
Alain Prévet

Hedy Reeds
James Reeds
Agnes Risom
Anne Rorimer
Louis Rorimer
Salvatore Scarpitta
Craig Hugh Smyth
Richard Sonnenfeld
Mark Sponenberg
Thomas Stout
Bernard Taper
Nancy Yeide

Interviews Courtesy of Actual Films

Harry Ettlinger
S. Lane Faison Jr.
Kenneth Lindsay
Charles Parkhurst
Seymour Pomrenze
Craig Hugh Smyth
Bernard Taper

Smithsonian Archives of American Art Oral History Interviews

William Constable
S. Lane Faison Jr.
Walker Hancock
Thomas Carr Howe Jr.
Charles Parkhurst
James Plaut
George Stout

ACKNOWLEDGMENTS

Thirteen years of awareness and curiosity, nine years of time invested, and five years of focused research: Unless you've given birth to a project of this magnitude, it's difficult to understand the importance of the acknowledgments section of a book. No matter the amount of personal sacrifice, such achievements are rarely singular. Many people, some kindred spirits, others who made a specific contribution, enabled me to tell this story.

No one person made more personal sacrifice to assist me in every way possible than Christy Fox. Her belief in this story, her love of the Monuments Men, and her unwavering support and encouragement on this long journey are present on every page. The calm and seasoned experience of my attorney and counselor, Michael Friedman, demonstrate why the "counselor" portion of his title is often more valuable than the "attorney." Peter McGuigan and his team at Foundry Literary & Media, including Stéphanie Abou and Hannah Brown Gordon, shared my vision about the magnitude of this story. He has ably represented me in the publishing world. He also introduced me to Bret Witter, whose professionalism and work ethic are matched only by his selfless commitment to tell a great story using words alone. Ours has been a joyous collaboration. Michelle Rapkin, my editor, loved the story of the Monuments Men from the moment she first knew of them. Her support and endorsement of my work has been exemplary, doubly so when considering the sudden loss of her loving husband, Bob. Her team at Center Street has been committed to this project every step of the way. In particular, Pamela Clements, Preston Cannon, and Jana Burson of the Center Street Marketing and Publicity team; Chris Barba, Chris Murphy, Gina Wynn, Karen Torres, and the entire Hachette Sales group, and Jody Waldrup, deserve recognition. Rolf Zettersten and Harry Helm have been enthusiastic about this book from the outset, and I thank them both.

When working in the subject area of World War II, the volume of documents, photos, and film images is staggering. Overlaid with translation issues involving, for this book, French, German, and Italian, the challenges that had to be overcome were at times bewildering. It was my good fortune to have two outstanding researchers at my side. Elizabeth Ivy Hudson cut her teeth assisting me with my first book, *Rescuing Da Vinci*, and was my lead researcher for all of this book. Dorothee Schneider joined our team for the last year of research and made invaluable contributions not the least of which were her fluency with German and ability to be wherever in the world we needed her. I am very proud of them both. James Early, Karen Evans, Jamie Lewis, Tom Rupreth, and Anne Edsel Jones also contributed. Full-time travel to archives and interview appointments is a daunting responsibility my assistant Michele Brown handled with patience and a smile. Assisting us with translations were Arlette Quervel and her husband, Yves, and Carol Brick-Stock.

The various archives we visited and their staffs were uniformly knowledgeable and helpful. The National Archives and Records Administration in College Park, Maryland, is a marvel to behold. I owe thanks to Drs. Greg Bradsher and Michael Kurtz and the many fine people at NARA. At the National Gallery in Washington, D.C., I want to thank Maygene Daniels and her assistant Jean Henry. Charles Perrier at the New York Public Library was also exceedingly helpful. At the Louvre Museum in Paris, we were fortunate to have the enthusiastic assistance of Alain Prévet, who was able to locate most any document from memory. Thanks also to Catherine Granger, Nicholas Jenkins, Laura Moore, Gene Fielden, Corinne Bouchaux, and Desiree Wöhler.

Dr. Bruce Cole, Dr. Edmund Pillsbury, Jim Mullen, Claire Barry, and Emmanuelle Polack each provided distinct assistance, but they all had something in common: a direct connection with the Monuments Men. No connections, however, were more important than the actual Monuments Men themselves and their family members. Some had their letters and family documents organized and readily available; others had to expend considerable time and effort to locate them. Making available letters of such a personal nature involves absolute trust, and for that we will always be indebted to their family members. In particular I want to say a special word of thanks to Deanie Hancock French, Anne

Rorimer, Tom Stout, Robert and Dennis Posey, and Dorothy and Elizabeth Ford.

During my watch, I knew and became friends with fifteen Monuments Men and their families. As I write this acknowledgment, nine are still with us. To those who have departed—Lane, Craig, Salvatore, Charles, Sherman, and Ken—and those still here—Seymour, Bernie, Anne, James, Horace, Richard, Mark, Robert, and Harry—and their families, thank you for believing in me and trusting me to preserve and put to use your remarkable legacy.

Special recognition must always be made of Lynn Nicholas, whose scholarly work in the field of Nazi looting during World War II continues to be essential source material for anyone working in this area.

Nine key figures took a risk to bring visibility to the Monuments Men. Their assistance was essential, each in their own way. For providing us with that chance I want to express thanks to Congresswoman Kay Granger, Steve Glauber, Charlie Rose, Randy Kennedy, Melik Kaylan, Eric Gibson, Susan Eisenhower, Dick Bass, and the late William F. Buckley Jr.

Several dear friends helped maintain my spirit. I extend thanks to George and Fern Wachter, Leslie Tcheyan, June Terry, Mike Madigan, Allen Cullum, and Rod Laver. Keith Jarrett's music soothed my oftentimes anguished soul.

Finally I want to express a special word of thanks to Kathleen Kennedy-Marshall, whose precise and persistent questioning of me years ago led to my discovery of how to tell this story.

Help Us Finish the Mission of
The Monuments Men

The Monuments Men Foundation for the Preservation of Art is a not-for-profit, IRS-approved 501(c)(3) organization that continues the mission of the Monuments Officers by bringing visibility to the hundreds of thousands of cultural objects still missing from World War II and assisting those seeking to return such items. If you have information about a work of art, document, or other cultural item you believe was stolen or "liberated" during the war, please contact us at monumentsmenfoundation.org.

For access to our Educational Program, a complete listing of the Monuments Men and women from all thirteen nations, and to read additional Nazi documents and letters from the Monuments Men not included in this book, please visit monumentsmen.com.

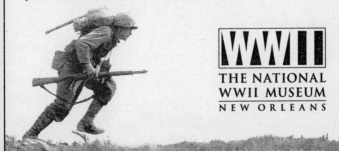

INDEX

ABOUT THE AUTHORS

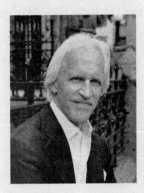

Jimmy Bruch

ROBERT M. EDSEL is the *New York Times* bestselling author of the non-fiction books *Rescuing Da Vinci, The Monuments Men,* and *Saving Italy,* which tells the dramatic story of the Monuments Men during the Italian campaign, the near destruction of *The Last Supper,* and a secret Nazi surrender that imperiled the nation's treasures. Mr. Edsel is also the co-producer of the award-winning documentary film, *The Rape of Europa.* He is the Founder and President of the nonprofit Monuments Men Foundation for the Preservation of Art, which received the National Humanities Medal. Mr. Edsel has been awarded the "Texas Medal of Arts" Award; the "President's Call to Service" Award; and the "Hope for Humanity" Award, presented by the

Dallas Holocaust Museum. He also serves as a Trustee at the National WWII Museum in New Orleans.

BRET WITTER has co-authored six *New York Times* best-sellers. His books have been translated into more than thirty languages and have sold nearly two million copies worldwide. He lives in Decatur, Georgia. bretwitter.com